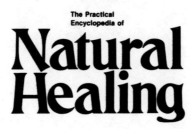

The Practical
Encyclopedia of

# Natural Healing

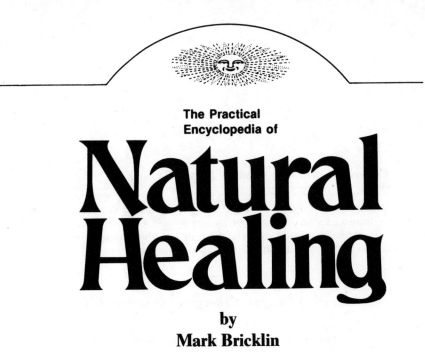

The Practical
Encyclopedia of

# Natural Healing

by
**Mark Bricklin**
*Executive Editor,* PREVENTION® *Magazine*

## With Special Contributions by

B. Joan Arner
Alan S. Bricklin, M.D.
Barry Bricklin, Ph.D.
Patricia M. Bricklin, Ph.D.
Michael Clark
Ara Der Marderosian, Ph.D.
Walter B. Dudley
Jim Duke
Stephen M. Feldman, D.D.S.
John Feltman
Esther C. Frankel

Theodosia Gardner
Grace Halsell
Ruth Heyman
Joan Jennings
Leslie J. Kaslof
Jane Kinderlehrer
Leonard Lear
Richard Lee Lindner, R.Ph.
Jean Rogers
Lois Stevenson
Major Judith C. Wood, USAF

Rodale Press, Inc. Emmaus, Pennsylvania 18049

**Library of Congress Cataloging in Publication Data**

Bricklin, Mark.
    The practical encyclopedia of natural healing.

    Bibliography: p.
    Includes index.
    1. Naturopathy—Dictionaries.   I. Title.
RZ440.B67      615'.535'03     76-26864
ISBN 0-87857-136-1

Printed in the United States of America on recycled paper

20   19

# Contents

# NOTICE

The therapies discussed in this book are strictly adjunctive or complementary to medical treatment. Self-treatment can be hazardous with a serious ailment. I therefore urge you to seek out the best medical assistance you can find whenever it is needed.

# How To Use This Book

In this book, I approach methods of natural healing by two avenues. One is to describe different schools or modalities of natural healing, such as naturopathy and music therapy. There are certainly more modalities of natural healing than I have been able to cover here, but I have attempted to include those which I think will be of most interest, most help, and can be adequately explained without going into excessive detail.

I also approach a number of ailments individually, discussing those therapies which seem to be most pertinent and useful. Most of the therapies presented are based upon studies published in medical journals or books and interviews with scientists and clinicians. Other information is purely anecdotal and is presented as such. Finally, in some instances I also present herbal or folk remedies. These are three dimensions that are quite distinct in many ways, and I have tried to structure each entry so that what I feel is the most reliable information is presented first.

In drawing upon the vast body of medical information about natural healing, I have greatly emphasized those findings which are relatively recent. I've done this both to conserve space and to recognize the fact that a good deal of the older material is available in other books.

In various places in the text, you will find references such as "Meyer suggests that . . ." or "According to Levy . . .". Those are the names of authors of herbal books, and their full names and books are listed in our annotated bibliography, included in the section on HERBAL MEDICINE.

Finally, this book is meant to be educational in nature and is in no way designed to instruct or prepare anyone in self-treatment, let alone diagnosis. Keep in mind that health problems are highly individualistic; similar symptoms in two people can mean two entirely different things. A therapy (natural or synthetic) that brings rapid improvement to one person may be of no help to another person and may cause serious side effects in a third. I not only urge that all potentially serious health problems be managed by a physician, but that you should be satisfied that your physician is providing you with the *best* medical care available to you.

# Introduction

Many people think of natural healing as a somewhat radical or perhaps mystical alternative to conservative medical care. There is a place for it—*probably*—they may feel, but when it comes to anything *serious* involving *health,* natural healing had better put on a look of proper awe, pack up its basket of herbs, whole grains, vitamins, and exercises, and slink out the back door—without slamming it.

Not very long ago, that was the concept I had of natural healing. In the course of writing this book, I discovered that the truth is just the opposite of what I had supposed.

Medical care, with its X-rays, laboratory tests, drugs, and surgical procedures, can be an invaluable tool when it's needed. But like that other tool, fire, medical care can singe the careless hand and—sometimes—utterly consume the innocent.

Natural healing cannot do certain things that medical care can. But neither can the best medical care do some very important things which natural healing can. As a doctor points out in this book, it is worth remembering that for nearly all of mankind's time on earth, we were able to survive and spread our kind without any medical care whatsoever. Even today, most people in the world have very limited access to modern medical care.

But the important thing is that natural healing and medical care are not mutually exclusive. They each have their strengths and limitations. In many areas, they overlap. And significantly, interest in natural healing today is perhaps greatest among young physicians who have graduated from some of the nation's leading medical institutions.

We might legitimately wonder why these young doctors, with their minds filled with the wonders of contemporary medicine, are intensely interested in natural healing. And that leads us to an understanding of why natural healing has not and must not be swept from the scene by the admittedly awesome presence of medicine.

Natural healing is basically a much more *conservative* approach to health care than medical practice. Medical practice aims for the quick cure, by means of introducing substances or instruments into the body which are highly antagonistic to whatever is causing the disease. Novelist Robert Gover says that a doctor is happiest when he "can jump on top of a disease and stomp it to death with his bare feet." He wants to see results, fast, and he wants *you* to see that *he's* the one who's giving you those results. Because of this desire for swift decisive victory, medical practice tends to be adventuresome, dramatic, risky, and expensive.

## An 'Organic' Approach to Healing

Natural healing takes a slower, more organic approach. It recognizes first that the human body is superbly equipped to resist disease and heal injuries. But when disease does take hold, or an injury occurs, the first instinct in natural healing is to see what might be done to strengthen those natural resistance and healing agents so they can act against the disease process more effectively. Results are not expected to occur overnight. But neither are they expected to occur at the expense of side effects and dangerous complications.

The natural healing orientation means that when you have a headache, instead of immediately reaching for aspirin, which may injure the lining of your stomach or cause even more serious side effects, you reach for a pillow and try taking a nap. Backache? Instead of reaching for Valium right away, which can cause fatigue, loss of coordination, and worse, try relaxing those muscles with local applications of heat. *Severe* back pain? Instead of going immediately to potentially addictive pain relievers, consider an osteopathic manipulation which will often remove the cause of the pain. *Chronic* severe backache? Before going to surgery, consider first an exercise program which in many cases can make surgery unnecessary.

Note that in each case, the natural healing approach is conservative. It says, simply, "Let's not do anything drastic until we see if something simpler, cheaper, and safer works."

Those who look upon medicine as the never-ending discovery of new drugs and new operations often consider natural healing to be an unwanted brake on "progress." Others seem to be so involved in their professionalism that they become highly agitated at the very mention of a word like "vitamins." There is no place for self-prescribed vitamins or exercises in good medical care, they may exclaim. And we have no argument with that. *But what is good for "medical progress" or "medical care" and what is good for human beings are two entirely different things.*

In fact, the record shows all too clearly that "medical progress" has in many cases spelled despair and even death for thousands of people who trusted their health to doctors and their "new, decisive answers" to just about everything. And it's this record of medical fallibility which has caused so many people, particularly some physicians, to give priority to conservative natural healing techniques whenever possible, and to use these techniques supportively when medical care *is* necessary.

## Doctors' Convictions Can Be Lethal

New drugs or operations are not always the cause of medical blundering. Benjamin Rush, the colonial Philadelphia physician, sometimes referred to as the "Father of American Medicine," was probably responsible for killing many people who might otherwise have survived the epidemics of his time. Rush was convinced that intestinal cleanliness was next to godliness, and his favorite medicine was a strong dose of laxatives. In cases of fever, especially, he insisted that the proper therapy was to "purge, purge, and purge some more." And if that didn't work, the patient could always be bled with leeches or other means. While it is difficult to imagine how a debilitated patient with a high fever could be helped by the swift production of dehydration and anemia, Rush once described the "sublime joy I now feel on contemplating the success of my remedies."

Significantly, according to a recent editorial in a medical journal, "Rush was far from being a fanatic; he was regarded by many as being very gifted, as an acute observer, and as a conscientious physician."

Thousands upon thousands of European women in the late 19th century died in the throes of childbirth fever after being infected by their doctors. Women who delivered the old-fashioned way, at home, with a midwife, were safe, because the hands of the midwives were not tainted with germs from the autopsy table. What is even more tragic is that many women *pleaded* to be allowed to have their babies at home. The fact that as many as four out of every five new mothers were dying in some maternity wards was no secret.

But doctors insisted that the women come to their wonderful modern hospitals or forego medical attention altogether.

More recently, probably within the memory of most readers, it was the habit of physicians to insist that following childbirth, a woman should be kept in a hospital bed for several weeks. After all, childbirth fever had been eliminated when doctors finally realized that they ought to wash their hands once in a while, so what healthier place for anyone to be than a hospital? Today, we know that this excessive doctoring or hospitalization probably cost many women their lives, as a result of fatal blood clots which arise most easily when a person is kept in bed day after day.

The story of medical interference with the natural course of childbirth is far from over. While most doctors still insist that a hospital is *the* place to have a baby, recent statistics still show that, in general, a woman is safer having her baby at home, attended by a midwife, than she would be in a hospital. The major reasons are the unnecessary or excessive use of drugs, the unnecessary use of forceps, and infection with virulent and highly resistant germs which, as Ashley Montagu puts it, collect in hospitals the way money collects in a bank.

Recently I heard a leading dermatologist scoff at the notion that a change in diet could help acne. Yet, that doctor was not so young that he could have forgotten the days when doctors gave X-ray therapy for acne. Possibly, cutting out candy and ice cream *won't* help some people with acne, but medical historians now say that X-ray therapy was of no use at all in clearing up acne, not even superficially, except perhaps for a few weeks following treatment. But one thing that X-ray therapy *could* do which a change in the diet couldn't is trigger the development of cancer.

X-ray therapy was also given for tonsillitis, and people who received this absurd treatment have been urged in recent years, like people who were given X-ray treatment for acne, to undergo careful examination for the presence of cancer caused by those X-rays.

The X-ray fad for tonsillitis was replaced eventually by the tonsillectomy-adenoidectomy fad. Like most other children of my era, I had my tonsils removed, and I remember my father telling me that the operating room was filled from one end to the other, and that the surgeon started at one end and worked his way expeditiously down the line. Apparently, he worked a little *too* expeditiously on me, because I had to undergo a second operation some years later for the removal of scar tissue. I could have been even more unlucky, however. It's conservatively estimated that at least 200 children die as a result of undergoing tonsillectomies every year. That's bad enough, but medical authorities now say that about nine out of every ten tonsillectomies are entirely unnecessary, which means that most of those deaths are entirely avoidable.

But the tonsillectomy is not the only operation which is performed excessively. It's now believed that a great many hysterectomies, hernia repairs, gallbladder removals, and operations for "slipped disks" are also unnecessary. Recent clinical research into the therapeutic effects of a high-fiber diet also suggest that a good many operations to remove hemorrhoids or inflamed (but not cancerous) portions of the low bowel could also be avoided if a dietary approach were tried first.

All that adds up to an enormous amount of unnecessary suffering, expense, and from several hundred to several thousand avoidable deaths every year. And the point is not that there is a certain amount of recklessness involved in selecting patients for surgery, but that a more *conservative* approach would be to exhaust all natural healing methods *before* deciding on surgery.

## The Other Side of Miracle Drugs

In all probability, drugs are misused even more frequently and with more disastrous results than surgical procedures. Estimates as to how many people are affected by drug reactions every year vary widely. One recent estimate put the *death* toll at 30,000. Another estimate says that 300,000 are made seriously ill every year by drug reactions. Personally, I feel that these figures are inflated, but whatever the real number might be, it is high enough to be embarrassing to the medical profession and certainly enough to give anyone second thoughts about taking a drug—especially when that drug may be unnecessary.

I find it especially discomforting to realize that the pharmaceutical industry spends in the vicinity of *one billion dollars* a year just to advertise and market its drugs to doctors. No matter how you look at it, that's a lot of salesmanship. And we may ask: If doctors are knowledgeable about drugs, if they have been trained in their use, if they have a scientific understanding of them, why is it necessary to spend one billion dollars a year on promotion and advertising to push these pharmaceuticals? If doctors prescribe drugs rationally and scientifically, why are certain very heavily used and highly profitable items like Librium promoted with full-page, full-color advertisements in what seems to be every single issue of every major medical journal? And what is the relationship between this heavy promotion schedule and the fact that Librium (prescribed for "anxiety") is currently the most heavily prescribed brand name drug?

Until just a few years ago, it was common practice for some drug companies to reward doctors who purchased large amounts of injectable products by giving them premiums such as tape recorders, stereo sets, and golf clubs. And does that, we have to wonder, have anything to do with the fact that a recent medical study revealed that more than half of all physicians presented with a patient who has a common cold will prescribe or inject him with an antibiotic—even though an antibiotic has no power at all to control the growth of the common cold virus?

It's not just a question of the overuse of drugs. Antibiotics can produce serious side effects. They can cause some highly sensitive people to die in a matter of minutes. I am familiar with the case of one young girl who was given the powerful broad-spectrum antibiotic tetracycline for acne. She was also advised by her physician to take sunbaths, as that may help acne. What the physician either did not know, or did not bother to tell the girl, was that tetracycline can make some people terribly hypersensitive to sunlight. In this case, the result was skin burns so severe and painful that the girl had a psychotic breakdown.

Besides antibiotics, it's likely that cortisone, tranquilizers, estrogen, and many other drugs are excessively prescribed. Often, the side effects of these drugs are not discovered until some years after they are widely introduced. Just recently, for example, evidence has been found that long-term use of estrogen significantly increases a woman's chances of developing cancer of the uterus.

A drug which is used only to snatch someone from the gaping jaws of death or a lifetime of suffering certainly should not be condemned because it may cause serious side effects. In other cases, the possible side effects seem entirely out of proportion to the benefits which the drug offers. Consider, for instance, the drug phenylbutazone, which is sold under several trade names to treat rheumatoid arthritis, osteoarthritis, bursitis, and similar conditions. *If* the drug relieves pain, which it does not always do, that relief is only temporary. Yet, here are just *some* of the possible side effects known to be caused by this drug, as listed by one manufacturer: ulcerative esophagitis; acute and reactivated gastric and duodenal ulcer with perforation and hemorrhage; ulceration and perforation of the large bowel; nausea, vomiting, and diarrhea; aplastic anemia; leukemia; bone marrow depression; metabolic acidosis; fatal and nonfatal hepatitis; anaphylactic shock; fever; kidney failure; high blood pressure; inflammation of the lining of the heart; optic neuritis and bleeding from the retina of the eye.

In all fairness, the manufacturer does clearly warn physicians that this drug must not be administered casually and that patients must be carefully evaluated and monitored. Nevertheless, it is awesome to realize that all those side effects, which sound like the collective result of an atomic holocaust, can be caused by a single drug.

That's why I believe so firmly that we must become increasingly aware of every possible alternative to drug therapy, from acupuncture to yoga therapy.

One weak point in medical care which is not generally appreciated is the relatively high degree of error in laboratory tests. Many of us probably have the idea that when results of an analysis of urine, blood, tissue, or some other bodily substance return from a laboratory, you are at that point presented with the ultimate truth of the matter. That would be a very pleasant state of affairs, but unfortunately, many laboratories both in and out of hospitals are too often very careless with their analyses.

In one recent year, reports the Center for Disease Control, clinical laboratories turned in "poor performances" in analyzing as many as 25 percent of test samples. That figure of 25 percent poor performance is even more remarkable when you consider that samples sent out by the CDC are clearly marked as having come from that federal agency. If that is the best that can be expected when the lab *knows* they have to be at their best, we can only guess at the quality of their analyses in performing routine tests.

All this is not presented here to besmirch the reputation of the medical profession. Rather, I mean to suggest that it is wrong to consider natural healing as a kind of high-risk, hit-or-miss approach and medical care as uniformly reliable and safe. Many readers, perhaps, realize the shortcomings of medical care all too well through personal experience. Now, I think, the time has come to incorporate a better appreciation of these shortcomings into our very expectations of what medical care has to offer.

But don't get the idea that the *only* good thing about natural healing is that it is relatively very safe. It can also be surprisingly effective, sometimes much more so than drugs. In this book you will read of many instances where something as simple as a slight change in diet or applications of an herb succeeded in clearing up problems which had resisted the onslaught of drug after drug. It was reports of this nature appearing in the medical literature that led J. I. Rodale to found PREVENTION magazine more than a quarter of a century ago. And it is the mission of the magazine's present editor and publisher, Robert Rodale, to discover and bring to light similar reports which continue to be published in the literature, but which are all too frequently ignored by the medical practice establishment. It's the hope of all of us at PREVENTION and Rodale Press that this book will serve to highlight some of these discoveries and give natural healing its rightful place in the total picture of health care and well-being.

*Mark Bricklin*

# Acne

The latest word from the medical pimple establishment is that acne has nothing to do with diet. If you believe that, you'll believe anything. It's interesting to note, in this regard, that the test which "conclusively" proved that chocolate has no effect on the skin was funded by a very large manufacturer of chocolate candy.

As I write this, the latest and greatest medical treatment for acne consists of application of vitamin A acid, which causes the skin to peel, followed by swabbing the skin with an antibiotic. A year or two ago, the latest-greatest treatment consisted of vitamin A acid plus *systemic* tetracycline, a powerful broad-spectrum antibiotic.

When I was a teenager and bothered by pimples, as most teenagers are, my family doctor advised washing with brown soap. As a result of that treatment, my skin became highly irritated. The outcome was happy, though, because when I quit washing my face with *any* kind of soap, my skin improved greatly.

Before the era of brown soap, X-ray therapy was all the fashion. Countless thousands of youngsters fell prey to this medical fad, which was not only without any lasting benefit, but in some instances caused cancer years later. What the latest and greatest medical treatment for acne will be *next* year is anybody's guess.

When acne is mild, the best thing to do about it is nothing except to keep the skin clean. Vigorous scrubbing and application of all manner of chemicals will probably do more harm than good. Eventually, when the hormones of puberty settle down, the acne will most likely subside. Squeezing pimples which have not pointed, or otherwise abusing your skin, may cause pitting and scarring which *won't* go away when the acne does, so keep that in mind. The pimples will most likely be with you for only a few years, but the results of bathroom surgery can linger a lifetime.

Despite the official word on what causes acne, many people observe that eating certain foods aggravates their acne. Chocolate, nuts, and cola drinks are the most commonly implicated foods.

As far as nutrition goes, it's my overwhelming impression that the best course of action is to adopt a sensible well-balanced diet in which sweet junk foods and rich desserts like ice cream are eliminated. Any number of nutritional supplements may be helpful, so the reasonable course is a balanced and comprehensive program of nutritional supplementation.

Here are some excerpts which are typical of the experiences readers of PREVENTION magazine have reported: "When my son was 14 years old, he was bothered with acne and his face was all broken out, until some friends told me to get him some yeast tablets. He took one after every meal and in no time he was cured of acne."

"When I began regularly taking a natural B-complex pill, desiccated liver, and brewer's yeast, my acne began to clear. I mentioned this to a friend and she got the same results."

A 16-year-old girl who had suffered with acne since she was 12 cleared up her face "in one month" after she began taking vitamin A, vitamin E, and yeast tablets.

A woman said that on the advice of a roommate "my daughter began taking vitamin A and in only two weeks had no more new eruptions on her face for the first time in five years! But her face had become so scarred it took several weeks to notice that the scars too were gradually disappearing." The woman went on to explain that they were supposed to go to a dermatologist to have him reduce the scars when her daughter was 21, but this proved to be unnecessary as her scars "had just about all disappeared."

Zinc gluconate, which was introduced as a food supplement only recently, seems to hold considerable promise for acne sufferers. One woman said she had had acne for 12 years and had been to innumerable dermatologists who prescribed "treatments galore, all of which produced only slight improvement in my skin condition. . . . First, I began taking increased amounts of vitamins A and B. However, most effective in my case, was the addition of dolomite and bone meal tablets (four to six a day) and zinc gluconate. Of these supplements, zinc produced the quickest improvement, and only 20 mg. a day has practically cleared up my acne completely. Of course, proper cleansing and a diet low in fats and carbohydrates must also be followed."

Another woman said, "For three years I suffered with acne and now after one month's supplementation with zinc, my face is beautifully clear. Friends too are getting astonishing results."

Still another woman said she had had acne since she was 14, and at the age of 22 began taking 30 mg. of zinc a day. After three weeks, she noticed that her skin had "considerably cleared up."

A few years ago, we published a letter from a woman who

achieved remarkable results with capsules of acidophilus, a concentrated form of the beneficial bacteria found in yogurt. She had suffered with acne, she said, for over 20 years. "Then I started taking acidophilus capsules and within a matter of days the acne disappeared, and I have remained free of it as long as I continue to take acidophilus."

Subsequently another reader said that she showed the letter written by the first woman to her dermatologist "who immediately dismissed the remedy as old-fashioned, a joke. The next day I went out and purchased those capsules and liquid and now, over one month later, I am convinced that the liquid acidophilus has caused the acne to cease and my skin to feel smooth."

There's a peculiar kind of acne which accompanies menstruation, and for this, Dr. B. Leonard Snider of Erie, Pennsylvania, suggests that vitamin $B_6$, or pyridoxine, can be helpful. He told a dermatology meeting in 1974 that he put 106 teenagers—none of whom was known to be taking oral contraceptives—on daily $B_6$ supplements for one week preceding and then during the time of menstruation, for an average of three periods. Seventy-six girls reported that the supplement reduced the acne flare by 50 to 75 percent, while the other girls could notice no difference. The report I have does not mention the amount of $B_6$ he used, but 20 to 50 mg. a day would probably be appropriate.

# Acrodermatitis Enteropathica

Acrodermatitis enteropathica is a rare inherited disorder which usually appears very early in life. It causes terribly serious skin lesions which refuse to heal, disrupted bowel function, poor nutrient absorption, and stunted growth. Unless controlled by a drug (which itself can cause serious problems), this disease usually ends in death.

In 1974, it was conclusively proven that the disease can be 100 percent controlled with zinc supplements. In that year, in *Lancet,* Dr. E. J. Moynahan of the Hospital for Sick Children in London related that he and his colleagues added a daily supplement of 35 mg. of zinc to the diet of children with acrodermatitis enteropathica. They were astounded by the results. Not only did the horrible skin problems vanish, but the bowel symptoms "which had stubbornly resisted a variety of dietary regimens and drug therapy" were also completely normalized.

After some months, the doctors reported that "all of the children are now completely free from symptoms and are thriving well with zinc supplements alone; furthermore, they enjoy a normal diet, without restrictions." As a bonus, nearly all the children (except those approaching puberty) also went into a growth spurt—which was most conspicuous when the drug they were taking was rapidly withdrawn.

The children are not "cured" in the sense that they no longer have the disease; rather, the disease is completely controlled as long as they take their zinc supplements daily. The problem, it turned out, is an inherited disorder in zinc metabolism which requires supplements of this trace mineral to maintain normal health.

Actually, zinc isn't the only nutritional therapy for this condition. The other treatment is an exclusive diet of breast milk.

The disease never appears in babies who are breast-feeding. If it strikes a child who has been nursed, it only comes after he or she is weaned. Restoration of breast milk immediately abolishes all symptoms. When any other kind of milk or protein food is given, the child becomes sick again.

Dr. Moynahan speculates that children with acrodermatitis enteropathica lack a vital enzyme needed to handle a certain protein. In the absence of this enzyme, the protein substance apparently binds all the zinc in the diet and makes it unavailable to the body. Curiously, the offending protein substance is *not* found in breast milk. When zinc supplements are taken, the protein still binds up a certain amount of zinc, but there's enough of the mineral left over to fill the body's requirements.

The maintenance dose first successfully used by Dr. Moynahan was only 35 mg. of zinc a day. However, he recommends to other doctors that they use about 150 mg. a day in divided doses, to allow for poor absorption which may occur in the event of intestinal infections or diarrhea.

Within months after this medical discovery was published, reports were coming in from all over the world of the miraculous healing achieved with inexpensive supplements of zinc sulfate or zinc gluconate.

As a footnote, let me add that one of the first cases of healing acrodermatitis enteropathica with zinc in the United States—possibly *the* first case—was achieved by a reader of PREVENTION. Coming across an early report about Moynahan's pioneering work, this reader, whose son had A.E., asked her physician what he thought of the idea. He told her to forget about it—calling it "just another pipe dream." But the woman persisted and wrote to Dr. Moynahan in London. He very generously gave the woman full instructions for the zinc regimen, and in short order, the woman's son was healthy and free of pain for the first time in his life.

As a footnote to that footnote, I think it's important to mention that at precisely the same time as this was going on, a well-known and widely respected nutritionist wrote in a syndicated column that *no one* needs supplements of zinc, and that on no account should anyone take zinc supplements except on the advice of the family physician.

I'm not mentioning this to denigrate that particular nutritionist in any way; only to illustrate that the often-heard advice that one should never do anything without the blessings of one's family physician is dangerously simplistic. It assumes that the family physician is sure to know the answer to every question about health or nutrition. Obviously, that isn't the case. Doctors realize this only too well, but some seem to loathe to admit it publicly. In the case of serious illness, if the treatment or advice of your primary physician does not satisfy you, the sensible course is to consult other health authorities who may know more about the problem.

# Acupuncture

I have a sort of funny relationship with acupuncture: this strange and ancient oriental art burst upon the American consciousness just about the same time that I entered the field of health journalism. In fact, if memory serves, the very first article on health which I wrote was on the subject of acupuncture. I titled it *"Acupuncture?"* By that, I meant to convey the idea that using the body as a pincushion to achieve healing was almost incomprehensible. But I concluded the article with a challenge to the medical profession to take an honest look at acupuncture to see if there was really something to it. The mere fact that Western doctors can't "understand" acupuncture, I charged, was no good reason not to give it a fair trial.

To be perfectly honest, I never expected that a fair trial would be given. Much less did I suspect what has actually occurred.

Why acupuncture caught on so fast among American doctors, I can't say, except to suggest that perhaps there is something about inserting needles into a patient which makes a doctor feel "right at home." In any case, when I wrote that first article, my research was based almost entirely on some rather hard-to-get books and a few accounts in relatively obscure journals. I was able to locate only two physicians who were practicing acupuncture in the United States, and one of them consented to be interviewed only if we agreed not to mention his name.

That was in late 1971. Contrast that situation with the picture of hundreds of acupuncture practitioners from all over the world converging on the University of Pennsylvania in Philadelphia in December 1974 for the World Acupuncture Congress.

Judging by what we learned at that meeting, the reason acupuncture has taken hold so fast in the United States may be nothing more than that it usually *works*. And as often as not, after everything else has failed.

That is an important point to remember when trying to assess the value of acupuncture. By and large, patients who present themselves for acupuncture do so only after a chronic condition has resisted long years of traditional medical care, including every conceivable kind of pain medication and surgery. It is likely that if the cases seen by acupuncturists were not of this desperate variety, the results they obtain would be even more impressive.

I will not attempt here to explain the physiological basis of acupuncture. For one thing, I don't understand it. Second, no one else seems to either. A great number of theories have been put forward and arguments have raged, but little is known for certain. What is generally accepted, though, is that the best results are obtained by following guidelines set down many years ago by Oriental practitioners, who believed that by inserting needles at various points along "meridians" of energy which course through the body, it is possible to "normalize" or "balance" that flow and restore health. I should add that contemporary Oriental practitioners in no way deny the existence of bacteria. But what many do insist is that the proliferation of bacteria—or whatever else may be present—is not the cause of the patient's disease, but rather the result of an imbalance of energies.

Let me also add that a number of doctors and scientists still maintain that acupuncture in fact has *no* physiological basis and works only through a placebo effect—the power of suggestion. The problem with that reasoning is that doctors have been able to perform operations on *animals* using only acupuncture techniques for anesthesia. It is doubtful, to say the least, that an animal is going to hold still and not cry out in pain because it has somehow been "psyched" into believing that it won't feel anything when the scalpel cuts.

As for the techniques of acupuncture, they too are still subject to a great deal of trial and error. Basically, very slender needles are used and are inserted in numbers usually varying from two or three to a dozen or more. A good many doctors now use a technique in which a very small amount of electrical current is fed into the needle to achieve greater stimulating effect. Some specialize in what is called auriculotherapy, in which needles are usually inserted only into various points in the outer ear. Still other doctors dispense with needles altogether and apply ultrasonic energy along the chosen acupuncture points, while at least one Oriental doctor practicing in the United States—he is also a surgeon—prefers to use a very slender hypodermic needle and inject mild solutions, usually vitamins, into acupuncture points.

So many conditions have been treated with reported success by acupuncture that we would need a considerable amount of space merely to *suggest* the therapeutic potentials of the art. Because we have conducted many interviews with acupuncturists, we have decided to limit ourselves here to relating what we have learned firsthand. A good deal of the information will come from interviews conducted at the World Acupuncture Congress by PREVENTION staff writer Michael Clark, and we will approach the subject from the point of view of specific diseases that have been treated by acupuncture and the reported results.

## Migraine Headaches

Doctors have reported tremendous success with acupuncture treatment of migraine headaches. As those who are prone to migraine attacks know only too well, the usual medical treatments for these severe headaches leave much to be desired. And all the drugs now in general use are designed to be taken only after an attack has actually begun. In contrast, acupuncture treatment seems to be very effective in preventing the attacks from ever occurring, or rendering them much less severe when they do hit.

Dr. Howard D. Kurland of the Northwestern University Medical School and senior attending psychiatrist at the Evanston Hospital in Evanston, Illinois, reported that he and his associates completed a two-year study of headache treatment with acupuncture techniques. Their patients had a variety of headaches, including migraine, histamine cephalalgia (cluster headaches), whiplash, and tension headaches.

Dr. Kurland said he usually administers needle acupuncture in the head area. Following this, the patient is often taught how to treat himself with acupressure on certain points on the ear. These points are massaged and pinched when the patient feels an attack of migraine coming on.

"My treatment for headache is either acupuncture or acupressure," Dr. Kurland told us. "I do not give any prescription medicine for migraine headaches."

**Far Fewer Drugs Needed** • Using these new techniques, Dr. Kurland reported that he and his associates have achieved great success, with a reasonable degree of relief in *all cases* where the patient adequately participated. The efficacy of acupuncture and self-administered acupressure treatment was verified, he noted, by the fact that prescriptions for narcotics, painkillers, and other drugs were eliminated entirely in most cases.

Some of Dr. Kurland's most gratifying success has come in treating cluster headaches, which many people consider to be the very worst kind. The headaches usually come in "clusters" of from five to seven and may last for several days. Ordinarily, a person affected with these headaches can do absolutely nothing for himself except lie down in a dark room with shades drawn and wait until the agony goes away. With acupuncture, followed up by acupressure at the first hint of an attack, some patients with a history of very severe headaches—who had been on some of the strongest painkilling drugs known—have over the two years had to resort to drugs only on a few occasions, Dr. Kurland said. And then, they only used aspirin.

Ralph M. Coan, M.D., who is not an acupuncturist, but is the Medical Director of the Acupuncture Center of Washington in Washington, D.C., reported that practitioners at his clinic had also achieved impressive results.

Dr. Coan said that when he looked at the results obtained from treating 40 consecutive patients with migraine headaches, he discovered that 23—or 58 percent—reported substantial improvement. The aveiage length of the remission of pain after a single series of five or six acupuncture treatments was 10.2 months. In 11 patients there was no relapse at the time of the Philadelphia meeting, an average of 15 months. In the majority of cases, Dr. Coan added, there is usually a marked reduction in medication.

"If the remarkable cure of acupuncture is related to a placebo effect, autosuggestion, or hypnosis, as some have speculated," Dr. Coan said, "this ancient form of therapy would have to be rated as an outstanding psychosomatic therapeutic adjunct. Acupuncture cannot be dismissed as something that works only on Chinese."

Another doctor reporting on acupuncture for migraine headaches at the Philadelphia conference was Dr. Lilia M. Palanca, a cardiologist and anesthesiologist on the faculty of the University of St. Thomas Hospital in Manila, the Philippines.

Dr. Palanca told us that she has been treating migraine headaches with acupuncture for about a year and a half. Her success, she claimed, after treating between 350 and 400 patients, is 100 percent.

Dr. Palanca uses several acupuncture points on the head, a technique she calls cerebral acupuncture. She noted, however, that many acupuncturists favor the ear for treating the majority of patients suffering from migraine headaches.

"I find that treating patients with acupuncture promotes a calming effect on them," Dr. Palanca said. "Initially they have a fast heart rate, but once the acupuncture treatment begins, the pulse slows down and the patient becomes very calm and relaxed." Dr. Palanca did not attribute the disappearance of the migraine headaches to this calming effect, but she did note that many doctors believe that migraines are caused by anxiety, and that in order to be cured, the patient has to somehow relax himself.

**Help May Be Related to Blood Flow** • Two researchers from the Departments of Anesthesiology and Biophysics at the Indiana University of Medicine believe that acupuncture may be connected with the blood flow to the head.

In an article in *The American Journal of Chinese Medicine* (October 1974), Dr. K. C. Kim and R. A. Yount reported on a series of acupuncture treatments they gave to 25 patients, 21 of whom were female, for migraine headaches. After six months of treatment, the pair reported that the frequency of headaches was reduced 68 percent and the duration 60 percent. Their results showed that 68 percent of the patients were able to completely halt their use of painkilling medications. Twelve of the patients were considered completely cured. Another impressive statistic reported by the pair was an 82 percent reduction of such common migraine symptoms as vomiting, absence from work, and the need to lie in bed.

In a discussion of their findings, they noted that other studies show that blood flow to the head is increased during the headaches. And the blood flow is increased even more to the side of the head in which the migraine occurs. The speculation of other researchers is that this increased flow is connected to the migraine. They hypothesize that acupuncture—in some way—affects the blood circulation in the head by balancing this "improper" blood flow to the head.

Although acupuncture seems, at this time, to be a very potent weapon in the fight against migraine headaches, it takes an expert acupuncturist to get the desired results. Even though patients may be taught acupuncture massage points at home, the person who suffers from this malady has to be taught the correct procedures to follow.

**Earlobe Massage ●** Dr. Ted Warner of Lancaster, California, a Doctor of Acupuncture who is president of the American Guild of Auriculotherapy, told us that for migraine headaches the main acupressure point is located on the lower part of the earlobe, or the tail of the helix. The point is massaged with the forefinger. Hold the thumb behind the lobe. Pinch the lobe between thumb and forefinger and rotate the forefinger in a circular motion.

"It's difficult to determine just how hard to massage the point," Dr. Warner said. "If the migraines are severe, the massage will be more vigorous. If they're mild, it will be more gentle."

Dr. Warner, who studied under Paul F. M. Nogier, M.D., of France, the man generally given credit for developing the modern auriculotherapy school of acupuncture, said that there are two other points just inside the opening of the ear canal. Practitioners stimulate these points with small glass rods bent in the shape of a small hockey stick, he said.

The points, he noted, are not in the ear, but on the structure of the ear known as the intertragic incisure, a layer of cartilage along the bottom of the ear canal opening.

"I've had good success with acupuncture and with auriculotherapy," he said. "It's an excellent adjunct to my practice."

## Psoriasis Treated

Dr. Desmond Beckett-George, of Grimsby, England, has used acupuncture in his practice a good deal longer than most Americans now experimenting with this ancient Chinese art. In the past several years, the British physician told the Acupuncture Congress, he's treated 36 patients who came to him specifically for acupuncture treatment of psoriasis. He was able to effect "some improvement" in all of them—and to cure 60 percent. "When I say 'cure,'" the speaker emphasized, "I mean that these patients have been free from symptoms for at least five years."

In an interview, Dr. Beckett-George elaborated: "You have no idea how much misery psoriasis sufferers experience. In 1969 I treated a 10-year-old boy with the worst case I've ever seen. The skin over his entire body was rough, cracked, and scaly. He had bleeding eruptions. His eyebrows were gone. He was losing his hair. The itching was intolerable."

The boy began receiving acupuncture treatment once a week. In nine months he was completely cured of any signs of the disease and has remained so since 1970. Less severe cases, Dr. Beckett-George noted, usually require only five to ten acupuncture treatments before positive results are seen.

Other Congress participants, besides the British doctor, also reported case histories of successful acupuncture treatment of psoriasis. They included Dr. Palanca and Dr. Kurland, whom we mentioned earlier, and Arthur L. Kaslow, an M.D. from Solvang, California.

## MS Crippling Reduced by Acupuncture

Dr. Kaslow, however, is not only experienced in psoriasis. His main interest is the treatment of multiple sclerosis. In combination with diet (one that emphasizes unprocessed natural foods), the California physician has found that acupuncture can definitely reduce some of the crippling effects of this disease.

In multiple sclerosis, the fatty substance, myelin, which normally sheathes the nerve fibers, has for unknown reasons degenerated. With many fibers deprived of all or part of their myelin sheathing, the central nervous system (brain and spinal cord) cannot always communicate properly with arms, legs, eyes, and other parts of the body. As a result of garbled or blocked messages from the central nervous system, crippling can be very severe.

"Some of my patients are what you call medical rejects," Dr. Kaslow told us. "Nothing else is being done for them, so they come for my acupuncture treatment as one last hope. They're 'basket cases,' some of them. I've seen them brought into the office on a stretcher. It really tears your heart out when they get enthusiastic after a single treatment and find they can move a thumb or a toe."

The California physician said that the first MS case he treated was a man so incapacitated that he couldn't wash or dress or feed himself. "After 10 treatments at my office and a series of treatments at home, the patient was able to take care of these needs without help. He's thrown his cane away," Dr. Kaslow said. "Another patient I have is now able to stand on one foot. That's a real accomplishment. It may not seem like very much to you or me, but for the individual who's been hobbling around and can't stand on both feet, let alone one foot, it's quite a triumph."

The "home treatments" Dr. Kaslow's patients receive are administered by the patients themselves. They are taught to use a portable electrostimulator—a device that emits a small electric current through a prod—to stimulate the "response points" located on the ear. The beneficial effect of the electric prod, apparently, is similar if not equal to that of expert "needling" at these points by the doctor.

Not only are the patients put in charge of their own simulated acupuncture, they are also encouraged to work out for themselves the appropriate times to self-administer this treatment. One patient, for example, at first found it necessary to stimulate the ear "points" 15 minutes before he noted any beneficial results. After a few days, however, he discovered that a few seconds' stimulation in the morning, early afternoon, and evening was enough to provide continuous voluntary control of his affected arm and leg.

**Diet Important** ● Diet, as we mentioned, is an important part of Dr. Kaslow's therapy—actually an equal partner with acupuncture. Patients are told to avoid all canned and preserved foods and to have everything on the table as fresh and unprocessed as possible. "There is no question in my mind," this physician said, "when one of my patients goes off the diet. The good response is lost. I won't even accept a patient for treatment unless he or she agrees to follow the dietary procedure along with the acupuncture procedure. Neither of the two seems to work alone."

He recalled one patient who phoned over a weekend because he had broken down and gobbled several ice cream cones. "All hell broke loose," the patient lamented. But immediate self-treatment with the electric prod and a return to the diet brought his disease back under control.

Like others, Dr. Kaslow cannot explain how or why acupuncture "works" to improve the symptoms of multiple sclerosis. But he does have a theory that MS is not purely a problem of demyelination of nerve fibers. If it were, he pointed out, the destroyed myelin sheaths would make it impossible for any procedure to eliminate symptoms—and yet the procedures he uses do just that, to a greater or lesser extent. Furthermore, he argues, MS patients typically go through periods of remission of symptoms—again something that couldn't happen if the destroyed myelin sheaths were the sole explanation of the disease. "Why and how an MS patient has any remission is something medical science cannot account for at this time," he noted.

"I have a feeling that we're dealing here with a metabolic problem as well as a problem of nerve degeneration," he added. "In that context I use acupuncture and diet, and have had positive results."

Another doctor, who only recently has begun to use acupuncture in treating multiple sclerosis patients—B. F. Hart, M.D., of Fort Lauderdale, Florida—theorizes that this therapy stimulates alternative pathways in the central nervous system, so that message impulses to the arms, legs, etc. bypass the nerve fibers whose myelin sheaths have been damaged or destroyed. He suggests that acupuncture treatment is not the ultimate answer for patients with this disease, but rather a "holding operation" till something better is discovered.

In his presentation to the Acupuncture Congress, Dr. Hart reported on 14 MS patients who were able to walk but who had foot drop (a falling of the foot due to muscular paralysis). Preliminary comparative tests showed that acupuncture treatment using "points" on the head (cerebral acupuncture) was more effective than the standard procedure. Given cerebral acupuncture, the patients' foot drop was corrected in all but two instances.

## Osteopuncture for Joint Pain

"One day, one of the leading executives of a major West Coast company appeared in my office," Dr. Ronald M. Lawrence said. "He had a herniated disk in his back and was ready to undergo surgery to correct it. There was no doubt about what was wrong. His condition had been proven clinically without a doubt. I had objective evidence.

"The man was 34 years old," the North Hollywood, California, neurologist continued. "That's awfully young to have a condition like that. But it was obvious that he was in terrible pain. You could tell by the way he walked. He was hanging onto a cane the way a drowning man clutches a life preserver.

"I gave him a treatment that lasted about five minutes," Dr. Lawrence went on. "It was an admittedly vigorous treatment—more so than I usually give. The man got up and walked out of my office free from pain and without his cane. He came back to me the next day and asked me to tell him how I did it. I explained the process to him, and he walked out of my office satisfied.

"That was two years ago, and I haven't seen him since. He's still free from pain," Dr. Lawrence told us.

The "process" described to his patient with the herniated—or slipped—disk is a special form of acupuncture that Dr. Lawrence has labeled "osteopuncture," or literally, acupuncture of the bone.

"We usually reach the bone by inserting the needle into one of the approximately 120 areas that are relatively accessible to us. We penetrate the periosteum (the outer layer of the bone) and then go slightly beneath it. We'll find those places where pain is relieved. We know exactly where to strike the bone in the knee to relieve pain in the knee. We know where to strike the shoulder to relieve pain in the shoulder. We know that the greater the stimulation, the greater the pain-relieving effect. And the more strength that is devoted to the treatment, the more potent the effect of the treatment."

After the needle is on the right spot for treatment, Dr. Lawrence rapidly moves it up and down on the bone itself a number of times ranging from one to twenty, depending upon the extent of the pain.

Following the treatment, he says, the patient's pain is usually completely alleviated or reduced considerably.

Dr. Lawrence has several examples of dramatic results obtained with this radical treatment. One such incident occurred the night before a marathon run.

**An Arthritic Runs a Marathon** • When we interviewed him, Dr. Lawrence was president of a group of doctors who run 26-mile marathons for recreation, the American Medical Joggers Association. On this particular night in Boston, a doctor from Denver approached Dr. Lawrence asking him about his treatment. The Denver doctor had been forced to give up running because of an arthritic knee joint.

"He came to me at a meeting we held in Boston before a race," Dr. Lawrence said. "He told me that he'd heard that I was practicing this new technique. Well, he'd had a few acupuncture treatments in Denver, and they had given him some relief, but nothing permanent."

After one treatment, which consisted of tapping the bone on the outside of the knee with a hypodermic needle, the patient was completely free from pain. And to top it off, he ran the next day's marathon meet in record-breaking time for a man of his age, 54.

"After 26 miles, he had no pain," Dr. Lawrence said. "His pain eventually did come back, but he never had the severe pain that he originally had with his arthritic knee joint. And," Dr. Lawrence added, "he had the pain for almost two years before he received that one treatment."

Dr. Lawrence was interested in acupuncture almost from the time it became popularized in the United States after President Nixon's trip to China in 1972. While studying with an acupuncturist, both of them noted an unusual phenomenon. Whenever a bone was accidentally hit by the inserted needle, there appeared to be some relief from pain.

"He didn't particularly want to go into it," Dr. Lawrence related, "but I thought that it was interesting enough to pursue it."

This pursuit led Dr. Lawrence to develop "osteopuncture," which he has used successfully over the past few years. In fact, Dr. Lawrence said, he and his associates have treated over a thousand patients with osteopuncture with good results. "We have found that by using this new technique, we can shorten the number and frequency of treatments needed for pain control and we note that effects seem more permanent."

**Life Made Easier for Amputees** ● One of Dr. Lawrence's most significant successes, he believes, has come in the area of a pain syndrome commonly called phantom limb pain. This is experienced by amputees who may be suffering severe pain which seems to come from arms or legs they no longer have.

"Almost all amputees are routinely, physically aware of the absent limb," Dr. Lawrence explains. "Pain researchers have said that the limb feels as if it is still there. And about one in seven experiences actual pain from it. This is why it is called phantom limb pain.

"I'd say that our success rate is as high as 80 to 85 percent of all the patients we see with this problem," Dr. Lawrence continued. "We get a lot of referrals from doctors treating these patients who don't know how to handle it. Many don't know how to treat it. Relief usually comes to our patients within 30 seconds to a minute."

Included in Dr. Lawrence's overall success rate, which he says runs between 85 and 88 percent, are successful treatments for low back pain, osteoarthritis, rheumatoid arthritis, and a whole cross section of disk problems.

**Disease Remains But Pain Vanishes** ● Dr. Lawrence noted that this treatment does not "cure" any disease in the classical sense of the word. Instead, it only eliminates the pain.

"The underlying reason for the pain is still there," he emphasized. "In an arthritic joint, the arthritis is still there. But the pain isn't. However, most people are satisfied that the pain is gone." Sometimes, as a side effect, when an arthritic joint is treated with osteopuncture, there is a reduction in swelling, he said.

Since the pain is gone, and pain is one of nature's ways of telling you that there is something wrong, people undergoing Dr. Lawrence's treatment still remain under the supervision of their own doctors. Often, however, by freeing the patients from the chains of pain, some healing does take place.

"We had a case of a man with an arthritic hip. I mean this was *really* arthritic. There was no movement in the joint at all, and X-rays showed that the joint was practically fused," he said.

"After he received our treatment for pain, he began moving his hip slightly. He said that he could almost hear the calcium deposits cracking up as they broke away. He came back for more and more treatments and eventually got a great deal of movement in the hip.

"Actually," Dr. Lawrence continued, "the object of the treatment in that case was to get more and more movement into the joint. The reduced pain allowed this to occur."

Dramatic achievements aside, Dr. Lawrence said that when an arthritic joint is eased of pain, the resulting freer movement sometimes brings on an increase in the blood circulation, along with an accompanying easing of the condition that caused the pain in the first place.

## Acupuncture and Pain Relief: Experiences at the UCLA Clinic

**Author's Note:** The majority of acupuncturists are engaged in private practice. I thought it would be helpful to get a kind of academic or institutional perspective on the subject, so I asked journalist Richard Cramer to look into an acupuncture research project being conducted at the University of California at Los Angeles. He discovered that the UCLA doctors were every bit as enthusiastic about acupuncture as the others we spoke with. His report follows:

The patient, a successful businesswoman, had already had disk surgery for back pain three times in her young life. Now she was in the hospital again, facing an even more traumatic procedure: cutting a section of the spinal cord to sever the pain pathways. But before resorting to such a drastic step, doctors tried something else— acupuncture. Fortunately, it worked.

"This is the type of patient we'd like to see before she's had any surgery," recalls Dr. Richard Kroening, Associate Research Physician and Director of Professional Training at UCLA's Chronic Pain Clinic. "But of course, we started acupuncture after she had two surgeries and a spinal fusion."

It took about 30 standard acupuncture treatments—needles to the low back, behind the knees, in the thigh—and today she's a functional person again. She's up, walking around, off medication, sleeping comfortably, free of depression related to her pain, even back at her old job.

Such are the results more than 50 percent of the time at this Los Angeles clinic where acupuncture is used for the treatment of intractable pain. Everything from cervical sprains and strains and musculoskeletal pain to osteoarthritis and tension headaches are being relieved, all after everything Western medicine has to offer has failed.

**Doctor's Migraine Relieved** ● Consider the case of a 42-year-old physician suffering from chronic migraine headaches. Weaving a trail of intense pain from the back of his skull over his scalp to his eyes, the headaches were as regular as clockwork—arriving almost nightly at 11 P.M. Although the doctor could prescribe the most potent and newest pharmaceuticals for himself, nothing helped.

After his first acupuncture treatment, his symptoms worsened. By the second, the attacks persisted but with less intensity. After seven treatments (each consisting of two visits per week), the frequency of migraine was markedly down, with pain moving from "excruciating" to "uncomfortable." The patient himself felt the difference: "It was like night and day."

By the end of six months of treatment at the clinic, the physician's migraine headaches slid from twenty per month to less than one each month.

Together with Dr. David Bresler, Director of the UCLA Acupuncture Research Project and Adjunct Assistant Professor in the Departments of Anesthesiology and Psychology, Dr. Kroening has administered over 18,000 acupuncture treatments to some 2,000 patients in the past two years.

At UCLA, a trial of acupuncture therapy consists of 10 or 11 acupuncture treatments. Each treatment involves two sessions a week. Evaluations are made after every 10 treatments by a staff physician and, naturally, the more chronic the complaint, the greater the number of treatments needed. In acute problems, such as muscle strains or sprains, only a few treatments are required for relief.

"We are interested in studying the effectiveness of techniques used by traditional Oriental practitioners," notes Dr. Bresler, "by bringing them into a clinical laboratory where they can be supervised and observed scientifically. By thoroughly evaluating the nature of each patient's problem and response to acupuncture, we can determine the true value which acupuncture may offer for the treatment of illness."

The Acupuncture Research Project at UCLA is interested in more than just the subjective reports from patients as to whether or not they are pain free. "We also want to see whether there are changes in their sleep patterns," says Dr. Bresler, "in the amounts of analgesic medication they require, and in their daily activities."

In addition, a number of functional tests are administered to complement the subjective reports of patients. "In the case of a low back pain patient," observes Dr. Bresler, "we want to know if he can put on his shoes and socks, cut his toenails, or climb stairs."

**Trying the Needle Before the Knife** ● One of the more interesting observations made by researchers at the California clinic is the relationship between lasting pain relief and related surgery. Simply stated, if a low back patient is helped with acupuncture and has *not* had any low back surgery, pain relief generally remains for at least six months. On the other hand, if patients have had back surgery, they generally do not remain pain-free for six months, although they may have received some short-term relief following acupuncture therapy. "Thus it's very clear," says Dr. Kroening, "that many low back pain patients should be given acupuncture prior to surgery, and not after all else fails."

**Help for Osteoarthritis** ● On the basis of their research findings, Drs. Bresler and Kroening believe that a significant number of pain patients—especially the elderly with osteoarthritis aches and pains—can benefit tremendously from acupuncture therapy. No hospitalization or constant medical supervision is needed, and it is not a traumatic procedure.

A 67-year-old woman had been living with generalized osteoarthritis for years. It had become especially painful in her hips and knees, making stair climbing, walking, even sleeping almost impossible. Medication did nothing, and only topical heat offered a modicum of relief.

Her first five acupuncture treatments failed to relieve her pain, but by the sixth, she felt results. She could stand longer, walk easier, and her pain was markedly less sharp. After some 13 or 14 treatments, she continued to improve and found her pain only "mild."

After six months of acupuncture treatments, she stopped going to the clinic. Six months after that, her pain returned once again, though not as badly as before acupuncture.

"We consider her a success," Dr. Bresler feels. "We don't promise complete pain relief, only that we can help a great deal."

Yet acupuncture is still classified as "experimental," and although physicians are legally permitted to administer acupuncture in most states, medical schools have by and large not established appropriate training programs for physicians and other health care professionals. At the present time, it is impossible to determine the competence of a given acupuncturist, whether he is a physician or not.

"Until the appropriate federal and state agencies recognize the value of acupuncture," states Dr. Bresler, "and establish clearcut guidelines for training and practice, it will remain unavailable to hundreds of thousands of pain sufferers who could benefit from this ancient healing art."

### Seeking an Acupuncturist

If you are interested in acupuncture treatment, don't rush out to the nearest practitioner who claims skill with the needles. Your local hospital may have an acupuncture clinic or be able to recommend one.

A nonprofit organization, The Acupuncture Information Center of New York, 127 East Sixty-ninth Street, New York, New York 10021, can help you in finding a qualified acupuncturist in your part of the country.

Referrals to acupuncturists who are M.D.'s may be obtained from the National Acupuncture Research Society, Suite 1508, 505 Park Avenue, New York, New York 10022.

In both cases, be sure to include a stamped self-addressed envelope.

# Arthritis

People who say that arthritis is incurable are correct in the sense that there is no "magic bullet" that can wipe out this chronic, painful, and often disabling condition.

In another sense, they are misleadingly pessimistic, because many cases of arthritis have been greatly—and often unexpectedly—improved when the individual decided to take action on his own.

That doesn't mean encircling your body with copper bracelets and eating nothing but raw fruits and coconut milk. It means a responsible and determined effort to seek out the best advice you can get and trying every conservative measure before resigning yourself to surgery or a lifetime of drug dependency.

A case in point. A woman whom I know well developed rheumatoid arthritis at the age of about 45 or 50 and went to a leading rheumatologist, or specialist in treating arthritis. He prescribed corticosteroids, which are considered the most effective anti-inflammatory drugs. Several years later, after moving, she went to another doctor who reviewed her case and kept her on the corticosteroids. Meanwhile, her condition became somewhat worse, and it was necessary for her to walk with a cane. Finally, when one of her ankles was degenerating and becoming quite painful, still another doctor, a surgeon, suggested an operation which he said would help her walk better.

At this point, the woman decided to consult another specialist, who informed her that the operation probably would not help her at all. He then asked if any of the other doctors she had been to had prescribed orthopedic shoes. He was surprised when she said they hadn't, and he then prescribed a pair for her. A few weeks later, she was walking without a cane for the first time in years.

Her pleasure in being able to walk better without surgery was given a bitter taste, however, by the realization that none of the other doctors she had seen even mentioned orthopedic shoes. The *Merck Manual* states that "Orthopedic shoes, with various modifications to fit individual needs, help many patients," so this is no great secret. Yet, had she not persisted in her search for a better treatment, she might have had to undergo entirely unnecessary surgery.

## Drugs Waste Bones

There is another aspect to her case which is both important for arthritis patients to understand, and revealing of still another failure of her doctors. One day, after having been on the corticosteroid medication for a number of years, she bumped her arm against a table and discovered a few days later, to her amazement and disgust, that she had broken a bone. At this point, her doctor informed her, "Well, that's what happens when you take corticosteroids for a long time. Your bones go."

That was the second or third doctor she had been to, all of whom were aware of her drug schedule, and yet none of them had warned her of this dangerous side effect of cortisone drugs. There is a curious outcome to this incident, though. Shortly later, she visited an orthopedic specialist who already had received her X-rays, and he mentioned to her that her broken arm seemed to be healing incredibly fast for a woman of her age and history.

Why was that? It seems that about a year or two before this incident, the woman had begun taking two dolomite tablets daily, supplying herself with a moderate measure of calcium and magnesium. Apparently, she didn't take enough of these minerals to reverse the calcium-wasting effect of her drugs, but it was sufficient to allow her broken arm to heal swiftly. Following that incident, she doubled her intake of dolomite in hopes of preventing future fractures.

From what I can gather, this is a common occurrence. Although the *Merck Manual*, for instance, warns that when a patient who is on corticosteroids complains of an ache in the mid-spine area, the doctor should immediately suspect osteoporosis and begin giving calcium supplements, there is not a word of advice to give calcium or other nutrients prophylactically so that the wasting is kept to an absolute minimum.

So again, if it had not been for this woman's own initiative, her condition would likely have been much worse than it was and her bones vulnerable to yet more fractures from only slight bumps.

Drugs may not be the only thing causing fractures in arthritis patients. An article in the *British Medical Journal* in 1974 points out that "Dietary vitamin D deficiency seems to play an important role in causing both the fractures and the osteopenia [bone frailty] of long-standing rheumatoid arthritis." The authors further point out that many people with advanced arthritis rarely leave the house, and so do not receive much vitamin D from sunlight. They recommend a daily supplement of vitamin D to help prevent these needless fractures.

## Diet and Arthritis

It is probably wise for the arthritic to take a full range of supplements, because of the stress produced by this condition. For the arthritic who is taking heavy doses of aspirin, a generous supplement of vitamin C is especially important, because aspirin depletes this vitamin from certain blood fractions and therefore lowers resistance to a variety of diseases. Large doses of aspirin can also cause ulcers, of course, but even if they don't, there is almost certainly a considerable amount of blood loss taking place from the stomach. Over the course of years, this loss could possibly produce anemia or near-anemia in the patient whose diet is not rich in iron.

Some doctors have suggested that a specific vitamin deficiency, such as pantothenic acid, is involved in arthritis, and that supplements are the answer. I am not impressed, however, by their evidence, nor by the responses of people who have tried the one-vitamin approach. Other doctors take a broader view and prescribe a diet which is high in protein, high in raw fruits and vegetables and their juices, improved with a full range of supplements, and which excludes all refined carbohydrates, saturated fats, junk foods, tobacco, and alcohol. Statistically, this approach—by itself—cannot be said to perform miracles, but it makes a lot more sense than simply taking one special nutrient.

An exception is $B_6$ especially for stiffness of the hands: 50 to 100 mg. daily plus magnesium and vitamin C.

In my own opinion, I would say the best diet that an arthritic can go on—if she or he is overweight—is one which will remove all the excess poundage. When weight loss is accompanied by gradually increasing daily exercise, which is continued until just before a sense of fatigue is felt, the results are sometimes astounding.

Although it may sound ironic, the same exercise or joint movement which can produce so much pain in the arthritic may also be his or her best bet to arrest or even substantially improve the problem. When a joint is not used over a period of months or years, it tends to freeze or lock up, and that is the worst possible eventuality. Surrounding muscles will simultaneously atrophy, which makes the problem even worse. An exercise program should be started when the pain is relatively quiescent, with every affected joint, whether it be in the toes or the neck, taken through the fullest possible range of motion. There will be some moderate pain or discomfort involved (don't do it to the point where it causes real pain) but when done gradually and progressively, and with a kind of dogged determination to keep those joints from locking up, the results can be most gratifying.

## Help for Morning Stiffness

If you wake up in the morning with stiff hands, you may find that wearing a pair of stretch gloves at night will help. At least, that's what one study reported in *Geriatrics* said in 1975. On the other hand, tight gloves may actually *cause* problems. Not long ago, a letter was published in *Lancet* from a woman surgeon who said that when she moved to a new hospital, she began to develop persistent aching pains in her right hand. "I attributed the pain to age," she said, "but I was puzzled by the rather abrupt onset." By sheer luck, however, the doctor discovered that at her new hospital, they used a different brand of gloves, in which the sizes were slightly smaller than the make she had used before. When she changed to a half-size larger, her joint pain ceased immediately.

If your whole body is stiff in the morning, try going to bed in a sleeping bag. That may sound slightly ridiculous, but one recent study shows that it can be remarkably effective. The discovery was actually made by a young Boy Scout, who had been suffering with juvenile rheumatoid arthritis. He noticed that after he slept in his sleeping bag during a camp-out, he did not experience the usual morning stiffness and pain. After the trip, when he went back to sleeping in his bed, the stiffness and pain returned. The following night he wrapped himself in his sleeping bag, which he had spread out on top of his bed, and the next day again enjoyed relief from his symptoms.

When his grandmother got the news, she tried it herself. She had osteoarthritis, an arthritis of the bone which usually afflicts people over 40. The next morning, she felt like a new person.

That's how Earl J. Brewer, Jr., M.D., chief of rheumatology service at Texas Children's Hospital in Houston says it all started. In *Pediatrics* (October 1975), Dr. Brewer writes that after learning how effective a treatment the sleeping bag was to the scout and his grandmother, he decided to let his other patients in on it. So the hospital staff asked all patients with morning stiffness to climb into a sleeping bag regularly. A number of them were so pleased by the simple remedy that they continued it at home.

The secret, of course, is that the sleeping bag keeps the body snuggly and uniformly warm during the night—much more effectively than an electric blanket, Dr. Brewer adds.

## Acupuncture, Arthritis, and the Mind

Under the entry on acupuncture, we mention a number of doctors who have reported considerable success treating various forms of arthritis (but not, to my knowledge, rheumatoid arthritis). Curiously, though, several recent tests of acupuncture for arthritis indicate that something rather peculiar may be going on here. In one test, one group of patients was given acupuncture on their backs for their arthritic pain. Another group of patients was merely pricked with pins which did not penetrate the skin and were not placed at the proper acupuncture points. Some weeks later, it was discovered that both groups had improved very considerably and that there was no real difference between the improvement in the two groups.

This suggests that in at least some, and perhaps many cases of arthritis, there is a psychological component which should not be ignored. It doesn't mean that the disease is necessarily caused purely by psychological or unconscious factors, but it does clearly suggest that when it comes to easing the suffering, psychology may be just as important as anything else.

A dramatic instance of this was reported in the *Journal of the American Medical Association* (December 9, 1974) by Forrest J. Cioppa, M.D., and Alan B. Thal, M.D., of Walnut Creek, California. They describe the case of a 10-year-old girl in whom a rheumatologist had diagnosed juvenile rheumatoid arthritis which responded only minimally to large doses of aspirin and physical therapy over a period of seven weeks. The child was "depressed, uncommunicative, and inactive." The doctors decided to try hypnotherapy. Four hours after her second session, the girl rode her bicycle "and was without pain, for the first time in twelve weeks. Two reinforcing hypnotherapy sessions were added. Schoolwork and social adjustment improved markedly. The child has remained well for 33 months," the two California doctors reported.

The moral of all this, perhaps, is that when it comes to arthritis, both doctors and the public must have a very open-minded attitude and be willing to try therapies such as acupuncture and hypnosis, despite the fact that they are still considered experimental. When the condition resists other forms of therapy, and when drug toxicity becomes a problem, it is downright foolish not to give these modalities an honest try.

I would also suggest keeping in mind this concept: Arthritis in person A is not necessarily the same disease as it is in person B. Even when the labels may be identical, and the symptoms similar, we must remember that the causes of arthritis are almost entirely unknown. A diagnosis such as "osteoarthritis" is only a word, and nothing more. It does not mean that the doctor understands why you are ill. Logically, then, he cannot be certain what is going to help you and what is not going to help you.

## Don't Scorn Folk Remedies

From this point of view then, and because the medical therapies for arthritis often leave much to be desired, folk remedies should not be scorned. And in fact, letters we've received from PREVENTION readers indicate that some people who have tried folk remedies and other treatments which lack scientific evaluation have been mighty pleased at the results.

First, we've received many letters describing often dramatic improvement of arthritic conditions when the person went on what some people refer to as the "PREVENTION diet," meaning the elimination of junk foods, sugar, white bread, alcohol, and other health destroyers; an emphasis on raw or lightly cooked fruits, vegetables, sprouts, and whole grains; and broad-spectrum supplementation with vitamins and minerals.

It would be easy to dismiss these cases as coincidences, or placebo reactions. Easy until you read the letters. One perfectly typical letter came from a woman who had arthritis in her knee for a year and a half. Her doctor recommended wearing a rubber stocking over her knee, which "had no effect at all." The pain was so severe that she couldn't sleep at night and walking was difficult, even with a cane. Going up and down stairs "became almost impossible." Finally, she said, she began taking vitamin C, vitamin E, bone meal, and dolomite. "In about two weeks the pain was entirely gone to my great joy and amazement! Gradually the stiffness disappeared and in a month's time I was walking freely."

Remember, I said that letter was typical, and I mean it. I'm not saying that the *response* is typical; only that one of the more common themes of letters we receive is that arthritis pain is relieved and mobility increased shortly after beginning a better nutrition program.

**Calcium May Be Important** • Be sure not to overlook calcium. I'm quite sure that calcium does not somehow "cure" arthritis, but my suspicion is that a good deal of what is called arthritis pain is either caused or aggravated by the demineralization of bones.

One reader told us that she developed arthritis four years before she wrote to us. She consulted six doctors but the only thing they could agree on was that she was going to have to "learn to live with it." This woman must have had real pain, because, as she put it, "at times it seemed the marrow in my bones had a toothache. At times I could not even turn a water faucet on. I prayed until I think even God must have tired of me."

One day, she related, she got hold of an old copy of PREVENTION and read about bone meal. "I got a bottle and started taking six to nine tablets a day. I set them by my chair. Within three days the pain had lessened and in a week it was all gone. I took the tablets for two weeks and then, being curious, I stopped. The pain returned. When I started again, it stopped. . . . I know three months do not make a cure. But I do not have pains, I can move easily now, and I am off painkilling drugs. I used to use about 200 Arthritis Pain Formula pills every five or six weeks, now I do not take any at all."

Another recent letter came from a registered nurse who said she had been "plagued with an arthritic neck for seven years. . . . After the same old story of thousands of dollars of ineffective treatment and years of incapacitating pain," she read in PREVENTION about the importance of calcium. At that time, she was taking three tablets of bone meal daily, but "I immediately began taking nine to twelve tablets daily and in one week was without pain! I told my story to a friend, a nurse anesthetist, who has osteoarthritis. She had refused a total hip replacement three years ago and has been living on aspirin daily since that time. Within 10 days she was totally free of pain—not one more aspirin!"

Finally, she related, the doctor she worked for, who happened to be an ear, nose, and throat surgeon, also suffered from an arthritic neck. She said they had always attributed their mutual plight to occupational position in surgery over the years. The doctor had used traction, muscle-relaxing drugs, painkillers, and finally had to cut down his surgery because of pain. He did not believe that bone meal or anything else could help him, because he had spurs on his cervical spine, but after beginning the bone meal regimen, the nurse reported, his pain was 50 percent better in just five days.

That's why I say you shouldn't overlook calcium.

**A Typical Folk Remedy** • Ruth Stout, the author of many books on gardening, wrote to us when she was nearing 90 years of age, and said that "Several years ago I got terrible pains in my back and legs. I went to see a doctor and he said I had a bad case of arthritis. He didn't need to tell me that! He sent me to another doctor for X-rays who corroborated the diagnosis and also recommended a heating pad and painkilling pills. No cure, both doctors said.

"Luckily I was just then reading a book about doing this and that for one's health. I turned to 'arthritis', where it said you can cure it by eating pecans, bananas, brewer's yeast, wheat germ, and avocados. Plus anything else you want to eat.

"Well, why not try it? I did. In a few days I abandoned the pills and heating pad, and in less than two weeks there was no more pain at all and has never been any since."

She said that she passed on this folk remedy to many others and has many "glowing reports of results."

**Alfalfa and Cherries** ● There are many herbs which are said to be good for arthritis, but going only by the letters we've received, the winner seems to be alfalfa. "For nine years I suffered with rheumatoid arthritis," one reader said, and then went on to list all the drugs she had taken. She had "quite a bit of crippling," was anemic, and was in constant severe pain.

Then, she received from a relative a recipe for alfalfa tea that had appeared in PREVENTION back in 1968. "I began drinking it every day for about three months," she said. "After that I drank it every other day and now I make it twice a week. Slowly but surely my health improved and the pain lessened each day. Today I live a nearly normal life (my wrists and shoulders are limited in function), my blood count is in the normal range, and my weight is 140 [previously she had weighed only 96 pounds at five feet nine inches]."

Additionally, she had altered her diet to exclude sugar, coffee, chemicals, overly processed foods, white flour, and to include fresh fruits and vegetables, vitamins, bran, less meat, and more protein and other foods. That's what you call alfalfa-*plus*!

The alfalfa tea recipe she referred to goes like this:

> Cook, but do not boil, in an enamel or glass pan, one ounce of untreated alfalfa seed (such as for sprouting) with 1¼ pints of water. Keep water moving but not boiling for half an hour. Then strain and squeeze seeds for more fluid. Cool and refrigerate, but do not keep for more than one day. To use, mix the strong base with an equal amount of water (or to taste), add honey if you wish. Use six or seven cups or four or five glasses a day. Try for at least two weeks.

That same recipe also did the trick for a California man whose arthritis in his back became so bad that he could hardly get in and out of his car. He enjoyed lawn bowling, he said, and the thought of having to give it up was very depressing. He then found out about alfalfa seeds, but rather than making a tea, he ground up three tablespoons of them every day, mixing them with yogurt or milk as part of his lunch. The results? "My back is in wonderful shape again, and I bowl three or four times each week."

Cherries have been eaten with gratifying results by many people suffering with gout, which is a form of arthritis. But they also seem to help other forms of arthritis. Some typical comments from readers: "I started eating cherries about a month and a half ago, after reading articles in PREVENTION about their helpfulness in similar cases. After about a week I woke up one morning and felt like a new person. Skin was clear, swelling was gone, and I could bend my fingers completely and painlessly. My wrists and ankles shrank, I wasn't even aware they were swollen before. Painful years of suffering and shame of unsightly splits and sometimes bleeding hands were gone. I couldn't believe it."

A New York woman said that she had bought some sour cherries to make a pie, "but sat around picking at them until I had eaten about a pound of them. Within a few hours, pain had left my shoulder and arm. I continued eating the sour cherries during their season and had relief the entire time. When I stopped eating them, the pain returned." Another reader with arthritic fingers started eating cherries and drinking cherry juice and after two weeks said that there was less swelling, and the pain was entirely gone. "I hadn't been able to make a fist before, but now I can."

Herbalists also value watercress and parsley for rheumatism, while Grieve says that the lemon "is highly recommended in acute rheumatism." Pokeweed berries are an old folk remedy for rheumatism, but no more than three or four should be taken at any one time, and only the ripe berries should be used. Unripe berries or too many of any kind of pokeweed berries can make you very ill.

# Asthma

One of the most encouraging recent developments in the therapy of bronchial asthma was the discovery that pyridoxine, or vitamin $B_6$, can help many people afflicted with this disease. Just as important, the large doses of $B_6$ required to achieve improvement do not—unlike asthma drugs—cause dangerous side effects.

In their report published in the *Annals of Allergy* (August 1975), a team of five physicians, headed by Platon J. Collipp, M.D., chief of the Department of Pediatrics at the Nassau County Medical Center in New York, describes results achieved in a trial with 76 young patients, all suffering from moderate to severe asthma and ranging in age from two to sixteen.

Earlier work of a biochemical nature suggested that asthma patients might have what is known as a pyridoxine dependency, meaning that they do not have a deficiency in the normal sense of the word but a greatly exaggerated need for the vitamin because of disturbed metabolism. The trial was therefore designed to be a scientifically rigorous one which would clearly demonstrate the results, positive or negative, of $B_6$ supplementation. To accomplish this, the youngsters were divided into two groups. Half received two 100 mg. tablets of vitamin $B_6$ daily; the other half took two placebo or dummy tablets. Neither doctors nor patients knew who was receiving the pyridoxine. This is what is known as a double-blind study, to ensure that the results would not be distorted by the power of suggestion or the eagerness of the doctors to see improvement in the test group.

The study was continued for five months. Each day, parents evaluated their children's condition using special forms to record wheezing, difficult breathing, coughing, tightness in the chest, and number of asthma attacks. Each month the children returned to the doctors for examination, and the forms were collected.

At the conclusion of the trial, doctors broke the code and discovered which patients had been receiving the vitamin and which the placebo. The results were impressive. During the first month of the trial both groups fared about the same. But beginning with the second month, the group receiving 200 mg. of $B_6$ daily experienced fewer asthma attacks than the other children, less wheezing, less coughing, tightness, and breathing difficulty. As a result, they required less medication—in the form of oral bronchodilators and cortisone—than the other children. These differences continued until the trial ended, being most significant during the second and fifth months.

"The data from these patients suggest that pyridoxine therapy may be a useful medication which reduces the severity of asthma in many, but not all, asthmatic children," Dr. Collipp and his colleagues concluded.

That is especially good news considering that some of the more widely used asthma therapies involve considerable risk. Prednisone, for instance, a steroid drug commonly prescribed for bronchial asthma, may produce such serious adverse reactions as convulsions, glaucoma, peptic ulcer, and psychic derangements. Steroids are even capable of suppressing growth in children. Another popular medication, isoproterenol, which is inhaled through the mouth when an acute bronchial attack strikes, can actually cause *increased* breathing difficulty in certain individuals. In some instances, misuse of such inhalers has resulted in abnormal heart rhythm and even death.

Pyridoxine therapy, on the other hand, produced no side effects at all. But keep in mind that it seems to take at least a month for improvement to appear. And although this particular study involved children, it may well be that adults would benefit equally.

The report on $B_6$ therapy is easily the most impressive piece of evidence for nutritional help in asthma. Other work I have seen suggests that some people may be helped by vitamins A and D. In general, do not take more than about 20,000 units of vitamin A a day or more than 800 units of vitamin D.

Anyone who has asthma should be aware that cold weather often brings on attacks. The emergency room of a hospital in New York City once plotted on a graph the number of cases of acute asthma attacks treated, and a dramatic spike was evident in the month of January. If the option is available, then, consider moving to a warmer climate.

## Herbs to Help the Asthmatic

The world of herbalism is not lacking in *materia medica* for the asthmatic. One of the most highly regarded herbs for this use is mullein, which grows in many places like a weed. The soft fuzzy leaves can be placed in a teapot with hot water and the steam inhaled through the spout to relieve symptoms. One reader wrote to us that after drinking eight ounces of mullein tea daily over a period of time—apparently several weeks—he gradually began to notice an improvement in his asthmatic condition. Previously, he said, he had spent thousands of dollars on prescribed medication that "at best gave but temporary relief." Now, he said, "I take no medication and feel wonderful. But I do drink mullein tea daily."

I have learned through experience that it is not of much use to describe an herb in print or even to present a drawing of it. Therefore, if you want to know what mullein looks like in hopes that it may be growing wild in your area (it used to sprout up all over my lawn until we began mowing regularly), I would suggest finding a book or a chart that has color photographs. You may be able to find mullein leaves or flowers in an herb shop or health food store.

Other herbs said to be helpful for asthma are elecampane, ephedra, eucalyptus, horehound, lungwort, and pleurisy root. Any combination of these herbs may be brewed into a tea and taken several times a day, especially at bedtime. A nice hot dish of garlic soup taken before retiring may also prove soothing. If the aroma of garlic is too powerful for you, folk medicine tradition has it that a tablespoon of corn oil or sunflower seed oil taken at night may be comforting.

## Beware of Aspirin and Additives

Too few parents of asthmatic children realize that a simple aspirin tablet can provoke a serious attack in many asthmatic children. If you have noticed problems following aspirin ingestion, consider yourself warned. Occasionally, the reaction can be very severe.

The artificial food coloring agent tartrazine, or Yellow 5, has also been reported to trigger asthma attacks in susceptible youngsters. Avoiding this additive isn't easy, because it is used in a great many artificially colored foods, some of which may not even appear to be yellow.

In light of the clinical and theoretical work of allergist Ben F. Feingold, M.D., who has been able to control both hyperactivity and allergic reactions such as itching, hives, and skin rashes by eliminating all artificially dyed and flavored foods from the diet, we could speculate that a purely natural foods diet might help asthmatic children. See HYPERACTIVITY, later in this book.

# Athlete's Foot

Athlete's foot is a fungal infection (actually ringworm of the feet) which in most cases can be controlled by keeping the spaces between your toes clean and dry with the peeling skin rubbed away. A dusting powder often helps. It's important to keep your feet dry, because it seems that the accumulation of perspiration may be more important in this condition than the fungi. Go barefoot as much as you can.

However, the condition sometimes resists every treatment in the dermatologist's bag, and it may spread to involve other parts of the feet and the toenails. According to one reference book, when the toenails become involved "cure is usually impossible." Note the word "usually"; sometimes, it seems, even the worst infections can be cured by natural means.

One woman told us she had had a severe case of athlete's foot for 20 years. It involved her toenails and even her heels, which began to split so that it became very painful for her to walk. "Finally," she wrote, "I decided to try mixing all the B-complex vitamins, backing them up with brewer's yeast, and putting them in a carrying agent that would make them adhere to my skin but that would be friendly to the B vitamins. The particular recipe I used was to crush up six tablets of riboflavin, eight tablets of niacin, and seven tablets of pantothenic acid and then mix them with two rounded teaspoons of brewer's yeast powder. Then I add two teaspoons of either crude sesame oil or rice bran oil. I mix them all together and apply once a day all over the feet between toes, on nails, etc. Then I put on a pair of clean white socks to keep it off good socks or bedding. Scrub feet once a day and remove any loose skin flakes. Reapply 'salve' *after drying feet thoroughly.* Keep 'salve' in the refrigerator. If it gets too thick to spread, add a little more oil or water. Be sure that water, if used, is not fluoridated or chlorinated." The recipe cured her case, at least.

A masseur said that he has had much success relieving athlete's foot by soaking a small piece of cotton in raw honey and placing it between the infected toes before going to bed. He covers his foot with an old sock to prevent soiling.

Another reader found that dabbing her feet with vinegar morning and night did the trick.

Another reader reported success after following the advice of nutritionist Adelle Davis, who said she cured her daughter's stubborn case of athlete's foot with yeast drinks and vitamin B supplements. In addition to this, this reader bathed her foot with goldenseal powder, dried her feet, and then dusted them with more powdered goldenseal.

# Back Pain

Everyone loves to talk about his or her diseases and I am no exception. So let me tell you about my low back problem and how I cured it—by accident!

The first time my back attacked me I was only about 12 or 13 years old. I had taken a "set shot" with a basketball from the half-court mark and I don't remember if a miracle happened and the ball went into the basket, but I do remember that I had to hobble home, crippled with pain. After several more such incidents, it seemed clear that I had inherited my father's bad back. His problem was quite serious, often laying him up for several days or more at a time, and necessitating, through the years, innumerable visits to doctors.

At 14, I took up weight lifting and concentrated on exercises for the lower back—notably, one called the "dead lift," in which you squat down with the back held absolutely straight. Then, with fully extended arms, one palm facing frontwards and one backwards, you lift a barbell to the standing position. Logically, perhaps, such exercises should have destroyed me, but they didn't. At that point, my back was still in good enough shape to respond to these exercises with rapid development of very powerful muscles along the sides of the spine. Generally speaking, the more powerful these muscles are, the more they will support your spine and prevent disks from slipping around. Throughout my teenage years, I continued these exercises until I was able to deadlift about 250 pounds. During these years, while I was working out several times a week, my back didn't give me much trouble.

In my twenties, I gave up weight lifting and every other form of exercise, and my back problem returned with a vengeance. once or twice a year it would "go out" on me, and as the years p these episodes became more and more painful and disabling. various occasions, I visited a chiropractor, an orthopedic surgeon, and several osteopaths, finding the greatest and quickest relief with the latter, who were able to snap my spine back into alignment whenever the occasion demanded.

During this time, several doctors recommended that I do certain exercises and I did do them—sometimes . . . for a while. The problem was that they didn't seem to do much good, even when I did them regularly, so after a while I just forgot about them.

Finally, after spending most of one day moving furniture and then washing and polishing my car (like many other victims of low back pain, I just wouldn't *learn*), I got the worst attack of my life. I was limping around with my knuckles practically dragging on the floor, and I still vividly remember propping myself up on a tabletop with one hand to make a phone call to the first orthopedic surgeon I could find in the telephone book. I was in such pain that I insisted he be paged at the hospital even though I didn't know him. I must say, though, that he was remarkably nice about it all, perhaps recognizing the suffering I had. I described my symptoms, my history, and he said he was quite certain I had a slipped disk. He instructed me to lie down on a firm bed and stay there, with a heating pad under my back and a couple of pillows under my knees. Then, as I recall, several times a day my wife was to remove the pillows, grasp one of my legs and firmly and steadily pull it for a few moments. Then the other leg, and finally, both legs together. I was also to take aspirin for a few days to help relieve the pain.

The improvement came quite quickly—in about two days, as I remember. In four days, I was just about as good as new, which surprised and delighted me.

So now I knew what to do *after* I had thrown my back out. But I still didn't know what to do to prevent these terrible episodes.

## Kicking Away My Pain

A short while later, for reasons having absolutely nothing to do with my bad back, I decided to take up karate—specifically, the Korean form of karate known as *tae-kwan-do*. Three times a week I worked out in a small gymnasium, for an hour and a half per session. About six months later I suddenly became aware of an amazing fact: my poor, weak, vulnerable lower back had turned into stainless steel! I could do *anything,* even carry heavy trash cans, without hurting myself. And most amazing of all, when I woke up in the morning, I never felt even the slightest twinge of discomfort as I rolled out of bed.

Naturally, I tried to analyze why practicing karate had achieved this remarkable effect. Curiously, there was not a single exercise or movement that we did in karate that had much resemblance to the standard exercises I had been told to do to strengthen my back. We did not, for example, lie on our stomachs and raise our trunks while someone held our legs down. Neither did we ever do any kind of sit-ups. But what we did do was kick—and I mean *kick!*

Korean karate, more than other forms of this martial art, emphasizes the use of the legs in self-defense. The Koreans feel there is no sense injuring your hand when you can use the heel or ball of your foot to do the job. So at every session, we practiced kicking endlessly. First, there were warm-up kicks with the leg held absolutely straight or as straight as possible, which loosens the massive, tight muscles in the back of the thigh. To complete the warm-up for these muscles, we would often hook our heels on a ledge about three feet high and then *gently* bounce forward. During our actual practice, we performed scores of front "snap" kicks, roundhouse kicks, side kicks, back kicks, and leg sweeps.

From a self-defense point of view, the purpose of all this was to give us sufficient control over our legs so that regardless of the position in which we were caught during an attack, we would be able to defend ourselves with our feet, striking the attacker anywhere from his knee up to his ear (after some practice, it is quite easy to stand directly in front of someone and deliver a kick to his ear).

But as far as my *back* was concerned, I became convinced that all this kicking and stretching was what had done the trick. Why, I didn't exactly know, since I had the idea at that time that the way to help your bad back was to do exercises which made your back muscles *contract,* making them stronger. All I had done was *stretch* the muscles in the hamstring area and perhaps stretch my back muscles too.

It also occurred to me that while we never did sit-ups, when you pick up your leg to throw a kick, your stomach muscles are responsible for most of the lifting. And, in fact, my stomach muscles had grown remarkably powerful, to the extent where I could be kicked (accidentally) in the stomach quite hard without feeling any discomfort.

A few years later, my suspicions were confirmed when I read a book called *Orthotherapy* (Evans, New York, 1971) by Dr. Arthur Michele, Professor and Chairman of the Department of Orthopedic Surgery at New York Medical College.

## A Surgeon's Explanation

Dr. Michele explains that the underlying cause of most back problems involves an extraordinarily large complex of muscles in the lower back known as the iliopsoas. He describes it as "Mainly a broad flat muscle in the lower back, but like an octopus, it has arms reaching out in many directions." Its lower segments are attached to the pelvis, hips, and thigh bones, while its upper extremities go to every vertebrae in the lumbar area of the lower spine, and even up to the lower thoracic (chest) vertebrae in the mid-back.

All too often, Dr. Michele believes, one of the many arms of the iliopsoas is abnormally short—either because of a birth defect or, more often, because of contraction resulting from lack of stretching and use.

The "arms" of the iliopsoas have a grip on so many bones, joints, and vertebrae, Dr. Michele explains, that a shortness of any one arm can result in a large number of symptoms—*which do not necessarily occur at the point of the underlying muscular problem.*

These typical symptoms, he says, include pain or stiffness of the spine, slipped disk, actual fracture of the spine or degenerative disorders of the spine, arthrosis of the knee or hip, and even a pain in the chest and poor functioning of internal organs.

Dr. Michele is convinced that many of his patients would never have had to limp into his consulting room or be wheeled into his operating theater had they followed a simple exercise regimen he has developed. Just as important—because the average person isn't interested in his back muscles until they desert him—Dr. Michele says that his exercises are equally potent as a cure, providing the spine has not become hopelessly degenerate. In fact, he says, after 35 years of orthopedic practice, he is certain that these exercises "can bring about what seem to be near miracles" not only with back problems, but other related muscular-skeletal problems.

A 27-year-old woman whose husband was a doctor came to Dr. Michele complaining of severe aching of the knees, hips, and lower back. During her menstrual period the pains were often so severe as to be disabling. After a bout of spring cleaning, she developed severe heartburn. Finally, she began to have headaches. She had already been to a gynecologist and had been X-rayed, but no cause for her problems could be found.

"Her case history is a perfect progression of the symptoms which can result from muscle imbalance," Dr. Michele explains. Her joint pains were caused by the imbalance, bringing about an uneven distribution of her body weight. "The symptoms of heartburn were caused when the esophagus, shortened from years of slumping posture, pulled the stomach up against it and partly through the diaphragm opening, making it possible for acid from the stomach to slosh back up into the esophagus." After following a regular exercise program, "most of her painful symptoms are gone," Dr. Michele reports.

Judy R., a woman of 25, had a severe pain in her shoulder radiating into her hand, a headache, and a miserable backache that simply would not go away. "Ultimately I was able to trace her various symptoms, head and back pain, to a rigid muscle in the hip. . . . After six weeks of an exercise program, she was able to report for the first time in two years that she wasn't in pain," the orthopedic surgeon declares.

In studying Dr. Michele's exercise program, I was struck by the fact that in respect to stretching certain muscles, it was very similar to what I had been doing in my karate classes.

So I recommend to you that if you don't want to take up *tae-kwan-do* (I'm not really sure if Japanese karate would have the same therapeutic effect) I recommend his exercises to you. In his book, he presents a complete program, with different exercises for different problems. Here, I would like to share with you a few basic movements which will give you an idea of what his program is like and may also prove quite helpful in themselves.

Dr. Michele gives two basic series of exercises. The first series is designed for people whose backs are in bad shape. The second series consists of exercises designed to maintain your back in good condition after you have remedied the fundamental lesions. Here, we are going to present a selected number of exercises of the first series—for those people whose delinquent back muscles need some basic disciplinary measures. If you're currently under treatment, you can ask your doctor about these exercises, Dr. Michele says.

If possible, set aside 20 minutes to a half hour, twice a day, for best results from these exercises. "Years of neglect, years of letting your muscles go unsupervised, cannot be atoned for in a few minutes of lackadaisical stretching every now and then," the physician counsels.

First, put on some clothing that will not impede your movement in any direction. If you really want to get in the mood, you can don a leotard or sweat suit, but underwear, old slacks, or pajamas are just as good. And take your shoes and stockings off.

The exercises we are going to describe to you are by no means a complete program, but we believe they will get to the heart of many muscular difficulties. In performing these exercises, it is important to warm up gradually and do the exercises in order, because the last ones act most directly on the iliopsoas itself.

**The Neck and Shoulder Uncramper** ● Here's an exercise designed

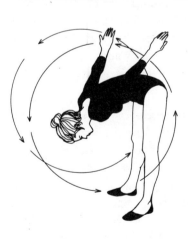

to relieve cramping and pain in the neck and shoulders. Stand with your feet slightly separated. Bend forward with your arms and head hanging loosely. Bring your arms forward, up and back in a free-swinging circle. If it is more comfortable for you, swing just one arm at a time. Make from 50 to 300 continuous circles with your arms at least once a day. This exercise is good for loosening the muscles of the shoulders, shoulder blades, and upper back. As the muscles stretch, you will be able to make larger circles and accomplish the stretching with fewer repetitions.

**For an Ache in the Middle Back** ● Moving down the back, the next exercise is designed to work out the muscles of shoulder blades and

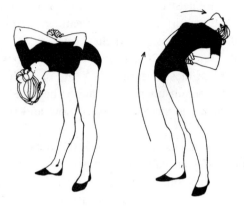

middle back. It also helps correct any exaggerated forward or backward curvature of the spine.

Standing with your feet wide apart and body bent forward at the waist, clasp your hands behind you. Let the weight of your head and shoulders pull your torso forward. Now, remaining bent at the waist, lift your torso by raising your head and arching your back while pulling your shoulder blades sharply together. Hold this position for a fast count of 10. Then relax and let your body droop forward again. Repeat this movement 10 to 20 times whenever your upper back, neck, or shoulders feel cramped. Otherwise, once or twice a day will suffice.

**The Low Back Stretcher** ● The next exercise is for stretching the low back and the hamstring muscles of the upper thighs. It accomplishes with orthopedic safety what the traditional toe-touching exercise was designed to do. Begin by sitting on the floor and putting your left leg out in front of you, toes straight up, and the leg swung over as far as possible toward your left side. Bend your right knee and bring the right heel in close to the crotch, keeping the left knee flat on the floor and holding your left hand in the small of your back. Sitting as erectly as possible, twist to the left until you're facing the outstretched left leg. Now reach out your hand and try to touch your left toes, bending from the hips. Bounce your torso up and down to loosen your muscles and get closer to your toes. Eventually, you

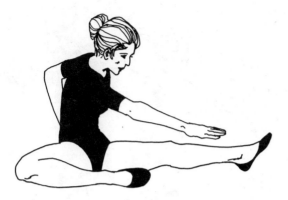

should work up to 100 quick bouncing motions. At first, you may not get too close to your toes, and probably won't be able to do 100 repetitions, but keep at it. It will get easier every day.

**The Knee-Chest Stretch** ● This next exercise is widely recommended by orthopedic specialists. If you've ever been to one, chances are he told you to do it. And chances are you didn't. Here's your big chance to make good.

Lie on your back on the floor with a pillow under your head and your knees bent. Keep your feet about 12 inches apart. Now grab your right knee with your right hand and pull as close to your chest

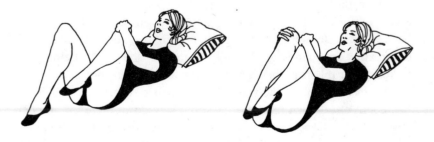

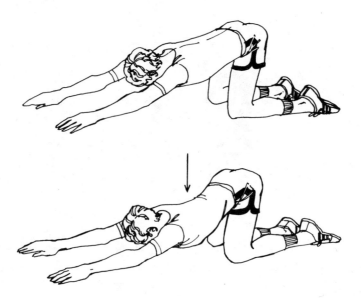

as you can. Bounce it toward your chest 20 to 50 times. Do the same with your other knee. To wind up, pull both knees up to the chest together and hold them as close to your chest as you can for the count of 10. It's sort of a boring exercise, but it teaches your quarrelsome muscles who's boss.

**Relaxing Your Uptight Spine** ● Here's an exercise which is a little more fun to do and is similar to one of the basic yoga exercises. Kneel on the floor with your knees about six or eight inches apart and bend forward from the waist, stretching your arms out over your head. Your elbows should be straight so that your forehead and lower arms and hands are actually resting on the floor. Being sure to keep your thighs perpendicular to the floor, press your chest down as far as it will go, all the way to the floor if possible. Hold it for a fast count of 10, then relax the chest but stay down there for another few seconds. Repeat as many times as you can in three minutes. This exercise stretches the hip joints, the entire spine, and the shoulder muscles as well; the perfect prescription for an uptight back.

**For Happier Hips** ● The next exercise, Dr. Michele says, "stretches the tight hip and thigh connector muscles and increases the range of motion, thus facilitating correction of hip and thigh disalignment." When you do it, you'll *feel* exactly what Dr. Michele is talking about.

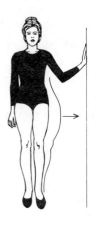

Stand at arm's length from a wall with your side to it. Place the flat of your hand on the wall for support, which you should be able to do without stretching. Now, bounce the hip facing the wall sharply toward the wall, so that your whole pelvis is jerked to the side. Repeat 20 to 50 times and then switch sides. If you can't do 20, which you probably can't, do as many as you can without straining yourself (the same goes for all the other exercises).

**And Finally . . . En Garde!** ● This next exercise gets right down to the nitty-gritty, which in orthopedic terms means the iliopsoas. "This exercise is a critical one as it stretches the iliopsoas and aids body flexibility and alignment," Dr. Michele comments.

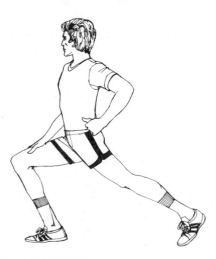

Get into a fencer's thrust position, as illustrated. Place your right foot forward, bending your knees and stretching your leg as far in front of you as you can. Turn your right foot in slightly, but try to keep the left one pointing straight ahead, with the heel lifted. Holding your torso erect, bounce your torso backwards until a pull is felt in the groin. To help balance yourself, keep your left hand on your left hip and your right hand on your right thigh. Do 50 bounces and then repeat with the left foot forward. Dr. Michele urges doing this exercise "as many times in a day as you have time and strength for."

## Some Personal and Practical Advice

At this point, I would like to add a few words of practical advice. First, if you know from experience that you will soon lose interest in doing exercises in your home, I strongly—very strongly—urge you to join a YMCA or health club. You will find that paying your dues up front will encourage you to visit your gymnasium regularly (three times a week is probably best) and more important, when you get in the habit of going to the gym, you will find that rather than being a nuisance, your exercises will be a lot of fun.

When you join a Y or health club, you may be tempted to forget about doing your exercises and just go for a swim in the pool or do some other more glamorous activity. Swimming and jogging are both good for the back, but in my own experience and from what I have seen in others, they will do absolutely nothing to help the person who has a *real* back problem. If you want to swim, fine, but first spend at least 20 minutes working on your back.

Since I began this essay on a personal note, I should conclude by saying that because I moved and was not able to find another karate club that I liked, I was forced to give it up. However, I found that by just kicking the air and otherwise stretching my hamstrings, I was able to keep my back in perfect shape. The one exercise I added was bent-leg sit-ups done on a padded incline board. I found these were remarkably helpful, but if you do them, be absolutely sure to get your knees way up in the air. *Never do sit-ups with your legs straight.* In fact, I don't even hold my back straight. I curl my head forward and pull it towards my knees, then I curl backwards until my shoulders—but not my head—touch the board. And then I spring forward again. If you have a padded incline board at your gym, I suggest beginning with the board prone, and only doing a few sit-ups in the beginning. Very gradually, over a period of weeks and months, you can increase the number of sit-ups you do and raise the board at the same time. I have found that combined with other exercises that gradually stretch and loosen the muscles in the back of the thighs, this particular form of sitting-up exercise, which is really more like a *curling* than the traditional sit-up, works wonders. It is especially good if you go to a health club during your lunch hour and don't have a lot of time to exercise. But if you're going to work out at home, where you don't have an incline board, you can get along fine without it.

Just a few more words.

Don't do any calisthenics at all. Push-ups and chin-ups are especially bad, and trying to bend over and touch your toes with your legs held straight is sheer insanity.

Joining a yoga class is a very good idea. It will stretch you just as much as karate, I've discovered.

Some people make a big fuss over the kind of mattress you should sleep on. In my case, I have found that compared to the effect of stretching your muscles, mattresses are meaningless. Neither do soft, mushy mattresses hurt my back, as they are reputed to. Of possible value though is sleeping on your side, with the legs well bent and raised. One leg should rest on top of the other.

# Bad Breath

Probably the most useless and self-defeating thing you can do for bad breath is to use a mouthwash. The more you use a mouthwash, the more you will *have* to use it because once the astringency and tart taste are gone, your mouth is apt to feel "fuzzier" than ever. That's why the mouthwash industry is so profitable.

The most basic approach is to practice good oral hygiene, using the Bass technique of brushing (see TOOTH LOSS), followed by flossing and thorough rinsing. The flossing is vital to keep the breath sweet. To help clean out your mucous-laden tubes in the morning, gargle, and snuff a little warm water into your nose, too.

Naturally, if you have a festering tooth in your mouth, with diseased gums, the bad breath is only a mild symptom of that pathology. In most cases, ordinary gum bleeding can be controlled by diligent application of the Bass technique and perhaps a visit to a dentist or periodontist. Extra calcium and vitamin C will also help. If you have a cavity, there is no alternative to having it filled.

Eating yogurt or acidophilus culture may help bad breath, and one woman told us that after suffering from "bad breath and a terrible taste in my mouth for over 20 years," and having tried mouthwashes and "all kinds of treatments," the problem disappeared shortly after she began taking 50 mg. of niacinamide.

John Gerard, the English Renaissance herbalist, who can always be counted on for elegant advice, said that "The distilled water of the floures of Rosemary being drunke at morning and evening first and last, taketh away the stench of the mouth and breath, and maketh it very sweet, if there be added thereto, to steep or infuse for certaine daies, a few Cloves, Mace, Cinnamon, and a little Anise seed."

Eating parsley and drinking fenugreek or peppermint tea are also said to help bad breath.

# Bedsores

A bedsore, as anyone knows who has ever suffered its special brand of torture, is very resistant to healing. But the flesh isn't all that suffers; one's medical bills skyrocket when bedsores complicate the prognosis. According to Dr. James W. Barnes, Jr., of Glenn Dale Hospital, Glenn Dale, Maryland, the cost of healing serious bedsores ranges from $5,000 to $10,000 (*Journal of the American Medical Association* [*JAMA*], January 8, 1973).

Bedsores can be a serious threat to life itself. Too many patients have survived major surgery only to expire later from the complications of bedsores during a long hospitalization. As blood, blood protein, and other vital nutrients are lost through the sore, anemia, debility, and lowered resistance set in. Dr. Barnes says that a study by the Veterans Administration showed that these persistent ulcers were the direct or major contributing cause of mortality in 10 percent of all paraplegics who died.

The medical term for a bedsore is decubitus ulcer. Decubitus is Latin for "lying down." Those who get decubitus ulcers have disabilities which confine them to a recumbent position. There are usually two causes of the sores: unrelieved pressure, especially at bony prominences (such as the hips), and poor nutritional status, which weakens the skin and natural repair mechanisms.

There's a whole catalogue of medicines, physical therapy measures, and nursing care practices designed for the comfort of the patient and the healing of the sore itself. Lately, however, there has been impressive progress in the treatment of bedsores—much of it achieved with relatively simple and inexpensive measures.

**Sugar and Honey Both Effective** ● Dr. Barnes has successfully been using common granulated sugar to help close up bedsores—with a healing rate of close to 80 percent. No, he doesn't feed the patients sugar, but rather he completely packs the ulcer with it, and then covers it with very thick airtight dressings.

Apparently, says Dr. Barnes, sugar does the job because the granules have an irritating effect which causes "local injury," which in turn stimulates wound repair processes. Also, the acidity of the sugar tends to increase dilation of the blood vessels, drawing more blood and lymph to the ulcer. Finally, all that concentrated sucrose actually kills bacteria, Dr. Barnes says.

For those natural food fans who may object to white sugar, even when packed into an ulcer, there is good news from Dr. Robert Blomfield of Chelsea, England, who prefers pure natural honey to do the same job.

In a letter to the editor of the *JAMA* (May 7, 1973), Dr. Blomfield says that when applied every two or three days under a dry dressing, honey promotes the healing of ulcers and burns better than any other local application he's ever used. (He adds that honey is also useful in promoting the healing of all cuts and abrasions.)

A registered nurse told us she had very good results dressing bedsores with liquid lecithin.

**The Air-Water Mattress** ● In Bridgeport, Connecticut, specialists in rehabilitation medicine have found that the best thing for patients with bedsores is the poor man's version of a water bed—an ordinary camping air mattress filled with warm water and kept warm with an electric blanket. Dr. Thomas F. Coyle, medical director of the Easter Seal Rehabilitation Center of Eastern Fairfax County in Bridgeport, says that—all other nursing factors being equal, especially turning schedules—ulcers heal about three times faster for patients who have these water-filled mattresses (*JAMA,* October 9, 1972).

Even better, says Dr. Coyle (admitting that "it sounds too good to be true"), of 500 patients who never used any mattress except the air/water unit, not one developed a bedsore.

But the chief problem with bedsores is not so much lack of suitable treatment or a water bed as it is the poor general condition of the patients in whom such sores develop. While the sore itself may be initiated because of constant pressure, particularly at bony areas, the rate of development and the severity of the sores depend on other factors, particularly undernutrition.

**Large Doses of Vitamin C** ● Just how important the role of nutrition can be in healing was demonstrated recently at the Manchester Royal Infirmary, University Hospital of South Manchester in England (*Lancet,* September 7, 1974). Dr. T. V. Taylor and a team of co-workers, in a double-blind trial of the effect of large doses of vitamin C on the healing of pressure sores, demonstrated that those patients who received supplements of vitamin C showed twice as much healing as patients who received a placebo.

Twenty surgical patients, each with a pressure sore, were included in the study. All were confined to bed with various conditions such as fractured thigh bone, stroke, and paraplegia (paralysis of the legs and lower part of the body). All the patients were using standard hospital beds and mattresses, receiving the same basic hospital diet and the same local therapy to the pressure areas. All the patients received identical-looking white tablets twice a day. Ten patients (group A) were given placebos. The other ten (group B) were given 500 mg. of ascorbic acid.

In group A the ascorbic acid levels in the blood before treatment were practically the same as those levels found in group B. After one month of treatment, however, the mean level in group B was *three times greater* than that of group A.

With the higher levels of vitamin C came a big improvement in the pressure sores—a reduction of 84 percent in size, compared to only 42.7 percent in the unsupplemented group. Six of the ten patients in the vitamin C group healed completely in just one month. (Three or four months is what it usually takes to heal a serious ulcer, according to Dr. Barnes.)

But vitamin C does not work alone. All nutrients are needed to promote health and healing, and in fact, the lack of almost any single nutrient can prevent healing. While collagen cannot be made without vitamin C, the strength of the connective tissue formed at the site of a wound depends upon the amount of vitamin A (*Journal of the American Dietetics Association,* 40, 97, 1962), as well as on the amount of protein obtained by the patient (*Nutrition Reviews,*

17, 144, 1959). A dietary deficiency of riboflavin ($B_2$) (*Journal of Nutrition*, 39, 357, 1949) and folic acid can delay and often retard the healing of ulcers and bedsores (*American Journal of Medical Sciences*, 221, 176, 1951).

The key mineral in healing appears to be zinc, required for the formation of crucial enzymes. Both oral supplements and locally applied ointments have been used with success in speeding the healing of wounds, with persons who have low zinc levels.

# Bed-wetting

Many doctors know what causes bed-wetting. The problem is that each one "knows" a different reason. The situation is actually quite revealing of the narrow and prejudiced thinking which too often pervades medical practice.

This was brought home to me first a few years ago, when two articles on bed-wetting (enuresis, if you want to be fancy) appeared back to back in a Canadian medical journal. The first article described a fiendish device that was placed between the bed wetter's legs at night. As soon as the very first drop of urine contacted it, the offender would get an electrical jolt where it hurts most and a loud alarm would be set off, waking up everyone in the house. Numerous case studies were described, and I was impressed not so much by the successes as I was by the failures. Some of the poor children on whom this damn thing was used continued to wet their beds for weeks, every night being shocked in their genitalia and embarrassed by their families running into the room. What the long-term psychological effects of this "treatment" would be I can only guess.

In any case, immediately adjacent to this article was another one, which claimed that the reason for bed-wetting was food allergies. The author of this article sounded convinced that he had found something important, but when I took a close look at his statistics, I could not agree.

The debate continues. Recently, letters and counter-letters from doctors, some of them almost hysterical with the conviction of their beliefs, have appeared in a few journals. In one case, a doctor who apparently had considerable experience with bed-wetting claimed that allergies were, in fact, the most likely cause. To this, another doctor answered that there is no evidence whatsoever, not a drop, that allergies have anything to do with bed-wetting. In a great number of cases, he declared, there is a physical abnormality in the urinary system of bed wetters, and when appropriate surgery is carried out, the problem ends.

I was just beginning to think that I was learning something about bed-wetting when I read a letter by yet another doctor who said that careful studies had shown that *less than three percent* of bed wetters had surgically correctible abnormalities of the urinary system, so it is absurd and dangerous to assume that bed-wetting is some kind of invitation for surgery. The most fruitful approach he said, was psychotherapy or simply a little more loving attention.

So now you know what causes bed-wetting.

But what do you do about it? First, if the child is less than about four years old, you should not even consider it a problem. And at any age, the worst thing to do is to scold or threaten the bed wetter.

A relatively simple hypnotic technique, which children can actually be taught to use themselves, is described under the entry of HYPNOSIS. I can't predict how much success you might have using this technique yourself, but I would strongly urge that you take the child to a clinical hypnotherapist for one or two visits and discuss that technique.

Nutritionist Adelle Davis once commented that a lack of magnesium causes "bed-wetting, sound sensitivity, and irritability," which led one reader to begin giving her bed-wetting son magnesium plus vitamin supplements. She found that it worked.

Another reader said that she noticed that when a fad started at school which involved soaking toothpicks in cinnamon oil and chewing them, her son (who loved cinnamon) swiftly stopped his bed-wetting (after M.D.'s and chiropractors failed to help). He was 11 years old at that time. She said that she shared this remedy with some other mothers and in one case, a nine-year-old girl who was a habitual bed wetter almost immediately ceased wetting after she began chewing on pieces of cinnamon bark purchased at the health food store.

Another folk remedy is a teaspoon of honey taken at bedtime.

Another woman told us about a remedy which she was given by a doctor as a child and which worked after all else had failed. The doctor said "to urinate and stop—over and over—until I was finished. This was to strengthen the muscle. It worked and I can contain myself even today much better and for much longer periods than my contemporaries and even my younger friends. I never have to get up at night as many of my friends say they do."

One doctor gives this remedy: tie a towel around the child's loins when he or she goes to bed. Be sure to knot the towel in front. Perhaps because it encourages the child to sleep on his back, it seems to work.

# Behavior Modification Therapy

Behavior modification therapy may be the most effective treatment approach devised for obesity, cigarette addiction, and other problems which involve the correction of ingrained habits. The behavior modification approach is described in detail in the entry, OBESITY.

# Biofeedback

The simplest way to explain biofeedback is to say that it attempts to give our conscious minds the same kind of profound control over body functions that hypnosis can give us in an unconscious state. Just as hypnosis has been used experimentally to produce "burn" injuries on the skin, cause warts to disappear, and reverse certain nervous reflexes that were once thought to be unchangeable, biofeedback has recently been shown to give us what had previously seemed an impossible degree of control over a variety of physiologic events.

Would you believe, for instance, that a person can be trained in a matter of days to cause the temperature of one hand to rise five degrees higher than that of the other hand, while not contracting the hand muscles? Would you believe ten degrees? Well, it's been done. It's even been done on animals: in one experiment, researchers trained a laboratory rat to produce a differential in the temperature of its two ears in order to receive a food reward.

At one recent scientific symposium, I watched with a mixed sense of fascination and revulsion as a man well trained in biofeedback techniques jab a large sailmaker's needle into the flesh of his upper arm until it came out the other end. There was not the slightest flinch of pain, and when he withdrew the needle (which was quite thick) there was no blood.

Two questions immediately arise. First, how are such apparent miracles accomplished? And second, why bother?

In the case of the hot hands, it's been found that when people trained in biofeedback cause their hands to quickly become warmer than normal, this can effectively short-circuit a migraine attack. One clinician has stated that in cases of "pure" migraine, he can often successfully teach this technique and stop headaches in a week or less. However, he said, in 90 percent of migraine cases, there is chronic tension that must also be treated over a longer period of time by biofeedback relaxation techniques. In any case, the supposed mode of action is that the blood which ordinarily engorges the blood vessels of the head in migraine is diverted to the hands and arms.

As for that grizzily needle incident, no one would learn biofeedback just to be able to stick needles in himself, but if someone can learn to block the pain from such an obvious injury, he can also be trained—theoretically—to block the pain of colitis, neuritis, and other conditions.

## How Does Biofeedback Work?

As for how biofeedback "works," no one really knows, but you can get some appreciation of what is going on by the following example. Suppose you had to explain to someone how to raise his right arm over his head. Try it. It's impossible. At best, you could tell him to tense the muscles of his arms, but this would only result in his arm going into a state of spasm. Yet, everyone knows how to raise his arm over his head.

It seems that at some early point in our lives, we all spontaneously and without any particular reason raised our arms over our head. At *that* point, we became aware that our arms were over our heads, and we "knew" what we did to get them up there. We made a . . . feeling.

Another example. How could you "explain" to someone how to ride a bicycle? Again, impossible. But when the person gets on the bike, and begins riding it, she can probably learn how to keep her balance very nicely in half an hour or so. What's happened is that she has learned how to control innumerable muscles involved in maintaining balance. But this learning experience is not something you could put down on paper or verbally explain to someone else. Somehow, certain pathways and reflexes that the rider never knew she had, become available to accomplish a certain task.

Now that you appreciate the importance of nonverbal learning, biofeedback training will not seem quite so peculiar. There are a number of techniques that can be used, but the most basic one is to attach a GSR device to the person's fingertips. This measures the galvanic skin response, or minute amounts of perspiration on the skin. The more tense you are, the more perspiration there is on your skin. As you become calm, there is less and less.

The electrodes are attached to a machine which converts the electrical information into an easily observable form, such as a light or a buzzing noise. The machine can be adjusted, so that the buzzing sound is moderately audible at the beginning of the session. As the device picks up more perspiration, meaning more tension, the noise gets louder. If the person becomes calmer and there is less perspiration, the noise becomes lower and is finally extinguished.

Rather than giving complicated instructions, the usual course is to simply hook a person up to a biofeedback machine and tell him to extinguish the buzz or the light. Naturally, he has no idea at all how to go about doing this, so what he does is simply experiment with himself. If he tenses his muscles, for example, he will find that the noise is getting louder. Then, maybe he figures that if he relaxes, the buzz will go softer. So he relaxes and the buzz does get softer. But it is not extinguished.

## Fine-Tuning Your Relaxation

Here's where it gets interesting. What usually happens next is that the person begins to put himself in various frames of mind that he believes will do the trick. There is a delay of several seconds between the feeling and the buzz, because it takes that long for the perspiration to appear on the skin, but he will soon enough find out if the machine is doing what he wants it to do. He tries other frames of mind. He imagines different scenes, different people, maybe different colors. Then, quite suddenly, he discovers that the sound is no longer there. What was he doing? He recalls it and keeps it up.

The next step would typically be to readjust the machine so that it has greater sensitivity. In other words, the buzz is going to sound when smaller amounts of perspiration are detected. In another session or two the person would probably learn how to counter this, and the process is continued until a satisfactory degree of relaxation is obtained.

The same technique would be used to teach someone how to warm his hands. But instead of measuring perspiration, skin temperature would be measured. The person would imagine whatever he found necessary to do the trick. And, incredibly, it's not only possible for some people to boost the temperature of one hand over the other, but to make *one part* of their palm warmer than the adjacent part! Further, researchers have found that when devices which measure very fine degrees of muscular activity are attached to a hand, it seems that unlike the reflexes involved in balancing a bicycle, this particular trick is not done with muscles at all. How it *is* being done, no one seems to know yet.

## Practical Applications

In any case, once a person has learned to become deeply relaxed, it becomes possible for him to elicit the same state of mind that he uses in the biofeedback laboratory when he is at home or at work. He simply relaxes and tries to precisely recall how he felt when he was keeping the buzzer or the light continuously extinguished.

Or, if the problem is blood pressure, he remembers how he felt when the monitor cuff attached to his arm revealed that his pressure was reduced to normal.

As with all therapies, results vary, but they are often impressive. Several researchers have reported promising results with asthmatics, pointing out that spasms of the airway passages involve muscular contractions, and that these muscular actions are amenable to relaxation training.

Many people suffering from headaches and chronic pain resulting from injuries or operations have learned to greatly reduce their dependency on drugs and sometimes give them up completely.

In an experiment with six patients with cerebral palsy, biofeedback training enabled all six to relax sufficiently to improve both fine and gross motor coordination. Four of the six also improved their speech, and a subsequent study confirmed these findings.

Sometimes, biofeedback training is used not to relax muscles but to gain active control over them. In such cases, devices measuring very slight muscular activity are attached to the target area and the trick is for the person to do whatever he finds necessary to make the machine go on, instead of off. Many patients discover that they do have some slight control over areas which were thought to be helpless or paralyzed, and with continuing work, a surprising degree of control can be regained. Rehabilitation of stroke and accident victims is one obvious application, although still experimental. One researcher has said that he has been able to train people with fecal incontinence, and no apparent nervous control over their anal sphincter, to become continent again with just one to four hours of training.

When biofeedback is given along with yoga or meditative relaxation techniques, the results seem to be especially gratifying. For one thing, when someone is practicing meditation for relaxation while connected to a biofeedback machine, he can immediately perceive if he is going about it in the proper way.

## Biofeedback, Meditation, and Your Blood Pressure

This combination approach was used by Dr. Chandra Patel and Dr. W. R. S. North of Britain in a study they reported in *Lancet* (July 19, 1975). They worked with 34 high blood pressure patients who were assigned at random either to six weeks' treatment by yoga relaxation methods with biofeedback or to a "placebo" therapy consisting of general relaxation.

Both groups showed some reduction in blood pressure. But while the "general relaxation" group went down from an average of 169/101 to 160/96 mm., the biofeedback group showed an average reduction from 168/100 to 141/84 mm. The drop of 16 points in the diastolic measurement, the second figure, is extremely significant.

Under the entry on MEDITATION, you will read of an experiment using meditation techniques alone which resulted in an average blood pressure drop from 146/93.5 to 137/88.9. Note that the results achieved by combining biofeedback with meditation were much better.

Actually, the technique used by Drs. Patel and North combined three methods of therapy which are discussed under separate entries in this book. They first relaxed people by using Jacobson's progressive relaxation techniques, discussed under the heading of RELAXATION. Once they had mastered this technique, a type of transcendental meditation was used, which is described under the heading of MEDITATION. To reinforce the successful practice of both these methods of relaxation, each patient was connected to one of two biofeedback instruments giving a continuous audio-signal whose pitch fell as the patient relaxed. First, a GSR device was used, followed by a second device which measured the electrical activity in muscles.

The doctors add that "Patients were also encouraged verbally and were shown their B.P. [blood pressure] records; they were also instructed to practice relaxation and meditation twice a day, and gradually to try to incorporate these habits into routine activities, the methods depending on individual circumstances. For example, each patient had a red disc attached to his watch to remind him to relax whenever he looked at the time, and some were told to relax before answering the telephone."

All the patients treated were already on medication, but it's obvious from their initial blood pressure readings that medication alone was not enough to achieve a really normal pressure.

From all this, it becomes clear that biofeedback potentially has a very important role to play in health care, and maybe an even more important role in preventive medicine. Presently, however, very few doctors have biofeedback equipment. Your best bet if you want to try it is to call your local hospital or medical school, which may have a biofeedback clinic or may use biofeedback devices in clinics specializing in headache, pain relief, hypertension, or rehabilitation.

Most doctors insist that biofeedback equipment should not be used without supervision. Although a number of devices are offered for sale to the public, some specialists claim that these devices do not have the required degree of accuracy. And at least one doctor has said that if "mail-order" machines *did* have this degree of accuracy, they should not be permitted to be sold, because they would be medical instruments.

I can't agree with that kind of thinking, and I suspect that an intelligent person could successfully use a good biofeedback instrument to teach himself to achieve greater relaxation. However, since such instruments are rather expensive, it might be foolhardy to invest $100 or more in a home unit unless supervision is available. It's likely, however, that high-quality but more moderately priced instruments will become available and may be genuinely helpful to many people.

I've just tried an extremely compact one-piece unit that sells for about $50 and found it works well. It takes a few minutes before any response from the machine is apparent, but using the techniques described under MEDITATION, I found I could extinguish the buzzing at increasing levels of sensitivity. Once extinguished for several minutes, I tested the device by imagining myself in an airplane that was about to crash. In 10 seconds, the buzzer was screaming.

I can't say for certain that using this device will enable me to achieve deeper relaxation than meditation alone, but my guess is that it will.

# Blood Pressure, High

High blood pressure, known in the medical trade as arterial hypertension, is a common ailment in the Western world, but very little is known about its causes.

Some people have an inherited tendency to become hypertensive and must severely limit their salt intake or take diuretic medications regularly to avoid disastrous complications. Many others gradually develop high blood pressure as they age, which may not be very threatening in itself but takes on a more sinister importance when it occurs along with a pattern of overweight, smoking, and clogged arteries.

Various authorities have singled out dietary components, especially salt, as the chief villains in the high blood pressure story. They point to people who live in areas where processed food is seldom if ever eaten and where high blood pressure is likewise low to prove that diet must be the culprit.

The problem is that these arguments are mostly theoretical, and with a few notable exceptions, which we will soon get to, there is no overwhelming evidence that adding or subtracting one or two items in the typical Western diet can bring about permanent remission of high blood pressure. Rather, the whole *pattern* of Western eating—heavy use of purified salt and sugar, heavy meat consumption, daily consumption of processed foods in which natural trace mineral balances have been disrupted—seems to set the stage for the emergence of hypertension as a major health threat.

## Eliminating Sugar May Help

Rarely do you read in the medical or popular literature that sugar may play a major role in hypertension. But one researcher who believes it does is Richard A. Ahrens, Ph.D., of the College of Human Ecology at the University of Maryland.

"The reason that I remain convinced that sucrose raises blood pressure is because we have been able to raise blood pressure at will in our laboratory by providing supplemental sucrose to both experimental rats and human volunteers," Dr. Ahrens wrote in answer to his critics in a letter to the *American Journal of Clinical Nutrition,* March 1975.

So far, Dr. Ahrens's work has only looked at the short-term effect of sucrose. As we write this, he is carrying out a study designed to last six months, which will hopefully determine if "the hypertensive effect of sucrose is really a long-term problem of public health significance."

## Meatless Diet Seems to Work Quickly

If sugar strikes you as a surprise villain in the high blood pressure story, you may think it even stranger that meat has also been indicted. Nevertheless, a Harvard research team led by Frank M. Sacks related some intriguing findings in the *American Journal of Epidemiology* in November 1974.

Sacks and his colleagues took a close look at people living in communal households in the Boston area, with a total of 210 participants from 17 communes. Most of the residents were young, but quite a few were in their 30s, and 14 were older than 40.

Most of the participants were "very strict vegans," the chief author of the study told us. Not only meat, poultry, and fish were out of bounds, but eggs and dairy foods as well. The less strict minority usually added fish or cheese to the communes' basic meals of a variety of grains, beans, seeds, vegetables, and occasional fruits.

The investigators found that blood pressure levels for the group were notably lower than what is usually found in Western populations —an average of 106/60, for example, in the 16 to 29 age group, compared to the average "healthy" 20-year-old American male's 120/75. Moreover, those who reported in their interviews that more than five percent of their food was of animal origin had higher blood pressures, both systolic and diastolic, than those who said their diet contained less than five percent animal foods.

No other factor considered by the investigators—including meditation, use of salt, use of sugar, smoking, coffee drinking, etc.—had a similar "highly significant" association with higher blood pressure.

The vegetarian diet, as the authors point out, seems to work "relatively rapidly" in establishing a pattern of below-average blood pressures. Most subjects grew up on the typical meat-eating diet of America's middle class and had followed vegetarianism for only about two years—in a few cases for only one or two months. Previous research by other scientists, the Harvard team notes, also indicates a fairly prompt response of lower pressure when dietary meat is eliminated—and a fairly prompt elevation of pressure if meat is added to a previously meatless diet. They cite numerous studies.

For example, a group of college students in California who were lacto-vegetarians (dairy products permitted) added meat to their usual diet and registered higher blood pressures within 11 days. (This finding was published 49 years ago!) In Yugoslavia, in 1963, elderly men and women were reported to have significantly reduced their blood pressures on a diet in which animal foods were restricted but not eliminated (meat, fish, and eggs provided no more than five percent of total calories); the pressure-lowering effect of this regime began to be noted after two months.

An astonishing study, conducted in the 1930s, found that a diet of fruit and vegetables could lower severe hypertension almost to the normal range. Fourteen patients kept on this strict regime reduced the mean blood pressure of the group from 218/122 to 158/94.

Whether or not going on a strict vegetarian diet is a worthwhile step for those who wish to control high blood pressure, I cannot say. On the other hand, it certainly makes sense to go vegetarian for a few months and see what happens.

In fact, if you were to change your diet so that you ate very little meat and dairy products, and practically no salt or sugar, you would be much the better for it regardless of your blood pressure. You would almost certainly lose a considerable amount of weight in the process—if you are overweight to begin with—and that in itself would reduce the risk of your high blood pressure problem to a significant degree.

## Nutrients May Help

When it comes to the possible use of nutritional supplements, there is some evidence, purely conjectural, stemming from the work of Henry A. Schroeder, M.D., that the heavy metal cadmium, an environmental contaminant, may lead to the development of high blood pressure in some people. Dr. Schroeder suggested that because of the antagonism between cadmium and zinc, some extra zinc in the diet might be of use. This is particularly true for people who have long eaten refined foods, because when grains are refined, cadmium is actually concentrated, while zinc is severely diminished.

Dr. Wilfrid Shute has said that vitamin E therapy often helps patients with high blood pressure, but he always makes certain that the condition has been stabilized before giving supplements. Patients with uncontrolled high blood pressure may have an adverse reaction. Few other investigators have noted any adverse reactions in hypertensive patients who take even very large doses of vitamin E, presumably because the condition is controlled with medication. In fact, a large but informal survey we recently took revealed that a surprising number of people had reduced their blood pressure significantly after taking vitamin E over an extended period of time, with the typical dose falling into the range of about 400 to 800 units a day.

Back in 1948, Dr. F. G. Piotrowski of The University of Geneva wrote in *Praxis* that, with a test group of about 100 patients suffering from hypertension, the use of garlic brought about a significant reduction in blood pressure. Dr. Piotrowski believed that the herb lowered the patients' blood pressures by dilating the blood vessels, which relieved symptoms such as angina pain, dizziness, and headaches. He claimed that in 40 percent of his sample cases, relief was obtained within three to five days.

Over the years, we have received a number of letters from people reporting that they were able to significantly reduce blood pressure by eating garlic on a daily basis, usually in an encapsulated form. How much garlic is necessary to hope to achieve a beneficial effect, I cannot say, except that it seems to vary.

Recently, several investigators have shown that high blood

pressure can be significantly reduced through various relaxation techniques, such as yoga or transcendental meditation, with or without assistance from biofeedback equipment. See MEDITATION and BIOFEEDBACK.

It would be unwise to suddenly give up medication and hope to control blood pressure through some other means. Rather, continue your prescribed medication and see if your doctor feels the improvement is sufficient to reduce or eliminate drugs.

# Body Odor

A Pennsylvania man came up with the slogan "Think Zinc— Don't Stink!" after ending a long battle with body odor (which no deodorant could control) by simply taking 30 mg. of zinc each day. He had no expectation that zinc would do this; he took it only because he felt that zinc would help his health in general. Two weeks later, he wrote that his body odor was gone. Not improved, just *gone.*

Another reader found that zinc did the trick for him too. He had "been troubled with underarm perspiration and odor, and with perspiring feet." He had tried various dusting powders on his feet and underarm deodorants (which gave him a rash) to no avail. Since taking zinc tablets, he reported, "I have no underarm odor, and my feet stay dry all day."

Why zinc should do this, I don't know, but it may be related to the fact that zinc apparently also helps—again unexpectedly—some long-standing cases of acne.

Let me also suggest, as an alternative to an aerosol spray, applying some common baking soda.

# Boils

Many people have begun their careers as amateur doctors by lancing boils, an unfortunate but probably inevitable practice. But please be aware of one fact: when a boil appears on or near the nose or cheeks, it should be treated carefully, only by a physician, because the risk of a serious systemic infection is high when such boils are not properly cleaned out.

Basically, boils respond to hot moist poultices, applied every hour or two. The heat encourages local immunity and also brings the boil to a point so that it can be lanced and cleaned.

Plain hot water may well be enough to soften and point a boil, but if you wish to use herbs, you can soak a cloth in some hot strong tea made from comfrey and flax (linseed). Flax seeds should be crushed before using. In making a poultice, the concentration of the herb is much stronger than when making a tea.

Traditional herbalism looks upon boils as a sign of internal impurities coming to the surface and recommends drinking teas made from such herbs as burdock, echinacea, goldenseal, barberry, yellow dock, and cayenne (capsicum or red hot pepper). Teas prepared from such herbs are strong and bitter, and after they are prepared (usually one teaspoon to a cup of water) they are taken a tablespoon at a time every few hours. Keep in mind, though, that when a traditional herbalist uses this approach, he or she knows exactly how to choose the most potent herbs and how to prepare them (echinacea, for instance, is much more soluble in alcohol than in water). Therefore, they must not be used as a home remedy for systemic infections.

# Bone Weakness

What follows should really be listed under the heading of osteoporosis. But I was afraid that some people would not realize the medical name for their frail, aching bones is osteoporosis or, perhaps, osteomalacia.

Osteoporosis is a slow, insidious affliction in which bones lose their substance faster than it can be rebuilt. Normal bone maintenance is a two-way street. New bone is constantly being formed at the same time that old bone is being resorbed into the blood. But, if calcium and other constituents of bone are drained away at a faster rate than they are being replaced, bones become porous, riddled with spongelike holes. Total bone mass shrinks, and along with it, bone strength. As a result, fractures are much more likely to occur—often after the slightest bump or stress. Bones may even snap spontaneously, just from carrying body weight. Pain in the spinal area is another common symptom.

"Osteoporosis in the early postmenopausal and elderly female is probably the most disabling, frequently occurring, and socially costly metabolic disease in the country," a team of bone specialists noted in the newsletter (February 1974) of the Jewish Hospital of St. Louis.

Osteoporosis is unlike most other diseases in that it is not a result of an infection, injury, or some other kind of "accident." In fact, after the age of 30 to 35, the total amount of bone in an individual actually shrinks "about ten percent per decade in women, and five percent per decade in men," mineral metabolism expert Dr. Louis V. Avioli explains.

There is a related bone disorder called osteomalacia, which is caused more by vitamin D deficiency than calcium deficiency, and which causes newly formed bone to become soft, pliable, and even misshapen. According to Dr. Avioli, "The usual symptoms of adult osteomalacia are weakness and generalized boneaches; of osteoporosis, localized back pain on arising or bending over, or pain in areas where the spinal vertebrae may actually have collapsed. The ordinary X-ray picks up only 30 to 50 percent bone loss or more. By this time, the horse is already out of the barn, so to speak" (*Medical World News,* October 19, 1973).

In the United States, osteoporosis is far more common than osteomalacia. The latter is not at all uncommon in Britain, however, and anyone—anywhere—who does not get sunlight or vitamin D supplementation is at risk of developing osteomalacia. It is not unusual for housebound elderly people to have osteoporosis *and* osteomalacia.

What can be done about these two conditions, especially osteoporosis?

That has always been a difficult problem to answer and has triggered many medical debates. One of the problems is that, as Dr. Avioli noted, osteoporosis can't even be detected on X-rays unless one-third or more of the bone mineral is already gone. That lack of sensitivity also makes it difficult to use X-rays to measure any improvement in osteoporosis unless the change is quite substantial.

Recently, a team of scientists and physicians in New York seem to have solved both problems, by devising a new method of measuring bone density and demonstrating that a natural therapy can be effective not only in halting osteoporosis, but even reversing it. Anthony A. Albanese, Ph.D., and four colleagues (including two physicians and one dentist), reported their work in the February 1975 issue of the *New York State Journal of Medicine*. They examined the bones of literally thousands of people and treated hundreds of people with extra calcium before publishing their results.

The first thing they did was test an ingeniously simple and reliable method of measuring bone loss—even *minimal* bone loss. By taking a low-intensity X-ray picture of the middle bone in the little finger, they were able to detect very tiny changes in bone density, while exposing the subject to a minimal dose of radiation. Thus, they could observe the onset, development, and reversal of osteoporotic bone disease just by keeping tabs on the thickness of the pinky.

**New Life for Old Bones** ● For their first patients, Dr. Albanese and his co-workers selected a group of 12 female residents of a home for the elderly and began giving them daily calcium supplements. These women ranged in age from 79 to 89—the years when the ravages of osteoporosis are most likely to catch up with and cripple the elderly individual. Calcium was prescribed because it is widely recognized that a negative calcium balance (in which the body excretes more of this mineral than it retains) is a major cause of osteoporosis. Other investigators had already shown that additional calcium can slow down or even halt the slow wasting away of bone. But the New York team wanted to do more than just arrest the progress of the disease.

The women in the experimental group were getting about 450 mg. of usable calcium daily from their regular diets, far short of the Recommended Dietary Allowance of 800 mg. The supplement provided an additional 750 mg. of calcium and 375 units of vitamin D (essential for calcium utilization by the bones), bringing their average daily calcium intake up to 1200 mg. At the same time, a group of 17 women (average age 82) served as controls. They were not given any supplemental calcium.

After three full years of daily calcium supplementation, finger measurements revealed that the bone density of women in the experimental group had *increased* from a coefficient of 90.6 to 96.1. Even though they were now three years older than when the experiment began, their bones were—for all practical purposes— actually younger. On the other hand, bone density in women who had not received extra calcium *decreased* from 90.3 to 84.2. Their bones, like themselves, had simply grown three years older.

Best of all, there were no undesirable side effects associated with prolonged calcium supplementation. Calcium levels in the blood and urine remained normal. There was no heightened risk of kidney stones or any other excess calcification problem, according to the authors. In fact, the only unexpected side effect was a beneficial one: a "striking" decrease in serum cholesterol levels occurred in the supplemented group within 12 months.

Next, the investigators turned their attention to a younger age group. They selected twenty-three healthy women hospital workers, ranging in age from 36 to 62. Fourteen received calcium supplements; nine served as controls.

"On the whole, little or no improvement was observed during the first six to nine months of supplementation," the authors relate. "Subsequently, some dramatic change occurred in four subjects." In one 62-year-old woman, the bone density coefficient shot from a little more than 80 to 120 in 36 months! Bone density of a 48-year-old woman increased from 93 to 122 during the same period.

Steady improvement was noted in eight subjects. And in six of those, bone density rose to levels normally found in *men* of the same age, whose fracture risk is usually lower. Again, no adverse effects were noted.

In two cases, women began taking the calcium supplements and for various reasons stopped. Measurements revealed that while the supplements increased their bone density, this effect was lost in a year or two after they stopped taking them.

**More Proof That Calcium Helps** ● The New York team also wanted to check out calcium in relation to estrogen. That hormone is frequently prescribed on a long-term basis in osteoporosis cases, because osteoporosis becomes much more serious after menopause. But when Dr. Albanese and his associates surveyed 50 women, aged 47 to 67, some of whom had been receiving long-term estrogen replacement therapy and some of whom had not, they found that there was no difference in the incidence of bone loss.

Checking further, they found that giving calcium and estrogen supplements, or calcium alone, reversed bone loss in 26 post-menopausal women. But estrogen alone had no effect on bone density.

Seeking the most severe test for calcium supplementation, the New York researchers decided to try the therapy on a group of five female fracture patients. Presumably these were subjects in whom bone-weakening osteoporosis had progressed furthest of all. (Incidentally, the investigators found that their pinky-measuring technique is highly predictive of future fracture risks in women 45 years of age or older. The lower the reading, the sooner they can expect a broken hip, vertebral collapse, or some other skeletal disaster.) After taking calcium supplements, all five women experienced a significant rise in bone density.

Four of the five had been on estrogen therapy for at least five years, but their response was no more favorable than that of the one patient who received calcium alone. This last, a woman of 73, had suffered a compound fracture of the lower spine. After 12 weeks of calcium supplementation, her bone density coefficient jumped from 92 to 110, the sharpest increase in the whole series.

All of this reminds me of the words of Dr. William Brady, a well-known physician and syndicated columnist who lived (and worked) until 91. In one of his columns, in 1965, he suggested to his readers that they start each morning as he did: by taking six capsules of calcium and vitamin D to help absorb it. "To this," he wrote, "I attribute the fact that I have no rheumatism, no nondescript ache or pain, no headache, no backache, and no other manifestation of calcium deficiency."

There are a few other important things worth mentioning about osteoporosis. First, like most conditions, it is probably easier to prevent it than cure it, so I would advise insuring adequate calcium in the diet throughout life, as well as as much outdoor activities as you can manage. Walking or working outdoors will actually help the calcium you eat form stronger bones, and the sunlight will enable your body to manufacture vitamin D, also necessary for strong, normal bones.

## Why It Took So Long to Find the Truth

Those of you who enjoy reading medical literature may have come across statements by doctors to the effect that calcium in the diet has little or nothing to do with osteoporosis. That assertion is based on the observation that in countries where people eat considerably less calcium than Americans do—Puerto Rico, for example— they do not have any more osteoporosis. There are three important fallacies in the conclusion drawn from these observations, however.

First, people in such countries (usually in tropical or semitropical areas) get much more sunlight than people living in North America or Europe. That means they get a lot more vitamin D.

Second, they obviously get a lot more exercise, which also results in stronger bones.

Third, people in these countries ordinarily eat much less protein than we do. And, it's recently been demonstrated, high protein intake actually causes calcium to be flushed right out of the system with urination. Helen M. Linkswiler and other members of a research team at the University of Wisconsin reported in *Transactions of the New York Academy of Sciences* (April 1974) that with a very moderate protein intake of 47 grams, young adult male research subjects were all "consistently in calcium balance" with an equally moderate intake of only 500 mg. of calcium a day. But when dietary protein rose to 95 grams a day—which is very close to the average American protein intake—*none* of the research subjects were in calcium balance with only 500 mg. of the mineral a day. At that point, they needed 800 mg. a day. And when protein intake was raised to 142 grams a day, "no subject was in balance at either the 500 or 800 mg. calcium intake, and only three of fifteen subjects were in balance at 1400 mg. intake."

We have to keep in mind that these experiments were done with relatively young men, not middle-aged women, who are most prone to osteoporosis. Nevertheless, the results do point to the very real possibility that men or women eating a diet high in meat, poultry, and fish, all high-protein foods, should pay particular attention to calcium intake.

It's also worth knowing that the long-term use of cortisone can lead quite swiftly to advanced osteoporosis and greatly increased risk of bone fractures. Dr. Theodore Hahn, a spokesman for the bone research team at the Jewish Hospital of St. Louis, which was mentioned earlier, has found that large, but carefully controlled doses of vitamin D, along with calcium supplements, can reverse this severe degeneration of the skeleton.

"Preliminary results from a group of 30 patients treated with this regimen indicate that bone mass can be increased by as much as 25 to 30 percent over a six-month period, thereby greatly decreasing the risk of bone fracture in cortisone-treated patients," Dr. Hahn said.

Smoking, by the way, can also aggravate a tendency towards bone loss.

We should add that it used to be thought—almost universally agreed—that a large amount of phosphorus in the diet interfered with calcium utilization. That has now been quite conclusively demonstrated to be not true. Apparently, what was being observed was the effect of protein, not phosphorus. (In the experiments with protein which we mentioned, the amount of phosphorus in the diet remained constant.)

For those who have osteoporosis, a reasonable amount of supplemental daily calcium is 1,000 to 1,500 mg. (or more on medical advice), along with 400 units of vitamin D. It may also help to insure magnesium adequacy, because that mineral is also found in bones. Based on everything I have read on this subject, I would suggest that a good way of getting these minerals is to take about half the calcium you want in the form of bone meal (which contains all the minerals needed for strong bones) and the rest in the form of dolomite (which contains a good amount of magnesium along with the calcium). To insure best utilization, it may be wise to use chewable tablets, or to mix powdered bone meal or powdered dolomite in with other foods.

For other bone problems, see LEGG-CALVÉ-PERTHES DISEASE, OSTEOGENESIS IMPERFECTA, and OSTEOMYELITIS.

# Brain Dysfunction In Children

**by Ruth Heyman**

Brain dysfunction is a tricky, admittedly controversial diagnosis. But whatever it is, Ron had it. Immature and sad eyed, he was the scorned classroom dummy in the fourth grade of his suburban school. He couldn't sit still in his seat—he would wiggle like a Mexican jumping bean until he ended up sprawling on the floor. He was disruptive, destructive, impulsive. He had a memory like a sieve and his attention span was about as long as a TV commercial.

But what parents of children like Ron are more concerned about than the semantics of a differential diagnosis is: What's to become of such children? How far can a child like Ron go?

Well, Ron is now in sixth grade and is miraculously up to grade level. He is also on the class football team and an enthusiastic Boy Scout.

But why the dramatic improvement in his learning ability? And what's the secret of his social acceptance after years of being an outcast? The answer to both questions is a program that improves the functioning of the brain—diet therapy and vitamins coupled with sensori-motor exercises.

Until he was 10 years old, Ron had all the symptoms of minimal brain dysfunction. Hyperactive, incoordinated, and plagued by perceptual problems, he couldn't concentrate and he couldn't learn. Out of frustration, his behavior became erratic.

Ron's parents stopped at nothing in their attempt to quicken his apparent slow mind and quiet down his supercharged body. Let Ron's mother tell the story: "We knew in our hearts that he wasn't stupid, that there was something else wrong. We helped him every night with his homework. His father thought he was lazy and stubborn but punishments and bribes were to no avail. The family pediatrician put him on Ritalin for his hyperactivity, but it was not effective and since we didn't want him on drugs anyway, we stopped it after eight months. Even the neurologist we took him to could find nothing wrong.

"Just about when we were accepting the fact that Ron was slow, we heard about the New York Institute for Child Development. The day we took him there was the turning point of our lives. After a battery of functional, neurological, biochemical, and educational tests, they discovered that Ron was hypoglycemic and had a perceptual disorder. They prescribed a high-protein, low-carbohydrate diet and megavitamins. They gave him eye exercises. The family pediatrician scoffed but within six months, Ron's report card improved. He's calm now and he can concentrate. In one year, he jumped two grade levels in reading, arithmetic, and spelling. What more can we ask for?"

Twelve-year-old Ron is happy, too. Offer him a piece of chocolate and he turns it down. "I'm sticking to the diet and the vitamins. School is easier for me now. The teachers and the kids don't pick on me anymore. I'm doing fine, getting better and better."

## The Chemistry of Achievement and Underachievement

While the New York Institute for Child Development treats the severely brain injured as well as those with minimal brain dysfunction, their primary thrust is with the underachiever and their results are impressive.

Alan C. Levin, M.D., medical director of the Institute and a member of the American Academy of Pediatrics, glowed as he discussed the program in his pleasant office at the Institute at 36 East Thirty-sixth Street.

"More than three quarters of all the children seen here have a basic biochemical problem or a physical problem, such as poor visual, motor, or auditory function. When a child comes here, he is put through a series of biochemical and neurological tests, including tests for low blood sugar, allergies, thyroid malfunction, hormone deficiencies, and trace minerals. Visual, auditory, and tactile perceptions are evaluated. The Institute treats the child, guides the parents, and keeps in touch with the school. About 80 percent of all the children show marked improvement, often within weeks. Many will reach their normal class level, depending on their I.Q.'s, of course."

The program is triple-pronged: a diet regimen plus sensorimotor therapy and treatment aimed at whatever other physical disorders are indicated. Dr. Donald L. Gutstein, the Institute's nutritionist, explained how they evaluate a child's dietary needs. "The diet regimen is determined by assessing the biochemical tests, monitoring for food allergies, and reviewing the child's dietary habits. Specific allergies are uncovered by charting the child's behavior and food intake throughout the day. Also, we ask the family to record for one week everything the child eats and from this we estimate the protein and carbohydrate content and the food additives."

## Allergies and Hypoglycemia Are Common

The results of the biochemical tests indicate that most hyperactive children suffer from hypoglycemia, have enzyme and mineral imbalances, and are allergic. The diet prescribed eliminates refined sugar, refined flour, and food additives. All preservatives and artificial sweeteners are excluded. The child is instructed to eat high-protein, low-carbohydrate meals and protein snacks. Fresh, raw juices and vegetables are encouraged.

In addition to the diet, specific vitamins and minerals are usually prescribed, initially consisting of niacin, vitamins $B_6$, C, and E, panto-thenic acid, and calcium, the dosage being determined by the levels found on the tests and by the child's age and size. When allergies are noted, complete avoidance of the food or foods is mandatory.

Just as important to rehabilitation, says director Judith Dowd, is sensori-motor therapy, since all these children have difficulty coor-dinating at one or more developmental levels. They may have prob-lems hopping, skipping, eye tracking, handwriting, or ball catching. Therapy includes balance training, gross motor organization (lateral and cross-lateral movements on command), fine motor organization (eye and finger exercises), and eye-hand organization (overhead ladder and eye-hand tracking). All exercise programs are designed individually according to the needs of the child. They are adminis-tered at the Institute but home programs are prepared for youngsters who cannot attend sessions in New York.

What causes minimal brain dysfunction? It is believed that there may be a biological or chemical change in the brain tissue that results in poor function. The brain, a most complicated organ con-sisting of millions of cells with intricate connections, may be injured either before, during, or after birth. Among the suspected causes of injury are incompatible RH factor in mother and child, poor nutri-tion, inherited defects in the genes, technical problems at delivery, trauma, and infectious diseases. Recent studies relate pollutants in our air, food, and water to brain damage.

It is estimated that about five percent of American children are afflicted with a minimal brain dysfunction. It manifests itself with difficulties in learning and making social adjustment. The child is often late in walking, talking, and toilet control. His hyperactivity is not the result of isolated incidents but is nonstop, capricious motion. He may have perceptual difficulties, reversing letters, or skipping lines. Sometimes he can't distinguish right from left. He may have a hearing problem, and the subtleties of sound elude him. He may find it difficult to communicate and is repetitive in speech. Often learning to ride a bike is a Herculean task. He rejects baseball because he is awkward with a ball and bat. Nothing can hold his attention for long, and he dissipates his energy in all directions like a lighted sparkler.

Of course, every child has growing problems and time may be the healer. But when several of these symptoms plague a child, minimal brain dysfunction is suspected, and early investigation is indicated.

## How Laura Recovered Her Self

Many of these children have high I.Q.'s. Laura is a cute nine-year-old perfectionist with a peaches and cream complexion, whose native intelligence withered under the burden of a malfunction of her adrenal glands, low blood sugar, and a perceptual disorder. Not too long ago, she lagged far behind her classmates in reading and writing because she reversed letters and skipped lines. Her sickly skin tone worried her parents who believed it was an indication of a physical disorder. Though a timid child who spoke in whispers and hid behind her mother's skirts, she shattered her family with constant crying spells and her inability to sleep.

"We finally discovered that her emotional and learning problems were biochemical in origin and we stopped using the Freudian umbrella," says Laura's mother, who took her child from doctor to doctor in an attempt to help her. "The New York Institute for Child Development found the causes of her difficulties. With the change in her diet, the megavitamin supplement, and the sensori-motor program, there was soon a noticeable change in her personality as well as in her schoolwork. Instead of getting up at the crack of dawn, she now sleeps nine hours a night and has to be awakened. She speaks up now and participates in discussion. Her coordination is better and there is improvement in her vision, although she still needs visual training.

"When Laura goes off her diet and eats junk at a party, she may get a crying jag. Then she starts reversing letters and her reading comprehension suffers. But this condition improves after she resumes her diet. Laura is now in the fourth grade and keeping up with her classmates."

The interaction between mind and body is an intuitive gut wisdom probably as old as mankind. Oriental philosophy postulated that the mind controls the body and current experiments with biofeedback prove it. But the body also controls the mind, and the vanguard of the medical profession is treating brain dysfunction through biochemistry. They believe that nutrition to the brain affects the nervous system which controls the learning process.

"We are aware that the approach to this problem is multifaceted," said Dr. Levin. "The treatment involves a medical, nutritional, functional, and educational assessment. We've treated over 1,500 children and we know that our therapy works. Parents, teachers, and the youngsters themselves have moved from a hopeless acceptance of their learning disabilities to a positive, dynamic program. Of course, the earlier you get a child the better, because psychological problems inevitably follow learning problems."

Many of the minimal brain dysfunctioned are hypoglycemic. They have abnormal glucose tolerance and the level of sugar in the blood is too low to nourish their brain optimally. Six-year-old Frank who wants to be a builder when he grows up used to put his fists into the sugar bowl. Ironically, the more sugar he consumed, the lower went the level of his blood sugar. He was so wild and destructive that no babysitter would ever take the job twice. Now he can sit quietly in front of the television set, tie his shoes, catch a ball and best of all, do arithmetic and read.

"Six weeks after he started the high-protein, low-carbohydrate diet for hypoglycemia, there was an unbelievable change," said his mother with a smile. "He quieted down. He's no longer the hornet in our household. Instead of smashing his toys, he plays with them and even puts them away when he's through. Now he wants to do his homework and learn. And believe it or not, he's lost his craving for sweets. He sold me all the Halloween candy he collected for a penny a piece."

If nutrition is so effective with the brain dysfunctioned, will it also increase the learning ability of the normal child? William T. Mullineaux, Clinical Director of the Institute, says *yes*. "We believe that harmful food additives, white flour, and excessive sugar are the culprits that upset the normal functioning of the brain. We tested the effect of controlled food and vitamins on normal children in a Harlem nursery and found a 20 percent increase in I.Q. over a period of a year. There is no doubt that diet affects learning performance."

# Bruising, Easy

When a fat person begins to lose weight, at first all is joy. But weight loss is sometimes accompanied by an unpleasant side effect, namely easy bruising. Even a small bump or the pressure of restrictive clothing can bring on those black-and-blue smudges—a poor reward indeed for virtuous exercise and calorie cutting!

"Outside of informing the patients that they may be more prone to bruising as they lose their additional padding, do you have any suggestions?" This is a doctor's query to fellow professionals in a column entitled "Ask the Practicing Physician" appearing in the November/December 1974 issue of *Obesity and Bariatric Medicine.* His weight-losing patients, this doctor explained, already were receiving a multivitamin supplement plus vitamin K and large doses of vitamin C. But still they bruised. What else might help?

Of the six practicing physicians who offered suggestions based on their own clinical experience, four recommended citrus bioflavonoids. This is the nutrient, especially plentiful in the white pulp of citrus fruit, which is widely recognized (except in the United States) for its role in strengthening the capillaries—those tiniest blood vessels whose rupture under the skin causes the discoloration of bruising. In the United States, the Food and Drug Administration (FDA) has "determined" that, when it comes to strengthening capillaries or performing any other useful function, bioflavonoids are ineffective.

But Dr. Frank W. Barr, Charlotte, North Carolina, one of the physicians answering the query about bruising and weight loss, writes: "I do feel that citrus bioflavonoid, in spite of the FDA's criticism of the product, does a beautiful job over a three-month period in strengthening the capillaries. My patients all receive subjective and objective improvement with their 'bruising problem.' " Dr. Barr says a bioflavonoid compound has other advantages in that "it has no toxicity, the dosage may be pushed quite high, and it is, basically, a food supplement."

As to why a tendency to bruise should accompany weight loss in obese patients, Dr. Barr and other physician correspondents explain that the capillaries lose some of their mechanical support or padding when the fat around them is broken down. A fat person's capillaries have become "lazy," so to speak, depending on the support of fatty tissue instead of maintaining their own full structural stability. Hence, to prevent easy rupture when fatty support is removed, these weakened vessels need extra help to bring their walls up to normal strength.

# Burns

Drawing the heat out of a burn by submersion of the injured part in cool water is one of the most important steps to be taken in emergency treatment. In serious burns, medical attention is always to be sought immediately, but even with a severe burn, "prompt cooling can mean a difference between extensive deep burns and more limited superficial injuries," according to Michael F. Epstein, M.D., and John D. Crawford, M.D., both of the Shriner's Burns Institute in Boston (*Pediatrics,* September 1973).

The water should be cool, not ice cold. The kind of water that first comes out of the cold water tap when you turn it on is just fine. If the hand is burned, plunge it into cool water in the sink. If the burn is on the foot, splash cool water over it or get into the tub. If the burn is on the trunk, pour pitchers full of water over it.

If you are going to take yourself or the victim to an emergency ward, take along something like a clean pillowcase soaked in cold water and then rung out. Wrap it around the injured area.

Cooling does more than relieve pain. As the doctors from the Shriner's Institute pointed out, cooling can actually prevent a burn from becoming worse. That's because the heat that initially burned the skin is still present after the removal of the flame or scalding water or whatever caused the injury. And that continued heat will go on causing tissue damage for some time. The sooner the injury is cooled, the better, but there is some experimental evidence that even several hours after the injury, some complications can be minimized by the cooling technique.

What should you put on a minor or moderately serious burn besides cool water? There is no simple authoritative answer to this question, which is still being debated by doctors. Some urge putting nothing on it except the sterile dressing, while others claim that the burn will heal much faster if nothing touches the injury except air. Still others recommend various ointments and sprays.

## Foods That Cool Burns

Dr. Robert Blomfield of Chelsy, England, who works in the emergency department of a hospital, published a letter in the *Journal of the American Medical Association* in 1973 pointing out that "I have been using pure natural honey for the past few months in the accident and emergency departments where I work, and I have found that, applied every two or three days under a dry dressing, it promotes the healing of ulcers and burns better than any other local applications I've used before. . . . I can recommend it to all doctors as a very inexpensive and valuable cleansing and healing agent."

If you don't have any honey in the house, and you want an ointment for a minor burn, you might try yogurt. A woman wrote to us that she had good results with yogurt applied to a rather severe burn of her hand. She had to apply it three times because it kept drying out from the heat of the burn, but relief was swift and the burn healed very quickly.

Really severe cases of sunburn require medical attention every bit as much as other burns. But for the kind of sunburn that is bad enough to keep you up at night but will go away in a couple of days, splashing apple cider vinegar over the burn may bring quick relief. This is an old folk remedy, and when I tried it on my daughter, who came home with her shoulders and back painfully reddened with sunburn, I found that splashing and lightly rubbing the vinegar on her brought relief in a matter of seconds. I had to apply it again several more times that evening, and it smelled awful, but it did work. We have some anecdotal reasons for believing that apple cider vinegar can be helpful in burns other than sunburn, but no real medical evidence. Possibly, some of the relief comes simply from cooling. But its high content of acid may also have something to do with its beneficial effect. It's interesting that yogurt and honey are also on the acid side, and that all three have the property of retarding the growth of some pathogenic bacteria. However, I would never rely on them exclusively to prevent infection in a really severe burn.

Speaking of infection in a burn, it's interesting to note that doctors at the Shriner's Burns Institute report good results with giving burned children daily baths in a solution consisting of one part Clorox to sixty parts water (for example, one quart of Clorox in fifteen gallons of water). Each child was placed in the bath for about 15 minutes and watched over by two attendants. The solution sometimes stings, but generally it is well tolerated. It may be that this procedure, designed to keep wounds bacterially clean, is primarily useful in a hospital situation, where there is a constant danger of patients cross-infecting each other.

## Vitamin E for Burns

I am not aware of any medical studies demonstrating the value of topical or oral vitamin E in burn therapy other than those of Dr. Wilfrid Shute of Canada, who has used it for many years with gratifying success. However, based strictly on a large number of incidents related to us by readers, it does seem that vitamin E can be helpful. A typical example of such an anecdote was that related by a woman whose mother-in-law's blouse caught fire while she was cooking, giving her massive burns from chest to waist. The woman broke open a number of vitamin E capsules, covered her with the oil, and then quickly took her to the hospital where she was treated. Application of vitamin E continued for a number of days (she also took some orally), and the result was that "she healed so quickly that the doctor told her he never saw a woman her age heal on the sensitive chest area so rapidly and never leave a scar."

Another anecdote from a reader: "My son had a second-degree burn on the back of his hand from a laboratory accident at college. He saw a doctor and after two days healing had not started. His hand pained him terribly and was all weepy. Only then he allowed me to put on a wet dressing of vitamin E oil and by next morning healing had started and the fiery pain subsided. It healed without a scar."

Lelord Kordel gives this German remedy for minor burns. Put equal amounts of wheat germ oil and honey in a blender and let it run at low speed. Then add enough comfrey leaves to make a thick paste, blending it at medium speed until smooth. Apply to the burn and keep the remainder in the refrigerator to keep it from going rancid.

A simpler home remedy is to apply a slice of raw potato or to squeeze on raw potato juice to help get the heat out of a wound. Follow with an application of honey.

Aloe vera is probably the best known herb used for burns. If you have a plant in the house, cut off the thorns, slit the plant open, and either squeeze on the juice or lay the exposed side of the herb onto the injury.

## Vitamin C for Burns

Back in 1951, David H. Klasson, M.D., a surgeon, reported in the *New York State Journal of Medicine* that he had used vitamin C with impressive success to treat burn patients. He used the vitamin topically in a one percent solution (a stronger solution could be very irritating) and also gave patients from 200 to 500 mg. of vitamin C by mouth or injection four times daily. He was particularly impressed with how this regimen reduced pain and often made it unnecessary to give the patient morphine, which was widely prescribed in that day for extreme pain, but which was known to be highly addictive.

Dr. Klasson told of one patient who was brought to the hospital in exquisite pain after having been badly burned over 30 percent of his upper body in an airplane crash. Although he was given morphine, this pain remained severe for an hour, until his wounds were sprayed with the one percent solution of ascorbic acid. "There was almost immediate relief of pain," the surgeon said, noting that the pain did not return and no more morphine was required. The patient made an excellent recovery.

In another case, two patients who had been badly burned in a gasoline explosion were brought in. The burns on their heads and necks were treated with the ascorbic acid solution and daily application of a two percent ascorbic acid ointment. The burns on their hands and wrists were treated conventionally with sterile Vaseline, gauze, and Furacin ointment. Three weeks later, the wounds treated with vitamin C had healed, while those treated "conservatively" continued to exude fluid for another month.

To the best of my limited knowledge, this use of vitamin C for burns has not been independently confirmed and is certainly not part of standard burn treatment today. That is unfortunate, but hardly surprising: even when they *are* repeated and confirmed, vitamin therapy programs are often totally ignored by the medical profession.

## Feeding the Burned Patient

Doctors do, however, recognize the great nutritional challenges during the long recuperative phase in the victim of a severe burn. In a 1973 review on "Nutritional Support for Burn Patients," Charles Crenshaw, M.D., a Texas surgeon, declared that "re-establishing adequate nutrition for the severely burned patient is one of the most difficult aspects of patient care, and an important responsibility for the attending physician" (*Perspectives in Clinical Nutrition,* Eaton Laboratories).

Dr. Crenshaw describes some of the outstanding problems relating to special nutritional requirements with a burn patient from the earliest stages to the fine points of wound healing. He is talking about the severely burned patient, so what he has to say has most relevance in the hospital setting. But some of the highlights of his advice are worth knowing. In the earliest stages of treatment, especially if nausea and vomiting occur, he advises administration either of a glucose solution or Holdrane's solution, which provides for critical mineral replacement and consists of one-half teaspoon of salt and 1½ teaspoons of sodium bicarbonate or baking soda in a quart of water flavored with lemon juice. An adult should be given two ounces of this fluid per hour, and a child one ounce.

Food is very important. In general, Dr. Crenshaw says, the over-all objective is to provide 5,000 to 6,000 calories a day, including about 200 grams of protein for a man of average size. This is a lot of food for someone who may not be able to eat well and may involve intravenous feeding as well as multiple small meals.

He emphasizes the importance of adequate vitamins to insure that this high-calorie diet is utilized to best advantage. "In adults, the basic daily regimen for peroral vitamin therapy should include at least two grams [2,000 mg.] of ascorbic acid, 50 mg. of thiamine, 50 mg. of riboflavin, and 500 mg. of nicotinamide [niacinamide]. Children should receive about one-third of these amounts." In addition, he says, attention should be paid to adequacy of vitamins A, D, $B_{12}$, K, $B_6$, E, and folic acid.

## Preventing Stress Ulcers

Dr. Merrill S. Chernov of Phoenix, Arizona, reported in 1972 that injections of vitamin A can be effective in preventing gastroduodenal ulceration in the severely burned patient. He found that serum levels of vitamin A dropped drastically in the burned patient, probably due in large part to the fact that the patient with severe burns is losing great amounts of protein, and protein is necessary to mobilize vitamin A out of the liver. So even a patient with a history of good nutrition, who would have plentiful reserves of vitamin A in his liver, cannot use vitamin A when he needs it most. When the patient is well enough to begin eating a high-protein diet, serum vitamin A levels swiftly return to normal.

Dr. Chernov told the Fourth Annual Meeting of the American Burn Association in San Francisco that stress ulcers developed in nineteen of thirty patients who were not given vitamin A shots. Fourteen of these patients had serious gastrointestinal bleeding, which in seven cases was massive. In contrast, in twenty-two patients who received anywhere from 10,000 to 400,000 I.U. of a water-soluble vitamin A preparation daily, bleeding occurred only in four patients, for an incidence of 18 percent, against about 65 percent in the untreated patients.

Hyperbaric oxygen therapy (see OXYGEN THERAPY, HYPERBARIC, later in this book) can be helpful in the treatment of burns. Dr. George B. Hart and colleagues of the Naval Regional Medical Center of Long Beach, California, have found that when given within the first 24 hours of injury, hyperbaric oxygen shortens healing time and reduces complications and even the death rate. The formation of skin ulcers and scarring are diminished. However, they caution that the presence of viruses in the blood is an absolute contraindication to such therapy.

In a series of 191 patients, those who were treated with hyperbaric oxygen had a death rate some 30 to 40 percent less than predicted, they said.

# Bursitis

Bursitis is the painful inflammation of any one of the body's bursas, which are fluid-filled pockets which absorb the friction of moving joints. While bursitis may flare up at a number of sites, such as the knee or elbow or even the little toe (a bunion is caused by the inflammation of a tiny bursa), it most commonly occurs in the shoulder.

The treatment of bursitis may be sharply divided into two phases: During the acute stage of the attack, the extremity—usually the arm—should be completely immobilized. Movement at this time will only increase inflammation. So putting the arm in a sling is often a good idea. Also during the acute phase, cold packs may reduce pain and tenderness.

Ordinarily, this very painful stage of bursitis begins to recede in four or five days, although it may take longer. When the pain is no longer acute, therapy must be radically changed. At this point, it becomes essential to return full, normal movement to the joint. Naturally, this should be done slowly and cautiously. Doctors recommend swinging the arm freely in every direction, at first very gently, with support from the opposite arm. Exercise for only a minute or two at first, but do so frequently throughout the day. As pain continues to subside and movement returns, keep moving the arm until it can swing freely and fully in every direction. If you find this difficult, a physician can help you restore movement to the joint by carefully manipulating it for you.

The importance of regular exercise following a bursitis attack cannot be overemphasized. If you simply quit using the joint, it will very likely develop crippling adhesions in which the joint freezes up, and you may have a permanent condition instead of only a brief though painful attack of bursitis.

Another major change in the direction of therapy from the acute stage to the improved stage of bursitis is that during this latter stage, applications of heat, not cold, are suggested. It is particularly useful to apply heat to the joint prior to doing exercises, as the rush of blood to the area brought by the application of heat usually reduces pain and therefore permits freer motion of the joint.

Medically, ultrasound therapy is often prescribed and represents a conservative and effective approach to easing bursitis. At home, gentle but persistent massage will also increase circulation in the area, and as the *Merck Manual* points out, "hot fomentations"—poultices—will also help.

## Hot Poultices

Here are a few relatively easy-to-make hot fomentations that may be applied to help ease the pain while recovering from bursitis. A comfrey poultice is among the best. If you have fresh leaves of comfrey, use them, although you can also use dried leaves or the chopped roots. Place a generous handful into a pan, cover with water, and bring to a boil. Remove the pan from the heat and let cool to the point where the mash is warm but not excessively hot. Sandwich the sopping wet herbal matter between layers of gauze and apply to the inflamed area. If you find after a few applications that this is causing some minor irritation to your skin, first rub on some olive oil or lanolin before applying the poultice. The combination of the heat and the marvelous soothing qualities of comfrey should prove very helpful.

Linseed (flax seed) poultices are another old favorite. While pouring a pint of boiling water into a warmed enamel basin, simultaneously sprinkle in a quarter pound of the crushed seeds. Stir until the mixture resembles a smooth dough, then stir in half an ounce of olive oil. When the mixture is comfortably warm, spread it on some clean linen which has been warmed in the oven, fold the linen over, and apply to the sore area. A variation of this poultice can be made by using somewhat less linseed and adding some slippery elm powder and marshmallow. All these herbs are very soothing.

To make a poultice which will be especially effective in bringing heat to the inflamed area, you can try a hot fomentation made from cayenne pepper (capsicum) and cider vinegar. Use one tablespoon of cayenne pepper in a pint of cider vinegar and boil gently for 10 minutes. When the mixture has cooled off, soak a small clean hand towel in it, wring out slightly, and apply to the skin. Again, be careful not to burn yourself, and protect the skin with oil or use a milder fomentation.

If you want to, there's no reason why you can't add some comfrey leaves or the powdered roots of marshmallow to this brew. After steeping, the comfrey leaves can be removed from the brew and applied directly to the skin along with the soaked towel.

You may want to try herbal teas to help ease the pain, especially at bedtime. A cup of strong camomile tea alone will help. For something which herbal literature indicates is somewhat more powerful, try making a tea consisting of two parts camomile, one part skullcap (the powdered herb), and one part lady's slipper (the roughly ground root). If taken at bedtime, you may also want to add some hops and passionflower.

## Bursitis and Diet

A word about bursitis and diet is now in order. Most people are aware that calcium deposits are usually present at the point of pain in bursitis. In fact, it is usually the granules of calcium pressing against the bursa which causes inflammation. However, all authorities are in agreement that these accumulations of calcium have nothing to do with the amount of calcium you eat. Furthermore, there are some cases of bursitis where calcium deposits are not present, and it has also been observed that many people have small calcium deposits in the tendon adjacent to the shoulder bursa and yet have no symptoms at all of bursitis. Therefore, unless otherwise instructed by your physician, it does not make sense to attempt to modify your calcium intake in order to prevent or cure bursitis.

A physician treating bursitis will often poke these calcium granules with a needle to break them up. Sometimes the deposit breaks up spontaneously, which usually causes severe pain. But the pain quickly subsides as the calcium is gradually removed from the site by the bloodstream.

There's no definitive information as to the cause of bursitis, but attacks are often brought on by a severe bruise. Occupations or other activities which cause great stress to the joints can bring on the development of chronic bursitis, which may be more difficult to treat than the acute variety. In such cases, the activity bringing on the pain should be stopped, if this is possible.

There is at least one report in the medical literature of a nutritional approach to bursitis. Back in 1957, I. S. Klemes, M.D., published an article in *Industrial Medicine and Surgery* entitled "Vitamin $B_{12}$ in Acute Subdeltoid Bursitis." Dr. Klemes described how he successfully treated large numbers of patients with acute bursitis with injections of 1,000 micrograms of $B_{12}$. He claimed that in most cases, relief was rapid, and subsequent X-rays revealed absorption of the calcium deposits. All in all, said Dr. Klemes, the $B_{12}$ shots only failed to help two or three people out of about sixty patients with acute bursitis.

However, the medical profession does not give this report much credence. The problem with evaluating *any* treatment for acute bursitis is that most cases, especially the worst, usually improve rapidly on their own within a few days. And since Dr. Klemes gave daily injections of $B_{12}$ for a week or more, and did not use a control group, it is impossible to say to what extent $B_{12}$ therapy is better than no particular therapy at all.

# Cancer

Natural therapies for cancer fall into two categories. The first includes a host of special diets, foods, and herbs which have been written about in many softback books sold mostly in health food stores. I confess that I don't know any more about them than what is written in these books, and there would be no practical purpose served by reviewing them here.

Scientists feel more at home with the second category of therapies—those consisting of individual compounds such as alkaloids from herbs and vitamins from foods. (They feel even more at home when the alkaloids and vitamins are synthesized.) Here, we find that while herb derivatives are in fact being used to fight a few forms of cancer, many barrels of the whole herb may be required to extract a single therapeutic dose. For that and other obvious reasons, such therapies do not fall within the purview of this book.

As for vitamins, there has been a tremendous amount of work done with vitamin A but only in laboratory animals, and, for the most part, only in *preventing* tumors or slowing very early growths.

There is one major exception to my finding that relatively simple and natural therapies for cancer—in human beings—do not have even *suggestive* medical or scientific evidence behind them. That exception is vitamin C.

Let me immediately point out that as we write these words, I do not know of any doctor in the United States who is using this treatment. And let me also admit that the statement that vitamin C can help cancer must strike many people as grossly exaggerated or even absurd. Am I really going to assert that vitamin C can help—that it can do anything at all—to combat an already-established cancer?

Answering that question is terribly difficult, even now that we have a detailed report from Scotland, where two doctors gave large doses of vitamin C to 50 consecutive advanced cancer patients. The general *impression,* though, of Dr. Ewan Cameron, a consultant surgeon at Dunbartonshire Hospitals and a nonresident Fellow of the Linus Pauling Institute of Science and Medicine, and Dr. Allan Campbell, a consultant physician at Lanarkshire Hospitals, is that "Our clinical findings support the general contention that large doses of ascorbic acid enhance natural resistance to cancer." Further, "We have found this form of medication to have definite palliative [symptomatic relief] value in the management of terminal 'untreatable' human cancer" (*Chemico-Biological Interactions,* 9, 1974, 285-315).

The first question that needs to be asked is *why* vitamin C should even be tried in treating cancer. Did the doctors get a research grant from the Secretary of State for Scotland on the wild guess that vitamin C might be helpful in cancer?

Not exactly. In another article in the same issue of *Chemico-Biological Interactions,* an international science journal, Dr. Cameron and Linus Pauling, Ph.D., director of the Linus Pauling Institute of Science and Medicine in Menlo Park, California, reviewed some of the highly suggestive bits of evidence that vitamin C, or ascorbic acid as scientists like to call it, may act in several ways to increase resistance to cancer. Chiefly, it's believed that vitamin C strengthens the natural defense mechanisms that help protect us not only against cancer, but all disease.

Drs. Cameron and Pauling underline the importance of this natural resistance to cancer by mentioning a 1973 study published in the bluntly named journal, *Cancer.* That report showed that while malignant cells were detected in the circulating blood of about half of all patients undergoing resection of colon and rectal cancers, this finding appeared to have no significance at all in predicting which patients were going to be alive at the end of five years. That's important, because some people still have the idea that to treat cancer, every last cell in the body which is cancerous must be destroyed. Obviously this just isn't the case, Drs. Cameron and Pauling point out. If it were, every last one of those patients in whom malignant cells were found in the circulating blood would have been dead from cancer at the end of five years. *Somehow,* their bodies must have been able to cope with those malignant cells in such a manner as to prevent them from establishing new malignancies.

## The Rationale Behind Trying Vitamin C

How does vitamin C fit into the picture of increasing these natural defense mechanisms? First, say the authors, the ability of the organism to encapsulate the spreading cancer in a "relatively impermeable barrier of dense fibrous tissue" may depend on the dietary availability of ascorbic acid, because this nutrient is necessary to build fibrous tissue. Vitamin C is also needed to give lymphocytes enough vitality to effectively attack invading foreign bodies in the system. And cancer may be one of the foreign bodies lymphocytes attack. Another area of possible importance for vitamin C is in the functioning of the adrenal and pituitary glands, which normally have a very high concentration of ascorbic acid. Under stress, however, the vitamin C is quickly depleted—and cancer certainly stresses the system to its very limits. By feeding these glands all the vitamin C they need to produce their hormones, the body may be better able to cope with such stress, Drs. Cameron and Pauling suggest.

Moving from theory to laboratory experiences, the authors point out that when laboratory animals are challenged with a powerful cancer-causing chemical, methylcholanthrene, this triggers a sudden upswing in their natural synthesis of ascorbic acid. In rats that develop tumors, the production of vitamin C goes even higher. On a body weight basis, they produce the equivalent, in a 154-pound man, of 16 grams (16,000 mg.) of vitamin C a day.

Man, of course, has lost the ability to synthesize vitamin C and must get it in his diet. But under the challenge of cancer, the dietary *intake* of vitamin C does not necessarily increase in man as the *production* of vitamin C does in most animals. (In fact, two British doctors recently reported, patients with malignant disease are apt to have extremely low intakes of vitamin C, to the point where they may develop scurvy. They therefore urge that all cancer patients be given vitamin supplements, according to a report in *Medical World News,* February 24, 1975.)

Scientists believe that a number of cancers may be caused by viruses, and if this is true, vitamin C may have an important role here, because several studies have shown that vitamin C tends to have a general antiviral effect. An antibacterial effect has also been described, which Drs. Cameron and Pauling point out could be important, because many tumors become ulcerated, making the patient vulnerable to a secondary bacterial invasion, which weakens him.

**Fifty Patients, All 'Beyond' Therapy** ● That brings us to the series of patients treated by Drs. Cameron and Campbell. Although only 50 patients are included in their joint report, the doctors actually gave vitamin C to many more patients, but excluded them from the study for various reasons. For example, because J. U. Schlegel, M.D., of the Department of Surgery of Tulane University has reported that extra vitamin C can prevent bladder cancer in animals, and is a "possible preventive measure" in regard to bladder cancer in man, *all* patients with bladder cancer were given vitamin C. However, they were also given standard methods of cancer treatment, so they were not included in the current study.

In some cases, patients who had originally been diagnosed as being "untreatable," and who were given vitamin C, improved so much on the vitamin regimen that it became ethically imperative to immediately give them established forms of cancer treatment as well. All these patients were therefore excluded from the study. That left only those patients who were considered by Drs. Cameron and Campbell, as well as at least one other independent clinician, as not having any chance at all of benefiting from any form of therapy. In most cases, they were considered "terminal." At best, they suffered from advanced cancer and were beyond the hope of any known therapy.

Most of the patients received 10 grams (10,000 mg.) of ascorbic acid daily, in four divided doses. Some received more. In the beginning, the vitamin C was administered by injection, but eventually, the doctors decided that this was no better than giving it orally.

**Vitamin C Isn't 'Harmless' to a Cancer Patient** ● One of the first surprises in this study was not a pleasant one. Long experience with vitamin C has led to the general impression that it is amazingly harmless, even in large amounts. In cancer patients, it turned out, this is not always true. Some patients proved not to be able to tolerate high doses of vitamin C in their stomachs, particularly those whose disease involved the upper alimentary tract. Some of these patients suffered from heartburn, nausea, and acid regurgitation. On the other hand, although fears have been expressed that when more than four grams of ascorbic acid are taken daily there is an increased risk of developing oxalate kidney stones, not one patient out of fifty developed any problems along these lines.

The biggest surprise, though, was that in four patients the large doses of vitamin C produced a catastrophic deterioration in a matter of days. In all cases, it seemed that the vitamin C had actually caused the tumor to hemorrhage and become necrotic (dead). Although the bleeding produced by this process proved fatal because the tumors were so large, Drs. Cameron and Campbell point out that this reaction "is in fact a manifestation of the very strong defense reaction, and would certainly be regarded as a very favorable response indeed in patients suffering from earlier and more localized lesions."

That was the outcome in four patients out of fifty. In seventeen other patients, nothing much of anything happened that could be attributed to vitamin C. Actually, that's not exactly true, because the majority of the patients in this study *felt* better after beginning vitamin C and suffered less from pain. But right now, we're just talking about the progress of the disease itself and not the subjective symptoms. For this purpose, then, the seventeen patients had "no response."

Ten patients had what Drs. Cameron and Campbell call a "minimal response." Some patients in this group seemed to take a slight turn for the better before going downhill, as expected. In other cases, the improvement was more dramatic but was eventually followed by a surprisingly swift state of deterioration.

In eleven patients, the development of the tumor or tumors seemed definitely to be slowed down. Case No. 29, a 67-year-old man, was typical. Suffering an inoperable cancer of the gallbladder and liver, he was expected to live not more than a few weeks. A week after beginning the vitamin C regimen, his appetite returned, he gained weight, and his obstructive jaundice problem improved. He died at home 209 days after starting on vitamin C.

**The Eight Most Interesting Cases ●** In three patients, the megadoses of vitamin C brought cancer to a standstill. A 56-year-old woman with adenocarcinoma of the colon underwent surgery but her condition had already spread to her liver. Curiously—perhaps significantly—when she began taking vitamin C, she experienced discomfort in the region of the liver but was encouraged to keep taking it, and the side effect eventually went away after about two months. "Now," the two physicians reported, "some 18 months later, [she] remains clinically well, with no evidence to suggest progressing malignancy."

Two other patients responded similarly: although they were hardly "cured," they simply stopped getting worse.

In five patients, there was actual regression, or shrinking in size of the tumor. But this didn't always mean that the patient recovered.

A 55-year-old man with cancer of the kidney that had spread to his right shoulder and left hip was put on ascorbic acid after undergoing surgery. At the time, he was not in severe pain, but was unable to work. He began taking 10 grams a day of vitamin C on April 10, 1972. There was steady symptomatic improvement with pain relief, and he was able to return to his job. Even more encouraging, X-rays showed that his bones seemed to be fighting off the cancer and were becoming recalcified where they had been eaten away with cancer growth. After one year, however, his condition took a turn for the worse. At this time, his vitamin C dose was doubled to 20 grams a day, and he again improved for a number of months. Following this improvement, however, the disease once again flared up and he died on January 25, 1974, 656 days after beginning ascorbic acid treatment.

Two other patients also died eventually, but not because of cancer. In both cases, autopsies showed that there had apparently been significant regression of cancerous growths.

Another patient had an extremely dramatic response to treatment. In a matter of weeks, his enlarged liver and spleen returned to normal size, and there were other signs of very significant regression found in X-rays and biopsies. Eventually, his dose of ascorbic acid was reduced and finally eliminated. Unfortunately, a few weeks later, the malignancy began to return, and he was again put on ascorbic acid therapy—which at the time of their report, the doctors say, seemed to be inducing a second regression.

Another man, 69, was operated on in 1969 for cancer of the colon. In 1972, he was readmitted to the hospital, deteriorating, with numerous signs that the cancer had returned in his liver. Six months after beginning the ascorbic acid therapy, all his liver function tests returned to normal. "More than 2.5 years later, [he] continues with his ascorbic acid and remains fit, active, and well in all respects, with no clinical or biochemical indication of neoplastic disease," Drs. Cameron and Campbell write.

**What It Means—And What Must Be Done** ● The big question at this point is whether or not the survival times of this group of patients were significantly longer than they would have been without taking vitamin C. The only way to pin down such an effect would have been for the doctors to have *not* treated another group of 50 patients whose conditions closely matched those of the treated patients. This wasn't done. And if it had been done, the doctors say, they would have broken the "control," because as their clinical experience increased, "we felt it to be ethically wrong to withhold ascorbic acid in otherwise hopeless situations, merely for the sake of obtaining observations of dubious significance for statistical comparison.

"However," they declare, "it is our opinion that most clinicians familiar with the practical realities of terminal cancer . . . would be inclined to agree that many of these patients survived much longer than reasonable clinical expectation."

Beyond the question of survival time, Drs. Cameron and Campbell report that in a number of patients they treated, giving ascorbic acid "produced quite dramatic relief from pain and opiate dependence in a matter of days." There were other benefits as well, one of which was that all patients who had malignant disease of the urinary tract experienced a significant reduction in the amount of blood in their urine, and a reduction in pain and distress as well. In at least six cases, the doctors say, "there is indisputable clinical and biochemical evidence to show that reversal of terminal malignant jaundice was induced for significant periods of time."

The doctors who made this report consider it to be a "pilot study" designed to see if there is any reason for conducting a more extensive and more carefully controlled test of vitamin C in cancer patients. The answer to this question, they believe, is definitely affirmative. If it does nothing more than relieve pain, it would be of great value. But there is good evidence to indicate that vitamin C may do more than this.

Drs. Cameron and Campbell say that they "expect it to have even greater value when used in the treatment of earlier and more favorable patients." Looking ahead, they declare that "We believe that, in time, ascorbic acid supplementation will come to be accepted as a standard measure in most, if not all, forms of cancer treatment. We conclude that large scale clinical trials along such lines are now clearly indicated."

## Diet and Malignant Melanoma

There's one more dietary approach to cancer that is worth mentioning. And that is a restricted diet designed to combat the progression of malignant melanoma of the eye.

A brief report on this diet describes the case of a 53-year-old chemistry teacher in Britain who had a malignant melanoma of the left eye. In his case, it was felt that surgery would result in the loss of sight because of the position of the tumor, which was also in a bad position for radiation therapy. He was then told about an experimental diet which had been tried in Denmark, consisting of a diet very low in two natural food chemicals, phenylalanine and tyrosine. According to S. L. Stevens of Addenbrooke's Hospital in Cambridge, "The basis of this form of treatment is that tyrosine, which can be formed from phenylalanine, is the basic amino acid in melanin production and a substrate for tyrosinase, the basic enzyme in melanin synthesis and essential for the respiration of the melanoma cell. These cells contain large quantities of tyrosinase, and when it is deprived of its substrate tyrosine, the growth of the melanoma is inhibited."

The diet was quite severe, initially consisting of only 10 grams of protein, including just 250 mg. of phenylalanine and a low tyrosine content. Eventually, additional amino acids were added to the diet to prevent a protein deficiency. Some problems arose with this diet, and it became necessary to use a low phenylalanine, low tyrosine commercial supplement.

The diet succeeded in drastically reducing the serum levels of both phenylalanine and tyrosine. The concluding sentence of the report is: "Meanwhile the patient has remained well and the Eye Consultant reports that the malignant melanoma has regressed."

It should be obvious from the nature of this diet that it must be supervised jointly by a physician and a dietitian. If you wish to discuss this diet with a medical professional, you may refer him to Stevens's report, "Low Phenylalanine, Low Tyrosine Diet for Malignant Melanoma of the Eye," which appeared in the British journal, *Nutrition,* vol. 28, no. 5, 329-330, 1974.

A psychological approach used in conjunction with the medical therapy of cancer is described under VISUALIZATION THERAPY.

# Canker And Cold Sores

When little fever blisters, cold sores, or canker sores flare up in and around the mouth, they stir up a kind of misery in their suffering victims out of all proportion to their diminutive size. Agonizingly tender to the touch, the tiny lesions stubbornly resist the many drugs, salves, and other treatments modern medicine has devised. About all most victims can do is patiently wait for the sores to run their natural course and disappear after seven to ten days, or longer. But they can and often do return with alarming regularity.

Fortunately, there is a remedy for fever blisters and canker sores that has been proved effective in clinical trials. But the therapy—which involves a concentrated food rather than a drug—is either forgotten or ignored by most of the medical profession. That remedy consists of a tableted suspension of living, beneficial bacteria from which yogurt is made.

Before taking a look at some of the results obtained using yogurt culture, let's try to get a better picture of the nature of the enemy.

## Canker and Cold Sores

The medical name for canker sores is aphthous stomatitis. Sometimes they are referred to as recurrent aphthae. Canker sores usually appear *inside* the mouth, often on the lining of the cheeks or the edge of the tongue. Each lesion is actually a tiny ulcer or open sore, whitish in the center and surrounded by a red border. Doctors don't know the underlying cause of aphthous stomatitis, but eruptions are often associated with allergy, emotional stress, mild local injury or irritation, antibiotic medication, and even menstruation. A severe flare-up of canker sores can be quite debilitating, because the discomfort makes eating and drinking difficult. Antibiotic mouthwashes and even cortisone have been used to treat canker sores, but as yet there is no treatment that could be called both safe and effective.

Fever blisters or cold sores often occur on the lips or *outside* the mouth, on the borders of the lips or nostrils. These blisters are caused by a specific viral disease, herpes simplex, which often lies dormant for years between attacks. Herpetic lesions often accompany fever—hence the name fever blister. But they can also be triggered by a cold, sunburn, or emotional upset.

## Beneficial Bacteria

Back in the 1950s, Don J. Weekes, M.D., associated with the Department of Surgery at Peter Bent Brigham Hospital in Boston, was treating several patients suffering from severe diarrhea. He prescribed tablets containing *Lactobacillus acidophilus* and *Lactobacillus bulgaricus,* beneficial bacteria traditionally used to culture yogurt and other sour milk products. Two of his patients were also suffering with severe aphthous stomatitis, and when they took the tablets, their ulcerous sores improved dramatically. Dr. Weekes decided to try the *Lactobacillus* treatment with other canker sore patients. The results of the first trials were reported in the August 15, 1958, issue of the *New York State Journal of Medicine:*

One patient, a 39-year-old woman and doctor's wife, had suffered from canker sores almost continuously since receiving an antibiotic two years previously. During all that time, no medication was able to bring her any relief. At Dr. Weekes's direction, she began taking two *Lactobacillus* tablets four times a day, chewed and then swallowed with milk. Her mouth ulcers promptly disappeared, only to return when she stopped taking the tablets. She resumed taking the medication with no subsequent recurrences and, according to Dr. Weekes, no undesirable side effects of any kind.

Another patient, a 42-year-old graduate nurse, was so plagued by canker sores that she was unable to take proper nourishment. She was admitted to the hospital suffering from severe dehydration. "Forty-eight hours after treatment with *Lactobacillus* therapy all ulcers had healed, she was taking fluids well, and urine volume returned," Dr. Weekes reported.

A third patient, a 38-year-old woman, suffered from herpes blisters on her lower lip as a result of sunburn. The lesions were just one day old, but when she began taking the *Lactobacillus* preparation, the blisters started to heal rapidly. However, Dr. Weekes noted that "When treatment was discontinued, the lesions which had previously been resolving, recurred."

**Larger Trial Successful** • Dr. Weekes continued his trials for a number of years before again reporting his results (*Ear, Eye, Nose and Throat Monthly,* December 1963). Calling his discovery of several years before "an instance of serendipity," he went on to describe clinical tests of the *Lactobacillus* preparation involving 174 patients. The subjects varied in age from less than two years to sixty-six years. All had painful blisters or sores in or about the mouth. In each case, the subject was advised to take four *L. acidophilus-bulgaricus* tablets four times a day with milk, the milk serving as an activating culture medium for the bacilli.

Among 64 patients treated for fever blisters on the lip, 37 obtained complete relief, while another 24 showed dramatic improvement and suppression of the lesions. In other words, 95 percent had favorable results. And the *Lactobacillus* tablets did more than just soothe and speed the healing of blisters. In some cases, they actually *prevented* the formation of new sores. As Dr. Weekes observed, "Of interest was the fact that when administered during the early burning and itching stage, therapy actually aborted imminent lesions."

The doctor also tried the therapy on 97 patients suffering from canker sores. The results were excellent, although not quite as dramatic as with the herpes patients. Forty were fully cured while 37 showed definite improvement within four days—a favorable response of approximately 80 percent. "Local soreness usually disappeared within 24 to 48 hours," he noted.

Dr. Weekes's findings were subsequently confirmed by a number of other medical researchers.

If you are frequently troubled by fever blisters, cold sores, or canker sores, the research we've seen suggests a daily dosage of from eight to sixteen tablets, taken with milk, taking a few tablets several times a day. Although eating whole yogurt is probably helpful, it doesn't deliver the potency of the concentrated tablets, and most yogurts lack the acidophilus strain. If you buy yogurt in the store, instead of making your own, avoid the pre-stirred varieties, in which the bacteria are no longer active. If you already have a mouth sore, you can allow the yogurt to completely cover it for a minute or two as part of the therapy.

When you purchase "lacto" tablets, make certain they contain living organisms. A product sold in drugstores is kept in a refrigerated case because the manufacturer guarantees viability.

## B Complex Can Also Help

While adding yogurt or yogurt tablets to your daily diet, it might also be a good idea to step up your intake of the B complex, particularly vitamin $B_{12}$ and folic acid. A recent study reported in the *British Medical Journal* (May 31, 1975) used large doses of $B_{12}$ and folic acid to heal aphthous ulcers in a group of 23 patients in Scotland. Unlike 107 other patients in the study, these 23 subjects— who, by the way, were all suffering from particularly severe and intractable mouth ulcers—were found to be deficient in $B_{12}$, folic acid, or iron.

A similar tie was cited by Carlton Fredericks, Ph.D., who noted a case of "persistent and very severe cold sores in a seven-year-old child who was taking numerous vitamin-mineral supplements, and which responded to no type of medical treatment, disappeared when 250 mcg. [micrograms] of vitamin $B_{12}$ were added to the treatment."

An experience with a nasty cold sore my daughter had seemed to confirm this. I gave her two 25 mcg. $B_{12}$ tablets and the cold sore was gone by the next morning.

To relieve the pain of a cold sore, try tincture of myrrh.

# Celiac Disease

Most of us have nothing to worry about. We can still safely, and somewhat quaintly, regard bread as the "staff of life." But for thousands of people—many of whom are unaware of their condition—a basic component of wheat, rye, barley, and oats can trigger a biological reaction that may devastate health—or go virtually unnoticed.

The same cereals which some people thrive on can cause depression, fatigue, infertility—or perhaps just a little rash—in celiac sufferers.

Celiac disease, also known as celiac sprue and nontropical sprue, has classical symptoms which are easy enough to recognize but are not always there *to* recognize. Someone who is "lucky" enough to display the symptoms will usually have diarrhea with pale, greasy, bulky, malodorous stools, along with any combination of weakness, weight loss, poor appetite, protuberant abdomen, pallor, bleeding tendencies, muscle cramps and spasms, scaling of the skin, bone pain, vomiting, or anemia.

But these symptoms do not always appear while the disease is doing its dirty work. Or they can appear or disappear more or less unpredictably. You can have celiac disease and eat loaves of bread and not feel the least bit ill—until one or two or all of the above miseries hit you. Or none of these may come your way at all. But your emotional ups may slowly get higher, while your downs sink lower.

Celiac disease hits you at one of your most vital spots, as far as nutrition is concerned—the villi of your small intestine. Villi are small, threadlike projections from the surface of the small intestine, which do the important work of absorbing fluids and nutrients. Celiac disease destroys villi by the millions. How? Why?

There are three pieces to the puzzle. Doctors have the first part and the last part. The first piece of the puzzle was found in 1953 when Dutch researchers proved that gluten, the protein portion of the grain which gives dough its tough elastic texture, is the villain which causes so much misery among celiac disease sufferers.

You might think that the connection between eating wheat (and barley, rye, and oats) and the symptoms of celiac disease would have been made long before it actually was. The Dutch doctors who finally established the connection explain this delay by "the unwilling-ness to implicate such a widely used foodstuff. . . ." We know all about unwillingness to implicate widely used foodstuffs in disease. In addition, the doctors go on to say, "In patients with celiac disease who are in good condition, the unfavorable reaction to wheat often does not occur until one or two months after ingestion" (*American Journal of Clinical Nutrition,* July 1965).

The last piece to the puzzle, the fact that celiac disease wreaks havoc among the villi of the small intestine, is well known. In fact, in the absence of other symptoms, celiac disease is diagnosed by examining a minute specimen of the surface of the small intestine. If the villi are ravaged, celiac disease is the culprit.

The *middle* piece of the puzzle is the one that's missing and mystifying researchers—*why.* Why does gluten trigger such a terrible reaction in certain people and act as the staff of life for others? And why is the terrible reaction so unpredictable?

While no one has the answer yet, there are lots of theories. The most prominent explanation is that celiacs are lacking a certain enzyme which breaks down and detoxifies gluten before it can damage the villi.

## Celiac Disease Turns Up Unexpectedly

Perhaps if the mechanism were clearly defined, we would under-stand some of the more sinister sides of the disease. For example, many more people might be celiacs than the reported statistics (one in 2,000 to one in 8,000) indicate. Not that they're hiding the fact that they have celiac disease: they just *don't know.* Their "allergy" to wheat, rye, barley, and oats might be severely impairing their intestine's absorption of nutrients. But because the overt symptoms have not developed yet, they don't realize they're malnourished.

In a Denver study, out of twenty-one consecutive patients with diagnosed celiac disease, only eight presented the classical symptoms. James Mann, M.D., who conducted the study, said that "celiac disease may be very minimal in symptomatology, or very devastating. The reported incidence of one in several thousand is probably reason-able, for cases with the classical symptoms. There may be a lot more. We have no way of knowing, since it's such a sinister thing."

Celiac disease is so sinister, in fact, that it has turned up in some places you would least expect it. The *British Medical Journal*

(October 3, 1970) said that "The disease may be difficult to recognize, especially by a doctor who does not specialize in this field. It cannot be overemphasized that celiac disease must be suspected in every patient with an obscure deficiency syndrome. . . . Though pathological changes in the bowel are probably present from childhood, the disease may present clinically at any time of life, including old age, and symptoms may sometimes appear in response to stresses such as pregnancy or gastric surgery."

But celiac disease has been turning up in conditions which are definitely not "obscure deficiency syndromes." Dr. Mann cited a Canadian study by Wilfred M. Weinstein, M.D., in which patients with dermatitis herpetiformis were fed large amounts of gluten. This skin inflammation is characterized by reddened patches of oozing elevations of the skin, accompanied by itching and burning. Every one of the patients developed the ravaged intestinal villi, which is the most dependable symptom of celiac disease (*Gastroenterology,* April 1974). According to Dr. Mann, "this form of dermatitis is not rare at all."

## Schizophrenics Aided by Gluten-Free Diet

Another even more sinister association links celiac disease with schizophrenia. F. Curtis Dohan, M.D., of the Eastern Pennsylvania Psychiatric Institute at Philadelphia, first suspected a connection between celiac disease and schizophrenia when he observed that certain substances excreted in the urine of schizophrenics were also in the urine of celiacs.

Dr. Dohan next observed that groups of schizophrenics had much greater than average incidence of celiac disease.

So he set out to compare results when one group of schizophrenia patients was put on a gluten-free, milk-free diet and another group was not. Release from the locked ward was used as the index of improvement. Milk was withheld because some celiacs will not improve unless gluten *and* milk are eliminated. Those on the cereal-grain-free diet were released in about *half the time* taken by the control schizophrenics on the high-cereal diet. To check the results, Dr. Dohan introduced gluten into the food of the cereal-free, milk-free patients, in the disguised form of a supplement. The difference in the rate of release disappeared immediately.

One year later, Dr. Dohan compared the rates of discharge from the hospital, not only from the ward, and found that after 110 days, *twice* as many people on the cereal-free, milk-free diet were released as those on the high-cereal diet.

Dr. Dohan stressed that while his results indicate that a gluten-free diet will help schizophrenics, long-term studies, involving much larger groups for six months or more, are necessary. "When talking about most people," he emphasized, "emotional ups and downs would be a more accurate and certainly less scary word than schizophrenia. Often, people don't know they haven't been feeling well until they're put on a gluten-free diet."

## Fertility Restored

Some people who could be helped by a gluten-free diet have been feeling bad for a long time *and have known it.* The best example of this is people who have celiac disease and who are infertile because of it. In separate British studies, strictly adhered to gluten-free diets enabled previously infertile men and women to become parents. In the case of the men (*British Medical Journal,* May 10, 1975) previous examinations had pronounced them *normal.* Not until biopsies of their small intestines were performed—a nonsurgical operation in which a small sample of the tissue is removed—were they diagnosed as celiacs. In the case of the women, (*Lancet,* January 31, 1970) each had developed celiac disease in childhood but had allowed the treatment to lapse as they became older.

## Lifelong Vigilance Is Vital

Apparently, childhood sufferers of celiac disease often neglect their treatment and reintroduce gluten to their diets. According to the *British Medical Journal* (October 3, 1970), "Childhood symptoms may vanish with the onset of puberty even though the bowel lesion is not cured, a phenomenon which remains unexplained, but indicates that therapy should be lifelong." Reviewing people who had celiac disease during childhood, W. Morrice McCrae and colleagues of the Royal Hospital for Sick Children, Edinburgh, Scotland, lament the fact that although the untreated celiac disease had affected growth and caused a high rate of anemia, "Had these patients been seen by a physician unaware of the past history of celiac disease, there would have been little to indicate, on routine investigation, the presence of a continuing disorder" (*Lancet,* January 25, 1975).

Maybe it's too tempting to speculate that if the treatment for celiac disease involved something other than avoiding the "staff of life," and required daily doses of some important-sounding drug, more doctors would be on the lookout for it and fewer celiacs would neglect their "treatment." But there is a positive aspect to treatment for celiac disease. And that is nutrition. Celiacs must do more than strictly avoid wheat, rye, barley, and probably oats. They must avoid the great number of processed foods that contain wheat "filler." They must even go beyond replacing the nutrients normally supplied by the foods they have to avoid.

With their intestinal nutrient-absorbing mechanism subject to lessened efficiency, celiacs must supply themselves with much greater amounts of important nutrients. Fat-soluble vitamins A, D, and K are liable to be excreted in the feces rather than absorbed, so they must be supplied in extra quantities in order to be sufficient. The B vitamins, especially pantothenic acid and folic acid which have been shown to be deficient in celiacs, must be generously supplied (*British Medical Journal,* October 14, 1972; *Lancet,* March 23, 1963). Mineral balances are usually upset by celiac disease, so iron, calcium, and magnesium intake must be increased.

Let's put this discussion in perspective and emphasize that chances are you *don't* have celiac disease, even in a mild form. But for some few people, the facts presented here may open a door of discovery. If you believe you are one of them, try giving up wheat, rye, barley, and oats for a month or two and see if there is any improvement.

# Chiropractic

You either love chiropractors or you despise them. Or you don't know them.

That is perhaps an absurd statement to make about a healing art, but I've found that it's generally true. Most M.D.'s have nothing but scorn for chiropractors, and many medical societies actively—one might even say viciously—attempt to deny chiropractors the right to practice. They constantly refer to chiropractic as an "unscientific cult" which has no basis in proven fact and is "therefore highly dangerous."

What apparently keeps the profession alive and gives it the vitality to fight back against the M.D. establishment is the thousands of people who swear by chiropractors and enthusiastically relate anecdotes wherein their troubles were solved by chiropractors after M.D.'s failed to help.

Basically, chiropractors operate on the theory that subluxations or misalignments of the vertebrae of the spine can produce a virtually unlimited array of symptoms, which may often be cured by a physical "adjustment" which puts the bony structures back into their proper place.

Some chiropractors will even tell you that they do not treat or cure disease; "All I do," said one chiropractor recently, "is to normalize the body."

Skeptical physicians point to one trial (structured by M.D.'s), in which a number of chiropractors were asked to bring in X-rays of spines with subluxations. The X-rays were posted, and a series of chiropractors brought in to identify the subluxation. Reportedly, none of them could agree on where the subluxation was—except on the X-ray each had personally brought in.

Be that as it may, most people base their opinion of chiropractic on personal experiences. Several people I know have told me those experiences have been excellent. Others were very disappointed and came away convinced that the chiropractor made them return to the office numerous times for manipulations which did nothing but induce pain. Others criticize chiropractors because at least some of them seem to be too eager to take X-rays.

Although many chiropractors would disagree, most people believe that they are most useful for treating musculoskeletal complaints such as stiffness and pain in the back or legs. In my own experience, I have found that taking a bad back to a chiropractor netted me an X-ray and numerous manipulations which were really more like massages or applications of pressure than true manipulations. Taking your bad back to an osteopath is more likely to get you a definitive manipulation, I have found. That is only my personal experience, but unfortunately, there is not much else to go on. Scientific studies of the ability of chiropractic to bring about improvement in illness are all but entirely lacking.

Recently, the government attempted to conduct a study which would appraise the true value of chiropractic, but they discovered that the physicians involved in the study could not communicate with the chiropractors and vice versa. They simply did not talk each other's language. So it must be admitted that nearly all the evidence concerning the value of chiropractic is purely subjective and anecdotal in nature.

## Chiropractors vs. M.D.'s

One exception to this is a survey conducted by Dr. Robert L. Kane and his associates at the Department of Family and Community Medicine of the University of Utah College of Medicine, who compared the effectiveness of physician and chiropractor care in 232 patients with back pain.

The patients were identified by scanning Workmen's Compensation records. The Utah researchers contacted and interviewed 232 persons who had been treated for back or spinal problems. Of these, 122 had sought the services of chiropractors, while 110 went to physicians. (Workmen's Compensation in Utah permits the injured worker to select his therapist from among physicians, osteopaths, and chiropractors. This ruling differs from state to state.)

The interviews revealed that patients who used chiropractors were slightly more satisfied with the care they received, more pleased with their improvement, and more quickly returned to their former status (*Lancet,* June 29, 1974). The differences were not very great, but the numbers clearly show chiropractors ahead by a slim margin.

They found, too, that in spite of the medical profession's disdain for chiropractic, more and more people are turning to chiropractors for assistance.

While those patients who were treated by a chiropractor required almost twice as many visits as the M.D.-treated patients, the average duration of their treatment was significantly shorter—6.5 weeks as opposed to 9.3 weeks for the latter group. (Physician-treated patients average one to two visits a week, compared to two to five visits weekly for those seeing chiropractors.)

Evaluating each patient's disability and improvement with therapy, Dr. Kane and his associates concluded that "the intervention of a chiropractor in problems around neck and spine injuries was at least as effective as that of a physician, in terms of restoring the patient's function and satisfying the patient." Chiropractic patients scored an average of 0.92 on the Utah researchers' ratio of improvement scale, slightly ahead of the M.D.-treated patients' average score of 0.86.

On the other hand, there was a tendency for M.D.'s to get the more serious cases, so the better record of the chiropractors must be seen in this light. Perhaps it would be fair to call it a tie—but a "moral victory" for the much maligned chiropractors.

In the area of personal relations, the chiropractors rated higher scores than the M.D.'s. As many as 6.5 percent of the patients were dissatisfied with the M.D.'s ability to make them feel welcome. On the other hand, no patient found any fault at all with the chiropractors in this area. Chiropractors also rated higher scores than the M.D.'s in ability to explain the problem and the treatment in terms which the patient could easily understand.

# Choking Emergency

You're seated at the table, enjoying a delicious meal, when suddenly your spouse or child begins to choke. A piece of food has lodged in the windpipe, cutting off oxygen and turning the skin blue. What do you do?

- Stand behind the victim and wrap your arms around his or her waist, allowing the head, arms, and upper torso to hang forward.
- Grasp your fist with your other hand and place the fist against the victim's abdomen, slightly above the navel and below the rib cage.
- Press your fist forcefully into the victim's abdomen with a quick upward thrust.
- Repeat several times if necessary, until the obstructing object is expelled. (If *you* are the victim, and no help is at hand, perform the above maneuver on yourself by pressing your fist upward into the abdomen as described, or use the back of a chair.)

If the victim has already collapsed, turn him so he is lying on his back. Then proceed as follows:

- Facing victim, kneel astride his hips.
- With one of your hands on top of the other, place the heel of your bottom hand on the abdomen slightly above the navel and below the rib cage.

• Press forcefully into the victim's abdomen with a quick upward thrust. Repeat if necessary.

The lifesaving procedure just described is known as the Heimlich Maneuver. It is named for its originator, Henry J. Heimlich, M.D., director of surgery at The Jewish Hospital, Cincinnati, Ohio. A specialist in the surgical and medical management of esophageal and swallowing problems, Dr. Heimlich set out to find a fast and effective method to overcome food choking, an all-too-common occurrence that kills approximately 4,000 Americans every year. Such asphyxiation is now the sixth major cause of accidental death.

## Soft Unchewed Food Is Most Dangerous

In many cases, the lethal item blocking the air passage is a piece of soft food that wasn't sufficiently chewed. Common culprits are beef, chicken, veal, spaghetti, lettuce, and clams. Apples, popcorn, cough drops, or pills are also potentially dangerous. When the food gets stuck, the victim can't speak or breathe. His complexion becomes pale and bluish. Then he collapses. Death occurs in four or five minutes. When such incidents occur in restaurants, bystanders frequently confuse the episode with a heart attack, leading to the tag "cafe coronary."

Attempts to remove the object with the fingers or by slapping the victim's back aren't always successful. And reaching into the throat with an instrument is extremely hazardous. Dr. Heimlich theorized that pushing out the food *from below* was the only logical approach. The maneuver he developed forcefully elevates the diaphragm, compressing the lungs and expelling air with great pressure.

Since Dr. Heimlich publicly introduced his technique in 1974, policemen, rescue personnel, and ordinary citizens have used it to save many lives. In addition to food chokings, three children and one adult were saved from drowning after other resuscitation methods had failed.

When the maneuver is properly applied, the food or other obstructing object is ejected from the mouth with great force. Expressions commonly used include—"it popped out of the mouth," "hit the wall," "flew across the garden," etc. Those who successfully revived drowning victims observed that water "gushed" from the mouth, and then breathing began once again. The important point, as the following true-life incidents demonstrate, is that the maneuver *does* work and is reliable.

## Case Histories

"My three-year-old daughter, Jo Ann, was eating a piece of chicken when all of a sudden she began choking," a police officer wrote to Dr. Heimlich. The family was camping in a remote area of western Massachusetts, three miles from the nearest telephone. "I tried to dislodge the chicken with my fingers but was unable to do so. At this time my daughter began turning blue, and I suddenly remembered a fellow officer describing your method to me. . . . After four or five attempts, the chicken was dislodged, and we all breathed a little easier."

Here is another report from a Marlboro, Massachusetts, man: "On the night of December 26, 1974, as we were eating leftovers from our Christmas dinner, a turkey vertebra bone wrapped in stuffing became lodged in my wife's throat and, if I hadn't read your article, I shudder to think of what could have happened. I cannot positively state that I did everything exactly right, but after several 'bear hugs,' with my left fist closed and my right hand covering the fist, the vertebra popped out of her throat like a cork out of a champagne bottle."

Sometimes the object causing the problem isn't food at all, as the mother of a one-year-old child discovered. "As I walked past Karen's crib," Carol Beckstead of California later recalled, "she was making an unusual sound. I realized that she was unable to cry and her airway was partially blocked. . . . I leaned her forward and applied pressure inward and upward between her navel and diaphragm. To my amazement, out popped a button-type eye with about a half-inch shank on it from a toy dog."

# Colds

If your health is disrupted by nothing more than an occasional common cold, count yourself lucky, for here is the very model of the disease which runs its brief course and goes away, *almost* regardless of what you do or don't do. On the other hand, the fantastic amount of hoopla which has been published on how to prevent and cure colds is eloquent testimony to its ability to make life plain miserable.

Because of this misery, some people take daily doses of vitamin C to help avoid catching a cold. But most people, I imagine, wait until they get the sniffles and then start bombing those nasty little viruses with the Big C.

And that makes sense, because vitamin C—it's recently been discovered—is something like a birth control pill for those viruses. That was discovered by Carlton E. Schwerdt, Ph.D., a biochemist at the Stanford University School of Medicine, and his wife Patricia, also a biochemist. The Schwerdts brewed cultures of human cells, added some vitamin C for two days, and then infected the cultures with a form of the rhinovirus responsible for the common cold.

As Dr. Schwerdt explained it to us, with the extra vitamin C in the culture, "The virus goes through one cycle of growth, but subsequent cycles seem to be inhibited." After the first cycle, 16 to 48 hours after the initial infection, virus yield dropped gradually until it was only $\frac{1}{20}$th that of the viral yield in the culture that did not get the vitamin C. After 48 hours, the treated culture had a yield $\frac{1}{40}$th as great as the unvitaminized cells.

Although the Schwerdts told us that "the mechanism of inhibition is not entirely understood," one of their experiments produced some evidence that vitamin C did its job in a manner similar to that of interferon, an infection-fighting protein produced by human cells.

He added that to produce the same concentration in the body that was used in their experiment, six to ten grams of vitamin C would have to be taken over the course of a day. He also mentioned that "the quantities used in the experiments did not adversely affect the viability of the human cells."

Those are some interesting findings, which, by the way, you and I paid for, since the experiments were funded by a grant from the National Institute of Allergy and Infectious Diseases.

Terence W. Anderson of Toronto, who has both a medical degree and a Ph.D., has probably done more work than any other scientist testing the ability of vitamin C to cope with colds in studies involving very large numbers of people. He has tried different dosage schedules, but in one recent study he apparently tried to cut down the daily maintenance dose to the most economical level. And he found that people who took just one 500 mg. tablet of vitamin C a *week,* but took three tablets on the first day of any illness, and two tablets on days two through five, have about one-third fewer sick days and suffer much less from chills, fevers, and all the other miseries associated with colds and sore throats.

How much vitamin C *you* need to beat a nascent cold back into oblivion no one can say. Taking several 500 mg. doses throughout the day is a good place to start. In my experience, some people will need a total of four or five grams (that's 4,000 to 5,000 mg.) to do the trick. The earlier in the course of the cold you take vitamin C, I've noticed, the better it seems to work. I've also noticed that when a cold has been hanging in there day after day, taking more vitamin C rarely seems to help.

Taking vitamin C, though, is not the only way to make life easier when you have a cold. Hot fluids seem to help, and there is no shortage of herbal brews which people have used successfully.

Dr. Bernie Rappaport, a California psychiatrist, told us that his favorite recipe is to "mix one-eighth teaspoon of cayenne pepper, the juice of one lemon, one minced clove of garlic, and one gram of vitamin C. Sip slowly."

Personally, I hardly ever get colds, but if I had one, I would try Dr. Rappaport's brew, because it includes many of the "tried and true" natural cold remedies. The cayenne pepper and the garlic both have germicidal properties, and both make you perspire, which seems to bring relief. Lemons are loaded with vitamin C (more so than limes) and are also rich in bioflavonoids, substances which seem to make vitamin C work better. If the mixture is too strong for you, feel free to cut it by adding water or an appropriate herbal tea.

There's a wide choice of teas said to be good for colds. My own favorite is camomile, but others swear by lemon balm, boneset (particularly good when fever is present), coltsfoot (good when the cold is complicated by a cough or congestion), elder, pennyroyal, and vervain, which Kloss calls "one of the most wonderful gifts of God in the healing of diseases" and recommends to be taken by the hot cupful every hour for fevers and colds.

Kordel tells the story of a young man in the far North who had a chronic congestion until, on the advice of an Eskimo, he plunged his nose into a wad of soft snow. Reportedly, the relief of congestion was dramatic, perhaps simply because the extreme drop in temperature caused his swollen tissues to shrink.

If the Eskimo cure sounds a little too chilly for you, or if you can't always get hold of some snow when you have a cold, Kordel passes along another ethnic remedy. In Poland, he relates, they heat a cup of milk until it's scalding hot. Then they add one tablespoon of honey, a teaspoon of butter, and stir until well mixed. Then they toss in half a teaspoon of grated fresh garlic. (If you have no fresh garlic, use garlic powder.) This savory concoction is then sipped slowly about an hour before retiring.

# Colitis

Neither the cause nor the cure for chronic colitis or ulcerative colitis is known. What *is* known, though, is that great care must be taken to distinguish true colitis from more common conditions which may produce very similar conditions: notably, diverticular disease, irritable colon, and spastic colon. In addition, the pangs produced by lactose intolerance in those who cannot properly digest milk sugar may be misdiagnosed as colitis, or become aggravated or even initiated by colitis.

It's important for the doctor to attempt to sort these conditions out, because true colitis involves considerable physical damage to the colon, while the other conditions are largely functional in nature and are much more amenable to treatment. Sometimes, however, a differential diagnosis isn't easy. A friend of mine, for instance, after several days of hospitalization and many tests, was told he had ulcerative colitis and would have to go on a very soft, bland diet. A few months later, when this treatment produced no results, he went to an outstanding gastroenterologist who in short order discovered that he did not have ulcerative colitis at all. His pain and diarrhea were caused entirely by his inability to digest lactose. When he stopped eating all dairy products, his symptoms disappeared completely and his colon returned to normal.

An example of an even more unfortunate misdiagnosis of ulcerative colitis was described in the September 1975 issue of *Radiology*. The patient was a 42-year-old woman whose X-ray signs indicated chronic ulcerative colitis and cancer, which can be a complication of ulcerative colitis. Sigmoidoscopy and biopsy seemed to confirm the diagnosis of ulcerative colitis, and the colon was removed because of the presumed cancer.

However, when the removed bowel was studied by pathologists, they found that the woman had neither cancer nor ulcerative colitis. What she had is a condition known as "carthartic colon," caused by the chronic use of stimulant laxatives. The woman had apparently been taking two laxatives daily for nearly 20 years, and her colon became so irritated that it appeared to be grossly ulcerated and even cancerous.

While I said before that the cause of colitis is not known, it has been suggested by several doctors that two antibiotics, clindamycin and lincomycin, can cause colitis. One estimate suggests that by 1975, these two drugs had been responsible for about 15 deaths (a result of hemorrhaging) and—perhaps—many thousands of non-fatal cases of colitis.

## Dietary Supplementation Required

Nutritional supplementation can be very important in preventing complications arising from colitis. The inflammation in the colon and the body's attempt to rebuild tissue can use up considerable stores of nutrients. At the same time, the inflammation may seriously interfere with absorption. Worse, many people with colitis eat a very bland or soft diet, which is probably lacking in a wide variety of vitamins and minerals. Where there is bleeding, there will probably also be anemia.

In severe cases, where absorption is seriously impaired, the physician may have to administer a good deal of these required nutrients by injection. In most cases, generous amounts of multivitamin and multimineral tablets will be beneficial. Chewables where possible are best.

Though I am not familiar with any studies pinpointing nutritional deficiencies or successful therapy with specific nutrients in human colitis, there is recent reliable finding that patients with regional enteritis, another inflammatory disease of the intestines, may have sharply reduced levels of vitamin C, particularly those patients with the worst cases. We know, too, that vitamin C is required for the regeneration of new tissue. Zinc is particularly important in healing chronic ulcerations of epithelial tissue. Vitamin A is equally important in maintaining strong epithelium. The amino acids of protein, of course, are the foremost requirement in rebuilding tissue, but they are also required to transport other substances, such as vitamin A, to the site where they are needed most. Therefore, a colitis patient should be on a totally high-nutrition diet to give his (more likely *her*) body every chance to heal itself.

### Eliminating Dairy Foods May Help

Probably the classic study of various diets for colitis patients is the one published by Ralph Wright, M.D., and S. C. Truelove, M.D., in the *British Medical Journal,* July 17, 1965. They looked most carefully at the benefits to be gained by excluding milk and all other dairy products from the diet and concluded that "the milk-free diet was superior to the dummy diet. There were twice as many patients on the milk-free diet who were symptom free throughout the trial period of a year as there were on the ordinary diet, while, conversely, fewer patients suffered from several relapses. From our figures, the best estimate appears to be that a milk-free diet is beneficial to about one in five patients with ulcerative colitis, with the suggestion that the proportion may be higher in patients in their first attack of the disease."

Finally, there is the possibility that the traditional soft, bland diet prescribed for colitis patients may—at least in some instances—produce more harm than good. During the acute stages of ulcerative colitis, of course, the diet must be soft. But some specialists are now beginning to think that colitis which is not in the acute stage might be benefited by the addition of some good water-holding fiber to the diet. I don't know of any tests that have yet been made with colitis patients on a high-fiber diet, but one doctor has mentioned that his patients with subacute and chronic ulcerative colitis "thrive" on about half a tablespoon of unprocessed bran and half a tablespoon of wheat germ taken with fluids daily. (See CONSTIPATION.)

# Constipation

Chronic, uncomplicated constipation, which is what we are talking about here, is not so much a matter of frequency as it is of comfort. The distinction is worth mentioning because many people who believe they are constipated are only on a cycle which may be slower than average. In true constipation, bowel movements may be irregular, but they are always uncomfortable and the stools typically small and hard.

In recent years, it has been demonstrated that the best treatment for the vast majority of cases of chronic constipation is the addition to the diet of unprocessed wheat bran. The idea really isn't new, but until recently, it had more of the status of a folk remedy than of a medically approved treatment. Its present wide acceptance as an unconstipating food can probably be attributed mostly to Surgeon Captain Thomas L. Cleave of the Royal Navy. Writing in the *British Medical Journal* in 1972, Captain Cleave recalled some of his early work with bran. As early as 1941, while he was Senior Medical Officer on a battleship, there was a scarcity of fresh fruit and vegetables and he "found such bran invaluable for correcting the constipation [of] the ship's company. . . . The sailors loved this stuff by comparison with purgatives. . . . I think it is a great tragedy of our present day that, with the Medical Research Council showing at least 15 percent of the population to be on regular purgatives, this precious material is ever lost through the manufacture of white flour."

Here is part of a letter published in *Lancet* in 1962, from Dr. Harold Dodd: "Constipation is an ailment of so-called civilization and it can be greatly relieved by the way we live. . . . I cannot speak too highly of Surgeon Captain Cleave's prescription—one tablespoon of unprocessed bran daily. It restores to the diet what the miller has taken out. For several years I have practiced and prescribed a dessertspoon of unprocessed bran and one of unprocessed wheat germ daily. It is moistened according to taste with milk, gravy, soup, coffee, or fruit juice. In most patients it insures a daily formed stool as smooth as with liquid paraffin. . . . Patients with diverticulitis and subacute and chronic ulcerative colitis thrive on it."

These letters tell us several important things. First of all, eating bran is not in any way like taking medicine. It is rather *putting back* what would normally be in the wheat if the miller had not taken it out (along with the wheat germ) in refining wheat to make white flour. Second, bran should be taken along with fluids. Third, it works beautifully.

In several carefully observed clinical trials, it has been found that on a bran-added diet, approximately 80 percent of patients are either completely relieved of their constipation or greatly improved. However, since most of these patients also had suffered from other intestinal problems for years, it is possible that an even greater percentage of success can be expected in most people. It has also been observed that along with the improvement in constipation, there is also a high degree of relief from cramping, abdominal pain, tender rectum, wind, incomplete emptying of the bowel, and even heartburn.

Why heartburn should be relieved by bran is not clear, but some of the leading investigators in the field are beginning to think that the addition of healthful amounts of bulk to the diet profits not only the bowels, but the entire alimentary canal.

## The Logic of Bran

Bran, of course, is a very concentrated form of food fiber or indigestible bulk. Many other grains, as well as nuts, fruits, and vegetables are also good sources of fiber, but what makes bran so special? It isn't simply the amount of fiber bran contains, but the fact that bran can absorb eight or nine times its own weight in water. As a result, it helps to form large, soft, moist stools which are easily passed.

Another big plus factor for bran is that unlike whole foods, it can be taken in regulated doses and mixed with a great number of other foods. So if you don't feel like eating a big bowl of oatmeal and some whole wheat bread and a couple of pieces of fruit every day, you can still get all the desirable bulk with a few spoonfuls of bran.

Bran, it must be added, is *not* a laxative. It is rather a normalizer or regulator of bowel function. In fact, studies have shown that chronic diarrhea is aided as much as constipation by bran. The bran apparently soaks up the excess water in the colon and forms normal stools out of it.

Some people object to bran on the grounds that it is "roughage" and "scratchy." Actually, once it's moistened, it isn't scratchy at all. It rather takes on the consistency of a sponge.

The kind of bran used successfully by doctors is not the kind that is sold as a breakfast cereal. This latter product is processed and usually contains sugar. Authorities in the field recommend unprocessed bran, which is a flaky-looking product that has little or no taste and is available at a very nominal price from health food sources.

When taking bran, it is best to begin with one or two teaspoons a day, always taken with some sort of fluid, and increase the amount until the desired effect takes hold. This may mean anywhere from two teaspoons twice a day to two or three tablespoons three times a day. At first, it often produces some wind and distention, but this condition almost always disappears within a week or two. It takes that long for your body to adjust to the added fiber. Expect this problem and don't give up just because you feel gassy for a couple of days.

Some few people are not able to tolerate bran. They may even be allergic to it. If this is the case, it is not very difficult to find other sources of useful food fiber. *Unbolted* white or yellow corn meal is rich in fiber, as is dark buckwheat flour and buckwheat groats. Fresh fruits such as apples, peaches, plums, and pears are all good sources of fiber—and contain a lot of water as well. Eat the skins and all. Fresh leafy green vegetables such as cabbage and spinach are also valuable, as are foods rich in unrefined starch, such as white potatoes, sweet potatoes, pumpkins, squash, and carrots. Almost any produce that comes out of your garden is going to help you.

Dried fruits are also an excellent concentrated source of fiber, but they should always be taken either with plentiful fluids or stewed. Prunes, by the way, are valuable both for their intrinsic fiber, and for a specific substance—which has so far resisted chemical identification—which has a direct laxative effect. Prune juice, because it works by virtue of this natural laxative substance, should not be taken regularly in place of real bulk. When bulk is consumed, the normal defecation reflex goes into action. With prune juice, you're depending upon an external stimulus, and just as with any over-the-counter laxative, the bowels soon become dependent upon this stimulation in order to work.

Blackstrap molasses has a mild laxative effect which many people will not even notice. It is best consumed for its nutritional value rather than for its laxative qualities.

## Check Your Living Habits

Bran and other forms of food fiber are not the complete answer to constipation. Regular exercise can be a great help. The more vigorous the exercise, the more it helps. Exercise which conditions the stomach muscles and back muscles is particularly valuable, but a nice long walk every day will also help. If the exercise makes you thirsty, as it ought to, take your fill of water. All the bran in the world won't solve your problem if you don't drink enough water to let it do its work.

It is also important to develop the right living habits. The most important thing is not to resist the call of nature when it comes. If you habitually refuse, nature will stop calling after a while. It's a good idea to visit your bathroom at the same time every day. A good time for this might be after eating a hearty breakfast which features an unrefined cereal product such as granola, wheat germ, or oatmeal. Corn flakes and similar products are totally useless, having been almost completely stripped of all their natural fiber. Also eat some fresh or stewed fruit and have at least one glass or cup of beverage. Two glasses would be even better.

Once in the bathroom, the trick is to relax. Pick up a magazine or a book. Just make sure you aren't reading about constipation, because the idea is to take your mind off what you are doing. Stay put for about 10 minutes, regardless of what happens. Repeat daily. Eventually, your colon will get the idea.

Some people have found that adding a supplement of brewer's yeast to their daily diet improves elimination. That is apparently because of the concentration of B-complex vitamins in brewer's yeast. Rice polishings are also valuable, as they contain not only the B vitamins, but fiber as well. Nutritionist Adelle Davis believed that the B-complex factor inositol is especially important in relieving constipation and recommended blackstrap molasses as a good source.

Herbalists recommend any one of a number of herbs for constipation, but we would advise that they not be taken on a regular basis for this purpose. If your bowels are to be retrained into developing a healthy defecation reflex, they need the bulk which results from food fiber. A tea made from something like licorice powder will have a laxative effect, but it works the same way that prune juice or a laxative does, by producing chemical stimulation of the nerves which control elimination.

In children, the most common cause of chronic constipation (remember, we're not talking about constipation that only lasts for a couple of days) is probably excessive milk drinking. It's not that milk itself is necessarily constipating but that it tends to replace solids in the diet. As a general rule, if the child is constipated and is drinking more than a quart of milk a day, the first step is to cut back on the milk and see that his appetite is filled with fresh fruits, vegetables, and whole grain products. If his appetite is very small, he can be given a teaspoon of mixed bran and wheat germ once a day. Although fruits and other foods contain some calcium, it is probably a good idea to insure adequacy of calcium nutrition with a supplement such as bone meal or calcium gluconate.

People commonly become temporarily constipated with a sudden change in living habits, a trip, or while under unusual stress. No particular treatment is required, but you might want to try adding some bran or stewed prunes to your diet to speed the return to normalcy.

On the other hand, if you suddenly become constipated and the condition does not clear up inside a week, you should by all means make an appointment with a physician, perhaps a proctologist. Likewise, any sudden change in bowel habits or the sudden onset of pain, bleeding, or a feeling that the bowels are not empty, even after you have had a bowel movement, should all be interpreted as definite signs that medical attention is in order. The chances are that nothing serious is wrong, but a number of potentially serious ailments of the gastrointestinal tract first make themselves known by such signs and symptoms. Early medical attention to these problems is often very rewarding.

# Convulsions

In preliminary tests on 23 patients, Danish doctors found that when vitamin D supplements were given to epileptics already on anticonvulsant medication, the frequency of the fits was reduced by about one-third (*British Medical Journal,* May 4, 1974). But those were only preliminary results, and confirmation is required with a much larger population.

On the other hand, every epileptic who has been on medication for a long time should discuss the prophylactic use of vitamin D with his doctor. Regardless of the frequency of seizures, anticonvulsant medication interferes with vitamin D metabolism, which in turn interferes with bone growth. The result can be bone wasting and fractures that become equally or even more serious than the epilepsy. Large doses of vitamin D may be required and guidance is needed from a doctor who is familiar with the continuing research in this field.

Antiepileptic drugs may also cause deficiency of pyridoxine, or vitamin $B_6$. At the 1975 International Congress of Pediatrics held in Buenos Aires, Dr. L. Reinken of Austria said that about half of the children who have epilepsy also have relative vitamin $B_6$ deficiency. He added that in some cases, therapeutic doses of the vitamin will deter seizures.

Severe deficiency of vitamin $B_6$ itself is sufficient to produce convulsions. This may occur if the child is fed an incomplete artificial formula or is born with a $B_6$ dependency, which means that he or she requires much greater amounts of this vitamin than other children. Dr. George W. Frimpter and associates, discussing $B_6$ dependency syndromes in the *American Journal of Clinical Nutrition* (June 1969), after discussing the brain damage which results in some of these cases, point out that "It is possible that had $B_6$ therapy been instituted from birth or earlier, retardation might have been prevented. . . . Whether pyridoxine should be given to an infant is a difficult decision; waiting until the first appearance of symptoms—notably of central nervous system degeneration—may be foolhardy."

In recent years, there has been considerable discussion about the relationship of the B vitamin folic acid to epilepsy. It's been found that anticonvulsant medications lower the amount of $B_6$ in the system, but it's also suspected that if $B_6$ supplements are given, the action of the drug will be hampered. It seems that folic acid is required for the transmission of nervous impulses and the effectiveness of antiepileptic drugs may even depend upon the lowering of folic acid.

The practical significance of this, however, is another matter. Although injections of folic acid in amounts 35 times higher than are permitted in any over-the-counter nutritional supplement have been known to produce seizure activity in epileptics, normal supplementation has rarely if ever been observed to give epileptics any problems. And in the case of a severe folic acid deficiency, which can produce megaloblastic anemia, death may result if folic acid is not given. However, the folate deficiency caused by anticonvulsant drugs rarely becomes this serious.

## Minerals Important

Magnesium and calcium are also important in some convulsive disorders. Cattle grazing on lush new grass which has been artificially fertilized may develop what is known as "grass tetany" or "grass staggers" unless they are given supplemental magnesium. And while deficiency of calcium can itself produce convulsions, magnesium even plays a role here, because an adequate amount of that mineral is necessary for the parathyroid gland to secrete a hormone which brings about a normal serum calcium level. A report in *Science* (August 18, 1972) by Dr. Constantine S. Anast and colleagues related that a teenage girl with convulsions and low blood calcium could not be helped until she was given injections of magnesium. Injections rather than the oral route were necessary because the patient had impaired intestinal absorption of magnesium.

A few anecdotes will show what can sometimes be done with convulsions, although we have no way of knowing if these anecdotes are relevant to any more than a tiny fraction of such cases. One woman told us that her son began having seizures at the age of six months, and after awakening, would go into a series of convulsions. Brain wave tests revealed epilepsy, but no brain damage or other particular reason for the seizures. The child "became slow and uninterested," having three or four series of convulsions each day. One specialist said the child would need to take Dilantin every day, while the other recommended phenobarbital.

The child was still having regular convulsions when the woman read about the importance of $B_6$ in convulsive states and began putting two tablespoons of brewer's yeast a day in the baby's bottle. "Within five days he showed a growing, gradual improvement. He was going all day without a single seizure, then two days, four days— I was thrilled!

"I told the doctor and he said I was 'grasping at straws.' When the brewer's yeast was gone, I began giving him 10 mg. tablets of $B_6$ daily. All of a sudden this child quit his twitching at night (sleeps all night), began perking up mentally, regaining what he had forgotten and learning again. His red, drowsy little eyes sparkled and he squeals with energy. But best of all, these arms have cuddled a serene little boy—without seizures."

Curiously, her doctor was probably right. She *was* grasping at straws. And as she learned, some straws turn out to be life preservers.

Another reader found that magnesium, in the form of dolomite, was what she needed. She said that she was 50 and had suffered with epilepsy since the age of 17.

"I went to dozens of doctors, had EEG tests and no results. I tried several drugs and at last had my seizures reduced by one of them. But still I was always tense, nervous, and lived with constant fear of the next attack."

Then, she said, she began taking two dolomite tablets a day, along with her regular medication, "And I have not had one petit or grand mal attack in 18 months."

## Watch Additives

It should be emphasized that convulsions may be caused by a great variety of underlying conditions ranging from high fever to physical injury. They may even, it seems, be caused by food additives. One recent report tells of several cases where the common flavor-enhancing additives MSG apparently produced strange shudders, but not seizures, in several children. Another child had attacks of migraine and vomiting when he ate MSG in foods, but only when tomato products were eaten at the same meal (Reif-Lehrer et al., *New England Journal of Medicine,* December 4, 1975).

One woman told us that her son began having periodic seizures at the age of two, and she noticed that the episodes frequently followed several meals of hot dogs. The question became a moot point when the child was put on phenobarbital which eliminated the seizures. However, when the drug was discontinued at the age of five, he began to have attacks several times a year until the family switched to organic foods containing no preservatives or additives of any kind. Following that change, the convulsions ceased entirely. The family attributed this to pure coincidence, but in checking over records they had kept of food intake, they noticed that "In every recorded incidence he had had a heavy dose of nitrites prior to the attacks." Nitrites are preservatives used in almost all hot dogs, bacon, sausages, canned hams, and luncheon meats.

# Corns

Corns really ought not to be treated only symptomatically, because they will probably return unless the underlying cause is corrected. In many cases, the problem is nothing more than the "typical" pair of shoes which throws the weight of the body forward against the front of the shoe, which is too constricted to begin with. The simplest answer to this is to try wearing sandals or negative-heel shoes.

Dr. Elizabeth Roberts, Professor Emeritus at the New York College of Podiatric Medicine, cautions against using over-the-counter "corn cures." The acid they contain can destroy healthy surrounding tissue as well as the corn, and that may lead to a dangerous ulceration. She is also opposed to corn pads that have an opening or depression into which the corn fits, on the grounds that pressure is built up in the surrounding area and the corn will bulge into the opening.

While she recommends that any corn should be treated by a podiatrist, there is something you can do to protect it until you have medical help. The best way to do this, she advises, is to purchase some spot-type bandages with sterile gauze centers. "Put the sterile gauze directly over the corn. Avoid the rectangular-type adhesive bandage that must be wrapped completely around the toe. The bulk may cause irritation and a constriction that may be too great for comfort" (*On Your Feet,* Rodale Press, Emmaus, Pa., 1975). For soft corns, which occur between the toes, frequently in facing pairs, she advises using strands of a good-quality lamb's wool. "Don't use the coarse type found in beauty parlors. The strands should be drawn out into a thin, even layer and then wrapped *loosely* around the toe. If two adjacent toes are involved, only one need be wrapped with the lamb's wool. Be sure to remove before bathing."

# Coughing

The active ingredients in many commercial cough drops, suitable for common, uncomplicated coughs, are wholly or largely herbal. One English brand, for instance, which is quite powerful, contains eucalyptus oil, cubeb (an extract of the berries, I presume), tincture of capsicum (an extract of red pepper in alcohol), extract of glycyrrhiza (licorice), and menthol (the essential oil derived from peppermint). All this is put together in some kind of sugar base, although they don't specify what kind. Many cough drops use honey instead of sugar.

For coughs and colds, Levy recommends gargling frequently with a strong brew of elder blossoms and sage leaves and tops. To this is added some honey, a small amount of oil of sweet almonds, and five drops of oil of cloves for every half-pint of gargle.

Clymer recommends a syrup made from comfrey, baked onion juice, and honey, taken as warm as possible. Kordel likes a strong infusion of the blossoms and leaves of honeysuckle for soothing the mucous membranes and expelling phlegm. Grieve remarks that "When brewed and boiled with garlic, [kidney] beans have cured otherwise uncurable coughs."

In addition to the herbs mentioned, teas and syrups, or even homemade cough drops, can be made from coltsfoot, horehound, marshmallow, red clover, the dried inner bark of white pine, bark of wild cherry, and elecampane. See also SORE THROAT.

# Cystic Fibrosis

Therapy in cystic fibrosis should ideally be continuous and may be quite intensive, as these children often have multiple problems and are highly susceptible to infection.

Diet is an important part of therapy, and according to the *Merck Manual,* includes sufficient calories to satisfy hunger (exceeding the usual requirements by up to 50 percent); higher than normal protein intake; half the normal intake of fat, and multivitamin preparations with added supplements of vitamins A and E. Some infants will also require vitamin K. In addition, because pancreatic insufficiency is very common in cystic fibrosis, supplements of pancreatic material known as pancreatin should be given with each meal in powder or tablet form.

For what it may be worth, we pass along an anecdote related to us by the parents of an infant diagnosed as having cystic fibrosis at the age of six months. The boy "had all the positive symptoms: body full of mucus, foul-smelling oily stools, couldn't be put down because of breathing difficulty . . . in short, he was a very sick baby that didn't respond to antibiotics and regurgitated his food. He also had the potbelly and skinny arms and legs.

"We decided to take the vegetable juice route to clear his body of mucus. We used white radish and carrot juice: one ounce of white radish juice and five ounces of carrot juice. These were freshly juiced in my friend's juicer and strained through cheesecloth into bottles."

The mother said her son "hadn't been interested in anything in more than a month, but in less than 15 minutes after that first bottle of juice, he was smiling and pulling at the buttons on my sweater. I was able to put him down in his playpen for the first time without his crying. In fact, he pulled himself up to the side and grinned at us, then forthwith started playing with his toys. Tears of joy came to my eyes. Until then he had been listless and lifeless. Obviously, it was the first time in a long while that his body utilized anything he ate.

"That day we gave him more carrot juice, mixed with cucumber, then beet juice, then spinach juice, all in small amounts with larger amounts of carrot juice." The mother said her son slept well that night for the first time in months.

Subsequently, they added to his daily diet some predigested liquid protein, a large amount of vitamin C, several hundred units of vitamin E (dry form), and several hundred milligrams of citrus bioflavonoids, as well as some defatted, raw, desiccated liver for B vitamins.

After a few days, the child seemed to be improving remarkably, but when the mother talked to her pediatrician about it, he was completely negative. They visited another doctor who insisted that the child be put back on his regular formula, and when he was, he began to regurgitate everything after two days.

At that point, the parents went back to their own formula, and the child continued to improve. "Shortly after returning to this routine, I began adding pancreatin to other normal foods such as oatmeal, millet, lamb, white meat of turkey and chicken, lean beef, and white fish. We avoided fats and greases. We gave him fresh vegetables, all blended in our own blender."

Several months later, the child was still improving and appeared to be virtually normal in every respect. The mother added that when "we heard of a 20-month-old baby who was diagnosed as having cystic fibrosis . . . we passed along our formula. He has been on the routine for just a month but is already free of mucus, and his second tests made only three weeks after starting on the program came out negative."

As the writer of this letter said, no one knows if these improvements or remissions will continue, but we share her belief that regardless of the "homegrown" nature of this therapy, it would be wrong not to share it with others who may be interested.

# Dance Therapy

## by Esther C. Frankel

"My aunt got measles from dancing." That was one mental patient's response to a dance therapist's first attempt to get a group involved in therapeutic movement. And it really isn't as absurd as it sounds.

From primitive times to our own century, magical powers, both curative and causative, have been attributed to dance. There are still many places where a witch doctor dances to exorcise the evil spirits inhabiting the body of the sick. During the Middle Ages, when people had become unnerved by disease, wars, and unstable conditions, groups of people danced hysterically to avoid the plague. That uncontrollable dance madness became a contagion, with dances lasting for hours until the participants collapsed in convulsions. This is the origin of the common name for chorea major, St. Vitus's Dance. In Italy, it was believed that the bite of the Apulian spider caused tarantism, for which the cure was a tempestuous jumping dance. The descendant of this dance is today's joyous, lilting Tarantella. And in our country, Ted Shawn, the father of serious American dance, gave as his credo, "I believe that dance has the power to heal mentally and physically." So dance therapy is a modern version of an age-old concept about the therapeutic powers of dance.

Today's dance therapist is a mental health professional who treats behavioral problems such as psychosis, neurosis, autism, regression, drug addiction, and alcoholism. Because dance is a primal response to rhythm and music, the therapist uses the dancer's techniques and vocabulary to put the patient in touch with himself—to help "get him together." Unlike the psychiatrist's method of working through language, dance therapy is nonverbal and action oriented. It is not a cure but is used as an ancillary method to the psychiatric verbal approach and medical therapy.

## Every Dance Therapist Is a Pioneer

The aim is to make the individual cognizant of his feelings through the direct sensation of movement. By translating emotional conflict into movement, problems become concrete. The ultimate goal is total body-mind integration to give the regressed, the withdrawn, the mentally ill a sense of self-identity and to build self-esteem.

Because dance therapy is a new field, everyone who has entered the profession is a pioneer. Each one has drawn upon his or her background and experience, and through trial and error has arrived at a personalized method.

It wasn't until 1966 that the American Dance Therapy Association was founded to establish criteria for professional education and competence in this specialized area. As a result, methods have coalesced into somewhat standardized procedures, based on a combination of dance and our present-day knowledge of the human nervous system and psyche.

We know that we are in touch with our environment through our five senses. Each one of our senses sends messages to the brain through a complicated network of nerves. The brain organizes the data and simultaneously determines the response we should make. Touch something hot, the brain commands, "Pull away!" We act as we feel and we feel as we act. The body speaks its own truthful language. We may be too polite to ask our hosts to turn up the thermostat when we feel cold, but we don't fan ourselves. What we do is hug ourselves. The body has spoken for us. We jump for joy and we slump when we're sad. We shrink back in fear and advance to show love. Mind and body are a unity, each affecting the other.

All of us project an image to which others react. That image is reinforced by body language. When feelings are blocked, the body is unable to externalize what we are feeling. Layers of social restraints hinder the recognition of our deeper feelings. When emotions continue to send messages to the body and the body cannot act on the impulse, the result is like an overloaded circuit. We blow an emotional fuse.

## How Dance Therapy Helps

What can dance therapy do? How does it work?

First of all, the group must be small enough to enable the therapist to give individual attention where and when it is necessary. During the most serious sessions some time is devoted to exercises for stretching and strengthening muscles. This is to give the body tone, so often lost by inactivity in mental hospitals. An observant therapist files a mental note of each patient's areas of tension— clenched fists, tight jaws, rigid arms, stiff gait, a head carried off center.

The formation most commonly used is a circle, because it creates a feeling of security and oneness. For withdrawn people, merely holding hands and facing other members of the group are healthy steps in the right direction. Appropriate music as accompaniment to movement may be selected by patients or the therapist. At times, patients may sit on the floor and keep time by striking beaters (bamboo reeds) against the floor. It is hoped that hitting the floor hard releases hostility.

Another method has participants respond to their *own* body rhythm rather than an imposed one. Daily routines are acted out—washing, dressing, brushing teeth, combing hair. They listen to their pulse beats and make sounds to the rhythm. Then one by one each body part moves to the rhythm—head, shoulders, arms, hips, knees, ankles. Finally the group moves around the room using simple basic steps—walking, running, hopping, jumping, skipping, sliding, leaping. Patients are encouraged to use their own imagery as they move.

**Learning to Touch** ● Tactile exercises, used so much in encounter groups, play an important part in dance therapy. We know that babies "make friends" with their bodies and also reach out to touch and feel everything they see. Most adults have the same impulse, or else why would museums have to put up signs saying, Please Do Not Touch? To our detriment, after many Do Not signs and No's, we become inhibited about touching things, even ourselves, and we're very careful about touching others.

The theory is that people who have lost a sense of their own identity may re-establish contact with themselves by feeling and exploring their bodies as babies do: they are encouraged to touch their hair, eyes, ears, lips, face, limbs. Then partners are selected and the participants touch one another all over—every part except sexual areas. That is explained to the group before starting, as obviously too stimulating and counterproductive. One of the benefits of this exercise is that patients who have kept their distance from others must get close in order to touch one another. Hopefully, improved sensitivity to others will result from this tactile experience.

Some therapists work best with no set plan. They feel that picking up the mood of their patients makes for greater spontaneity. Helene Lefco relates how she handled a tense situation when she returned to work, with a group of mental patients, after an absence due to illness (*Dance Therapy,* Nelson-Hall, Chicago, 1974). One 200-pound patient menacingly backed her into a corner. It was only after Lefco reassured her that the doctor didn't want anyone to catch her sore throat that the woman released her. Other patients showed their anger by sullenly refusing to respond to the therapist, although she had established a good working relationship with them.

Spontaneously, she called words for group reaction. "The magic word is 'Revenge!' " she shouted. One young man pointed an imaginary sword at her throat. Two patients pretended to strangle one another as others screamed, "Kill 'em! Get 'em!" One patient bumped Lefco with her shoulder and hip. This aggressive movement was turned into the game children play called "Cock Fight." The game entails two opponents, each standing on one leg, trying to bump the other off balance.

One of the most common movements found among emotionally troubled people is rocking. Not only the mentally ill, but grief-stricken people seem to have a need for the soothing effects of this prenatal movement. While rocking back and forth may appear to be atypical behavior, don't we have rocking chairs? How about repetitious finger drumming? And who has never bounced a crossed leg? We also repeat prayers when we are frightened. Repetitious movement is a clue that a disturbing fear or anxiety may be at the heart of the action.

The therapist may handle the compulsive behavior pattern such as foot stamping, floor pacing, fist pounding, and rocking, by imitating the movement alongside the patient. When the patient is comfortable with a partner in movement, the therapist begins to apply the dancer's skill—varying the tempo, dynamics, and rhythm. By speeding up or slowing the original movement, by changing the accents or the pattern, another movement is created. Rhythm and movement are contagious. Seeing the change, the patient feels freer about altering his pattern. At this point, it is to be hoped that the compulsive, atypical behavior will start to change and in time, disappear completely.

**Acting Out Hidden Hurts** • The effectiveness of dance therapy depends on the therapist's ability to create a tension-free atmosphere, allowing patients to "let it all hang out." It is hypothesized that by acting out past hurts and frustrations, the individual can come to terms with his emotional problems and learn to deal with them on a more mature level. The objective is to get beneath the veneer of outward composure acquired as a result of cultural restraints.

One method, called "Psychomotor Training," allows impulses— even killing and destroying—to happen, but only muscularly (Albert Pesso, *Movement in Psychotherapy,* New York University Press, 1969). A facsimile of a past event, or a fantasied one, is re-enacted with the person who has chosen the situation as the enactor.

Two other members of the group, called "accommodators," supply the necessary reactions to the enactor's actions. This is called a "structure."

For instance, in a structure based on childhood experiences of pain and repressed anger caused by a parent, the child enactor goes through the act of punishing the negative parent by striking the floor with a belt next to the parent accommodator. The parent figure must supply the necessary feedback, reacting as if he's being hurt. The child enactor's anger may be so extreme that he has to act out killing the "parent."

If the enactor is still too inhibited to attack the parent figure, an ally intervenes, grabs the belt, and "beats" the "parent," hoping to give the enactor the courage to do the same. Then the positive parent accommodators step in and provide all the love and approval the enactor needed but didn't receive as a child. They hold him or her and offer comforting words and soothing gestures. Such rituals are not used with mental patients because of their inability to distinguish between fantasy and reality.

The purpose of rituals or structures is to help the participants gain new insights into themselves. Hopefully, the outcome will be an improved self-image for both the enactor and for the accommodators. Once the debris of old festering hurts and angers has been cleared away, the rational, stable, "together" person should emerge.

Common to most methods is the "group hug" at the end of each session. Members form a close circle, and to the strains of soothing music put their arms around one another. This is to create an atmosphere of love and acceptance as the participants relax.

## How the Aged Are Helped

Dance therapy can be a boon to the aged living out their lives in nursing homes. Old people confined to bed or those who spend their days just sitting and waiting for the inevitable, suffer not only physical infirmities but psychological erosion of their self-esteem. Time has robbed them of their strength, their possessions, and their lifestyle. All too often, they are abandoned by relatives who are too busy to visit them. The sad result is a destroyed self-image. "I'm no longer a *mensch* (a person)," is the heart-breaking way one old woman phrased it.

Dr. Charles Taylor, Professor of Human Development at

Pennsylvania State University, believes that idleness in nursing homes can hasten senility. People who enter a home with normal social behavior patterns deteriorate and become withdrawn unless opportunities are provided for social interaction and exercise. Enter the dance therapist. His or her job is to change the patient's negative self-image as old and worthless. By providing opportunities for freedom of expression through movement, old people can regain some positive attitudes about themselves. To be able to come out of a stimulating session and think, "I'm alive and still able to move meaningfully," is a great feeling for old people.

Again, the formation most often used is a circle or a semicircle. The following is a sample of a session for geriatric patients:

1. Warm-up: deep breathing, stretching, head circling, etc. to stimulate circulation.

2. A dance situation: arm movements derived from folk dances such as the Hindu Gesture Dance, Japanese Fan Dance, or the Samoan Sitting Dance. While the patients are exercising arms, wrists, and fingers they are encouraged to sway, to move their heads and their shoulders. Props such as scarves, fans, rhythm instruments, balls, and balloons give patients something to hold on to and manipulate. Moving to music and singing makes for fun, sociability, and much needed laughter.

3. Relaxation: slow, quiet movements.

Although there is no one approach to dance therapy, members of the American Dance Therapy Association agree that the therapist's training should include a wide range of dance-movement experience. Such dance training enables the therapist to communicate ideas and feelings through movement, posture, and gesture. In addition, a psychological understanding of movement and body mechanics is essential for analyzing movement patterns of patients. A knowledge of the behavioral sciences, group dynamics, and human sexuality, some pedagogy, and psychology are among the recommended courses.

## Sensitivity Plus a Thick Skin

Above all, the therapist must be sensitive to the needs of others and have the ability to respond spontaneously to those needs—when to raise an inviting hand (palm up) to a withdrawn patient, when to put a comforting arm around someone in a deeply troubled state, when to change an activity before boredom, fatigue, or danger actually occurs. It requires flexibility to discard a prepared plan and structure a session around the prevalent mood of patients. To be able to "shift gears" automatically also requires knowledge and experience.

Just as sensitivity is a prime requisite for a good therapist, so is a thick skin. Dance therapists have been spat upon, vilified, punched, and knocked down if they weren't "on their toes." None of this behavior can be taken personally, and sessions continue despite individual outbursts of violence. At times, a good sense of humor can save the day, and the therapist as well.

To be tolerant and refrain from making moral judgments about unusual behavior, no matter how shocking, requires a person who has come to grips with his or her own hang-ups.

Trudi Schoop sums up the job of the therapist in her compassionate description of psychotic people. She regards them as "fascinating foreigners who communicate in another language. The challenge to the therapist is to penetrate their country and customs, to see and feel the world as they do" (*Won't You Join the Dance?*, National Press Books, Palo Alto, California, 1974). She further states, "Rather than suppressing the fantasy of a psychotic individual, we should fly with him for a while, then descend with him for a soft landing on earth."

Dance therapy is still in its infancy, its true potential yet to be realized. Lacking a scientifically tested and codified method, it may be said that it is many techniques in search of a theory. Does it work? Can it help? It's too soon to predict the full benefits of movement therapy in the absence of research with control groups. However, just getting mentally regressed people to relate to others in a group certainly beats sitting in the dayroom and staring into space. If it only provides an emotional release for long pent-up, repressed feelings, it may put the patient on the road to improved mental health.

As one patient put it succinctly in a note he slipped into the dance therapist's pocket, "Dance therapy is better than a straightjacket."

The following is a list of places that offer programs in dance therapy:

## California

Ms. Alma Hawkins
University of California at Los Angeles
405 Hilgard Avenue
Los Angeles, California 90024

**New York City**

Hunter College
Dept. of Health and Physical Education
695 Park Avenue
New York, New York 10021

New York University
School of Education
Division of Creative Arts
675D Education Building
Washington Square
New York, New York 10003

**Texas**

Texas Institute of Child Psychiatry
Children's Hospital
Houston, Texas 77025

Dr. Claudine Sherrill
Texas University
Box 23717
Denton, Texas 76204

**Washington, D. C.**

Ms. Anna F. Lohn
Chief of Dance Therapy Section
St. Elizabeth's Hospital
Washington, D. C. 20032

**Wisconsin**

Felise B. Levine, Advisor
Dance Therapy Program
University of Wisconsin
Lathrop Hall
1050 University Avenue
Madison, Wisconsin 53706

For further information about dance therapy, contact:
American Dance Therapy Association
1000 Century Plaza—Suite 216E
Columbia, Maryland 21044

# Dandruff

Probably the worst thing you can do for dandruff is to use one of the "medicated" dandruff shampoos. I say this based on personal experience. When I was young, I followed the advice of advertisements and began using one of the medicated shampoos once a week. For a few days after shampooing, there would be no dandruff. After that, I noticed that the dandruff would return with a vengeance. It became necessary to shampoo twice a week, then three times a week. The benefits became less and less while my dandruff became worse and worse.

Finally, I took a different approach. I threw out all the medicated shampoos and began shampooing *daily* with an extremely mild unmedicated shampoo. For many years, this has proven to be 100 percent satisfactory in eliminating—completely—both dandruff and oiliness.

Dr. John Yudkin of England believes that a high sugar intake can be a major contributing cause of dandruff. That observation may be related to the fact that dandruff is actually a mild form of seborrheic dermatitis, and various components of the B complex are often known to clear up this condition. The connection is that while sugar contains no B vitamins, it requires them to be metabolized, and may therefore cause depletion of these vitamins. One woman who tried eliminating refined sugar and taking B-complex vitamins told us that "I was delighted when after about a month, the ugly dandruff which had plagued me for many years vanished."

If you want something that may be better and more natural than a mild commercial shampoo, you might want to take a tip from another reader whose itchy scalp had driven her to a dermatologist who charged $40 for two treatments. When the condition returned, she applied vitamin E oil to her scalp like a hair tonic. "I used it heavy, to let it soak in good before going to bed. One hour after applying it, the itching stopped. I use it about twice a week now and the itching and scabs have disappeared."

For very oily hair, you might want to try a dry shampoo with either cornmeal or bran. One reader who had "profuse seborrhea" and "spent a fortune on dermatologists" who failed to help her, tried rubbing cornmeal into her scalp and hair and brushing it out. "It's like a miracle, walking around with a dry head," she said.

See also DERMATITIS, SEBORRHEIC.

# Depression

An enormous quantity of drugs are dispensed to treat depression, and it is difficult to say in how many cases such treatment is justified.

What you may think is depression may be nothing more than a bad case of boredom or the blahs. In other cases, depression is a feeling of "what's the use?" that seems to hit people at a certain time in their life, typically the forties. Executives and professional people may fall into this kind of depression not long after they have entered the very peak of their careers and become overwhelmed with the feeling that all their efforts have somehow not been personally rewarding. A person whose interests are home centered may become depressed after the children are grown. What I am trying to get at is that depression is, in a certain sense, sometimes "natural," and a few sessions with a psychologist may be more appropriate than drug therapy.

We should also add that depression can be a kind of nonspecific result of generally bad nutrition and may respond to a more sensible diet that cuts down on junk food and maximizes foods with honest nourishment. Multivitamin and multimineral supplementation (including trace elements such as zinc) should be used as a routine dietary measure.

The naturally occurring mineral lithium is widely used to treat certain types of depression. But although lithium is natural and is present to some extent in everyone's diet, it is far from being nontoxic. In fact, the effective dose of lithium is at the same level where toxic side effects begin to appear.

The amino acid tryptophan has recently been used with success to treat certain forms of depression. When six grams a day of this amino acid were compared to the drug imipramine in a controlled double-blind study, the imipramine produced improvement more quickly, but the tryptophan also produced "highly statistically significant improvements" (K. Jensen et al., *Lancet,* November 8, 1975, p. 920).

Although the reduction of symptoms was more rapid with the drug route, there were fewer side effects in the tryptophan group.

Some foods are rich in tryptophan, but the therapeutic dose used in these trials represents about 10 times as much of this amino acid as occurs in a 3½-ounce serving of soybeans, which are very rich in this protein component.

Women who become depressed after taking oral contraceptive pills over a period of time may have an easy answer for their problem: vitamin $B_6$ or pyridoxine. All women who take the Pill don't become depressed, and all women who *do* become depressed while taking the Pill are not necessarily suffering from a $B_6$ deficiency. On the other hand, from several trials already carried out, it's estimated that many thousands of women taking the Pill have become needlessly depressed because the hormones are depleting their bodies of vitamin $B_6$. Naturally, most women don't associate the depression with the Pill. A reasonable approach here would be to take 50 mg. a day of $B_6$ for several weeks, and then go to a maintenance schedule of 10 to 20 mg. a day.

To perk out of the blues, herbalists value a hot cup of rosemary tea, perhaps with a pinch of valerian.

# Dermatitis

We will define dermatitis as an inflammation of the skin that is caused by some environmental agent. In common usage, chronic dermatitis, which may last for years, is known as eczema, and is covered under that heading.

All of us are daily exposed to an incredible number of synthetic materials and chemicals in the environment. Some, however, are more sensitive to these substances than others. The *Merck Manual* lists some of the most common causative agents as plants and trees such as poison ivy and white pine; citrus fruits and onions; chemicals; medications such as antihistamines and antibiotics; cosmetics of all kinds; household detergents and polishes; and a number of fabrics, including wool, silk, synthetic fibers, leather, fur, and dyed goods.

Unless you want to go to a dermatologist for patch testing, the smartest thing is to be your own detective. Notice where the rash has appeared, and then try to think of every substance which touches your skin at that point. If the rash is on your hands, it's obviously going to be difficult. If the rash is on your back, and you perspire quite a bit, think first of detergent residue in your underwear or the fabric itself which is touching your skin.

If the rash occurs along the belt line, think of the elastic in your underwear. Recently, it's been discovered that laundering these elastics eventually causes chemical changes which can render the elastic very irritating to the skin. In this case, get underwear without elastic, or put some kind of cloth between the elastic and your skin, or simply throw out all the old underwear and start over. It will take some time until the elastic becomes offensive again.

If the irritation appears on the feet, take a good look at your shoes. Shoes today are built almost entirely from synthetic materials and in addition, some of them do not let the perspiration of the feet evaporate.

One woman told us that her husband broke out in a rash every time he put on a "perma-press" pair of pants or shirt. She said that "We solved this problem by washing them first, and after they spun dry, we put them in a solution of two quarts of vinegar to three gallons of water. We then let them soak for three or four hours and then took the bucket out to the line where we hung them up without wringing. After they were dry, there was no vinegar smell. We have no problem now."

If the dermatitis is not too unsightly and does not cause itching or other discomfort, probably the best thing to do is to be very casual about it unless it gets worse. In many cases, it will spontaneously subside. It may return after a year or two, subside, reappear, and so forth. The rash may even return, perhaps in a modified form, long after the irritant has been removed. In my own experience, I developed dermatitis on a finger while I was working in a restaurant as a teenager and had to wash dishes with a very cheap caustic detergent. However, for years after I graduated from the ranks of dishwashers, the rash would sporadically return, its appearance triggered apparently by nervous tension. Such are the vagaries of the human skin.

A number of natural remedies for dermatitis are discussed under ECZEMA. See also DERMATITIS, SEBORRHEIC and ITCHING.

# Dermatitis, Seborrheic

Seborrheic dermatitis in its mildest form is common dandruff. In more serious cases, the scales and itching may extend to the hairline, eyebrows, nose, and ears. In the worst cases, it may involve other parts of the body as well, particularly in areas where skin rubs on skin, as in fatty folds.

Supplemental B vitamins are always indicated in this condition. That doesn't mean that they are going to help everyone, or even the majority, but from a practical point of view, they are definitely worth trying. The preparation should include *all* B vitamins, including $B_6$, $B_{12}$, even PABA and biotin. This last vitamin, which the body ordinarily manufactures itself, has been repeatedly observed to help infants with seborrhea. If the mother is nursing, she would be well advised to eat goodly amounts of liver. Failing this, she may take biotin orally or by injection.

The importance of taking a complete B supplement was underlined by a letter we recently received from a woman who had had severe seborrheic dermatitis for 20 years, during which time she consulted no less than 10 dermatologists. She tried everything, from hot olive oil to medicated creams and salves. Some doctors told her she had a defective glandular condition. Others said it was nerves, and "all said it was incurable."

Although she had taken vitamins for years and had been quite conscientious about her diet, the big change came when she added 100 mg. of PABA per day to her regular vitamin intake. She reported that "My dermatitis, dandruff, nose scales, itchy eyebrows completely vanished in about three weeks." In the four years since she added PABA to her regimen, her skin has been perfectly normal.

# Diabetes

The life of the average diabetic is at least 25 percent shorter than that of the nondiabetic, according to the U.S. Public Health Service. Diabetics are especially susceptible to heart disease and stroke (two killers that loom large for *all* Americans), as well as blindness, kidney failure, and gangrene caused by poor circulation. Even simple infections pose additional risk. Yet, against these nearly overwhelming odds, thousands of diabetics manage to live normal, long lives—by taking care of themselves and, most importantly, by watching their diets.

First, let's clear up once and for all the widely held notion that a diabetic diet has to be unappealing and harshly restrictive.

In the book *Feast on a Diabetic Diet* (McKay, New York, 1969), naturalist and wild-foods gatherer Euell Gibbons tells the story of his brother Joe, who was first diagnosed as a diabetic while in the Navy during World War II. After learning how to give himself daily insulin injections and follow a diabetic diet, Joe was discharged and sent home.

"Our paths diverged," writes Gibbons, "and it was many years before I saw Joe again. Then I was invited to spend a week at his home in New Mexico. I arrived, prepared to conceal my dismay at the way he must by now look, and all that he must have to endure on a diabetic regime."

Gibbons was in for a surprise! "I found that the years had changed Joe less than they had changed me," he writes. "My love of good food was beginning to show around my middle, but he was still slender and flat-stomached." That night the brothers dined on a delicate, herb-flavored consommé, broiled sirloin, asparagus spears, tossed salad, hot rolls, and for dessert: fresh melon balls.

"Dinner was a revelation," Gibbons discovered to his delight. But his pleasure turned to outright amazement as the wholesome, delicious meals continued. "Early in the week," says Gibbons, "I became aware of the curious fact that Joe was actually eating far better than he had before becoming a diabetic; indeed he was eating higher-quality food than 95 percent of the nondiabetics I know."

## Weight Control Is Crucial

The most important factor in Joe's and every other diabetic's diet is weight control. By carefully calculating the proper daily calorie intake for their particular body weight and activity level *and never exceeding it,* diabetics are usually able to bring their weight down to an optimum level which is actually 10 percent less than standard height-and-weight charts recommend. The reward for such diligence is great.

"The overweight diabetic who successfully peels off enough pounds to get his weight back to normal usually experiences a dramatic improvement in his condition. Indeed, the symptoms often virtually disappear," says Charles Weller, M.D., in his book, *The New Way to Live With Diabetes* (Doubleday, New York, 1966). "Weight reduction and control can bring this incurable disease closer to complete remission than any medication." In many cases, the newly slender patient can stop taking insulin.

One facet of diabetic therapy that almost everyone is familiar with is the strict ban on sugar. When diabetes strikes, the victim loses the ability, normally provided by the hormone insulin, to keep the sugar or glucose level in his blood within bounds. Depending on the severity of the disease, he may have to take insulin injections or oral drugs to get the glucose out of the blood and into the cells where it is needed. Too concentrated a source of sugar will quickly overtax the diabetic's insulin reserves and send the blood glucose skyrocketing out of control.

"One of the first dietary rules for all diabetics is to avoid all sugar and foods containing sugar, such as pastry, candy, soft drinks, etc.," says Dr. Weller. "Although giving up sweet desserts may be inconvenient for relatives of a diabetic, they can console themselves with the knowledge that apple pie and fruitcake are not essential to the human diet and, indeed, their excessive consumption can be dangerous."

## Enjoy the 'Honest' Carbohydrates

While refined sugar and other simple carbohydrates like white flour must be carefully watched, diabetics are actually encouraged to eat more *complex* carbohydrates—the same bulky, fiber-rich un-processed foods that all Americans should be eating more of. Vegetables are ideal. For example, ". . . a diabetic can eat a large plate of spinach, which contains as much carbohydrate as a table-spoonful of sugar—which itself is specifically prohibited," says Dr. Weller. "Spinach is a bulky food, and this bulk slows down the body's absorption of carbohydrates."

Spinach, asparagus, broccoli, cabbage, string beans, and celery are among the so-called "Group A" vegetables which the American Diabetes Association says can be generously included in diabetic diets. Served raw, most "Group A" vegetables can be eaten almost without limit.

What makes these complex carbohydrates so special? "It's true that starch, honey, syrups, carbohydrates in fruit, vegetables, berries, and cereals all end up as glucose," writes Lawrence E. Lamb, M.D., in *Metabolics* (Harper & Row, New York, 1974). "The difference is in the speed with which the conversion is accomplished. . . . Most of the bulky vegetables will delay emptying of the stomach and smooth out the absorption of sugars into the blood." Whole grain cereals also have this ability, he adds.

Because, as Dr. Lamb points out, "Diabetics are particularly prone to atherosclerosis with the complicating problems of heart attacks, strokes, and poor circulation to the feet," they must also limit the amount of fat in their diet. They are also urged to substitute polyunsaturated fats for the saturated type when possible. Fish and poultry are especially recommended, instead of fatty cuts of meat. Greasy, fried foods are discouraged.

Many diabetics eat smaller, more frequent meals, rather than the two or three big meals most people consume daily. Researchers have found that multiple frequent feedings tend to keep blood cholesterol levels lower, for diabetic and nondiabetic alike. Again, we would all do well to follow the diabetic's example: Heart disease is the number one killer in the United States.

"The most efficient and the fastest way to develop atherosclerosis," said trace nutrient authority Dr. Henry A. Schroeder in his book, *The Trace Elements and Man* (Devin-Adair, Old Greenwich, Conn., 1974), "is to drink much coffee all day with three or four spoonfuls of sugar and cream; use marmalades and jams on breakfast toast, with sugar thickly spread with cream on processed breakfast foods; eat a couple of ham sandwiches for lunch on white bread, followed by a slab of pie; and for dinner take large portions of pork with rich gravies, deep-fried potatoes, and a lemon meringue pie for dessert, followed by a sticky sweet liqueur or two. Such a diet will almost surely result in an elevated serum cholesterol, a depletion of chromium, and atherosclerosis." *This is precisely the kind of diet the conscientious diabetic avoids like the plague!*

## How to Make Every Calorie Count

Since diabetics eat less than most of us, they are advised to make every calorie count. Fish liver oil for vitamin A is a recommended daily supplement for diabetics, Dr. Angela J. Bowen told the Southwestern Diabetes Symposium in San Diego (*Pediatric News,* June

1974). Diabetics and others on low-fat diets often need supplemental amounts of this fat-soluble nutrient, and tasteless fish oil capsules are an ideal source, the Seattle, Washington, physician said.

She also recommended that diabetic patients be given a vitamin E supplement, ranging from 300 to 600 mg. (equivalent to approximately 400 to 800 I.U.) per day. Diabetics, like everyone else, need *all* the known nutrients, including 12 vitamins and 17 minerals, Dr. Bowen said. To be sure of getting the full range of trace elements and other nutrients, she encourages her patients to eat the widest possible variety of permitted foods, in addition to taking supplements.

## Eat More Raw Foods

Diabetics who make an effort to eat more raw foods may be able to decrease or eliminate their need for insulin, according to Dr. John M. Douglass, of the Southern California Permanente Medical Group and Kaiser Foundation Hospital in Los Angeles.

One of Dr. Douglass' patients, an elderly man, had been taking insulin twice a day. When he started eating more foods in their raw, uncooked state, his insulin requirements began to fall. After four years he was able to get by with just half his usual amount of insulin a day.

A second patient, a young Mexican-American man, complained to Dr. Douglass that he would rather die than continue taking insulin "shots." By shifting to an 80 percent raw diet, he was able to control his diabetes with oral drugs alone.

What led Dr. Douglass to try the raw food regimen? "My rationale was that since early man lived entirely on raw food, perhaps such a diet would be less stressful to the human system in general and less diabetogenic than a cooked food diet," he writes in *Annals of Internal Medicine* (January 1975). Raw vegetables, seeds, nuts, berries, melons, fruits, egg yolks, honey, oils and goat's milk are the mainstay of Dr. Douglass' program.

Brewer's yeast is another familiar natural food supplement that's now being recommended for the diabetic patient. The yeast is a rich source of chromium-containing GTF (glucose tolerance factor), which is able to potentiate the insulin in our bodies. When biochemist Richard J. Doisy and co-workers at the Upstate Medical Center in Syracuse, New York, gave brewer's yeast extract to 12 elderly persons with impaired glucose tolerance (a major factor in maturity-onset diabetes), half regained a normal ability to metabolize their blood sugar within two months (*Medical World News,* October 11, 1974). Brewer's yeast also lowered the insulin requirements of some diabetic patients.

## Extra Doses of Vitamin C

Dr. George V. Mann of Vanderbilt University believes diabetics need extra-large doses of vitamin C. "The hallmark of chronic diabetes is accelerated vascular disease," he says (*Perspectives in Biology and Medicine,* Winter, 1974), and he suspects that the lesions that so often develop and impede circulation in the blood vessels of diabetics are a form of scurvy, or vitamin C deficiency.

Extra vitamin E can also help. Dr. Robert W. Hillman, of the State University of New York Downstate Medical Center in Brooklyn, says that "diabetics with small-vessel disease of the extremities may benefit from a daily dose of 300 to 600 mg. of alpha tocopherol" (the same amount recommended by Dr. Bowen, which translates to approximately 400 to 800 I.U. of vitamin E).

Diabetics who wish to minimize the ill effects of their condition should also eliminate cigarette smoking and alcohol and follow a program of moderate but regular exercise. It's also important to wear shoes which do not cause abrasions of the feet. A small sore that may be a nuisance to most people can lead to gangrene in a diabetic. We advise seeing a first-rate podiatrist if you have even the slightest problem with your feet.

Traditional herbalism places great value on blueberry leaves as a natural method of controlling or lowering blood sugar levels when they are *slightly* elevated. Some 50 years ago, the herbalist-physician Clymer relates in his book *Nature's Healing Agents,* two doctors from the Psychiatric Institution of Morristown, New Jersey, reported results showing that the leaves of the common blueberry plant had an active principle with "remarkable potency to reduce excess sugar in the blood," which they named myrtillin. However, they also found that it could not replace insulin when that hormone was needed. Clymer recommends that those who have moderately elevated blood sugar should steep some leaves in hot water for half an hour and drink a cup of the tea two or three times a day. Make the infusion fresh each time you use it.

# Diaper Rash

Most mothers know that a baby should have frequent diaper changes and the skin kept as dry as possible. When diaper rash is severe and you are using cloth diapers, they must be boiled. Zinc oxide ointment is effective, and one popular ointment contains vitamins A and D.

All these and many more methods, however, failed to work on the 15-month-old baby of a registered nurse. Despite all the treatments, the child had "three or four dime-sized raw bleeding areas on his buttocks, scrotum, and penis." The nurse then decided to try liquid lecithin, which she had used in her kitchen to prevent foods from sticking to the pan. "I applied a heavy coating of the oil to the diaper area that night and the next morning the areas which had been raw and bleeding each time I had removed the wet diaper, were no longer raw. At each diaper change I used the lecithin and within three days the rash was completely cleared up, leaving only a slightly darker area where permanent scars might have been."

# Diarrhea

Diarrhea is only very rarely a disease entity which exists by itself. It is usually a symptom of an underlying condition, and it is vitally important to try to find out what is causing the diarrhea. In many cases, you can do this for yourself.

Antibiotics often result in diarrhea because the normal bacteria in the gut have been killed off by the medicine. Food poisoning, which some authorities state is much more frequent than most of us imagine, is another common cause of sudden but short-lived diarrhea, and serves the good purpose of ridding the body of toxic bacteria as rapidly as possible. And of course, anxiety can produce diarrhea, just as it can constipation.

However, if there is any question about it, and if loose or otherwise abnormal bowel movements do not disappear by themselves in a matter of days, a thorough medical checkup is indicated. Diarrhea could be a result of anything from a food allergy to a major disease of the colon.

Aside from its importance as an indicator of an underlying problem, diarrhea can become a major problem in itself when large amounts of fluid are being lost. That is especially critical in an infant, where a dangerous state of dehydration can develop in a matter of hours. In these cases, swift medical attention is required.

Although most cases of diarrhea do not last very long, there are a number of natural methods which will alleviate the condition to some extent. Following a regimen of antibiotics, generous amounts of *Lactobacillus acidophilus* yogurt can be eaten. For an even greater effect, take about a dozen tablets of *L. acidophilus* culture every day, along with some whole yogurt. Foods rich in unrefined carbohydrates and fiber will help these beneficial bacteria get established in the colon and help end the diarrhea. However, it may not be of much use to do this while you are taking the penicillin, because the bacteria will be wiped out before they can get started.

Carob flour, frequently used as a substitute for chocolate, is very rich in a binding substance known as pectin and can be of considerable help in normalizing the loose bowels. A number of medical studies have proved its effectiveness.

Bananas are another traditional and effective therapy for diarrhea. Like carob products, they are rich in pectin, but they also contain magnesium, potassium, and other important nutrients. These minerals help replace those which are lost in diarrhea, while the easily digested carbohydrates in bananas help keep the child's weight and energy levels normal.

There are some few cases of diarrhea in adults which are chronic and habitual, much like habitual constipation. In such cases, there is ample evidence that the bran regimen will do as much for diarrhea as it does for constipation. One study showed that patients having chronic diarrhea, with half a dozen or more bowel movements a day, were helped by adding bran to their diet even more than those suffering constipation. Typically, after adding small amounts of bran to their diets, the patients had only one or two bowel movements a day. For more detailed information on bran, see CONSTIPATION.

Just as sudden-onset diarrhea needs medical evaluation, chronic diarrhea should also be evaluated before beginning any regimen, dietary or otherwise. That is because the diarrhea may be a symptom of a malabsorption syndrome, in which case there could well be long-standing vitamin or mineral deficiencies which will have to be corrected. In some cases, it may be impossible to bring nutrition levels up to normal with the usual forms of supplementation. Here, the doctor who understands nutrition can be of great help.

# Diverticular Disease

Diverticulosis is the presence in the lower bowel of small herniations or out-pouchings of the mucous membrane through weak spots in the muscles surrounding the colon.

These diverticula, as they are known, are not at all uncommon, particularly in older people, and they may not cause any problems. But during an attack of diverticu*litis*, in which these herniations apparently become inflamed, life can be miserable.

A condition known as spastic colon (or the irritable bowel syndrome) is very similar to diverticulosis. According to Franz Goldstein, M.D., chief of the Department of Gastroenterology at Lincoln Hospital, and professor of medicine at the Jefferson Medical College in Philadelphia, "The two conditions often cannot be differentiated on clinical or radiologic grounds and seem to blend into one another until the complication of diverticulitis arises" (*Journal of the American Dietetic Association,* June 1972). The irritable bowel syndrome, Dr. Goldstein points out, seems to be occurring with increasing frequency from the third decade of life on.

Because of the similarity of these conditions and the similarity of treatment involved, we will discuss all of them under this heading.

We must assume that if you have this condition, you have been diagnosed after a careful examination by a gastroenterologist or proctologist, who has probably ordered X-rays. Certainly, any persistent pains or cramping or other abnormal occurrences in the bowel demand swift medical attention.

The interesting thing about diverticular disease and spastic colon is that they are mostly *functional* diseases. This means that there is nothing wrong with the colon—except that it doesn't *work* right. Even when diverticula are present, it is not at all certain that they are anything more than *symptoms* of the disease, rather than the cause. Oddly, patients can be freed from all symptoms of this disorder without having these herniations removed or in any way altered.

Unfortunately, the path to freedom from symptoms may be

blocked by outmoded medical advice. One standard suggestion is to eat a low-residue diet. That seems to make sense, because if the colon is very sensitive, why stress it with high-residue foods like fruit, raw vegetables, and whole grains?

Another common recommendation is that the patients should seek psychiatric help, and there does indeed seem to be a definite emotional factor in spastic colon.

In light of the best research and clinical trials conducted in recent years, it can be said with some confidence that the first recommendation is *almost* always counterproductive. (Counterproductive means doing more harm than good, and most health care researchers find numerous opportunities to use this word.)

The second recommendation, for psychiatric or psychological help in cases of spastic colon, probably has much merit to it, but with the knowledge we now have about the operation of the colon, this recommendation is best made only after dietary therapy, rigidly adhered to, fails to bring about improvement.

## Recent Insights and Better Therapy

For what we *do* know now about diverticular disease, we have to thank a handful of British physicians. Basically, what they have found is that diverticular disease seems to be the result of eating a low-residue diet, typically high in meat, white flour, and all sorts of sweets, including plain sugar. In parts of the world where the diet consists largely of various whole grain cereal products, as well as fiber-rich vegetables and fruits, diverticular disease (and many other chronic alimentary canal problems) is extremely rare.

Bulk is important because in order to expel the scanty and hard waste matter which results from a low-residue diet, the muscular wall of the colon must contract with extreme force. When the bowels are relatively full of waste matter, as they are in those who eat a high-residue diet, much less contractive power is needed and much less *pressure* is built up in the process. And it is this pressure in segments of the colon which researchers feel causes the lining of the gut to herniate through the muscle, and also causes the awful discomfort associated with diverticulitis.

In a number of clinical trials, it's been found that adding small amounts of unprocessed wheat bran to the diet, along with sufficient fluids, is often just what is needed to restore the correct amount of bulk to the diet and relieve many of the symptoms of diverticular disease.

A major study of the effects of bran on people suffering from diverticular disease was published in the *British Medical Journal* in 1972 by Dr. Neil S. Painter and colleagues. After a clinical trial which lasted several years, the doctors declared that of 70 patients with *severe* diverticular disease of the colon, 62 enjoyed marked relief of symptoms. The patients were instructed to take some unprocessed bran every day, but also were told they could add other forms of food fiber to their diet from fruit, vegetables, and whole grain bread. In addition, they were all told to reduce their intake of refined sugar in all forms. Among the symptoms which were relieved in the great majority of cases were constipation, severe colic, abdominal pain, tender rectum, wind, heartburn, nausea, bloated feeling, and incomplete emptying of the rectum.

These patients had been taking anywhere from a few teaspoons to a few tablespoons of bran every day, adjusting the amount taken to suit their own needs.

## Soothing the Irritable Bowel

In the United States, an interesting test of bran for patients with the irritable bowel syndrome was described in the *American Journal of Clinical Nutrition* in 1974 by Dr. Joseph L. Piepmeyer of the United States Naval Reserve. Dr. Piepmeyer selected 30 patients with the syndrome, typified by a cycle of constipation followed by the passage of hard, small stools, followed in turn by diarrhea. Many of them had varying degrees of wind and frequently suffered from abdominal bloat and cramping.

Each patient was instructed to take eight to ten rounded spoons of unprocessed bran every day, either alone or mixed with other foods. They were also warned that there is an "adjustment period" of from one to four weeks when taking bran, and they should not discontinue it if at first it made them gassy or gave them diarrhea.

It's interesting to note that Dr. Piepmeyer took the time to explain to his patients the importance of roughage in terms of the anatomy of their bowels and to describe to them exactly what wheat bran is, emphasizing "the uniqueness of unprocessed bran vs. other cereal products."

Improvement in their symptoms was reported by 23 of the 30

patients after four months on bran. Four patients withdrew from the study because they didn't like the taste of bran. So of those who actually took it, 90 percent improved. As expected, their stools increased in volume and there was also a "marked decrease in abdominal distention and cramps which was associated with some decrease in anxiety."

But why bran instead of apples or nuts or raisins or prunes? There are several advantages to bran, but probably the most important one is that it actually absorbs about eight times its own weight in water, which according to surgeon T. G. Parks "results in the passage of more bulky, softer stools, particularly in patients previously troubled with constipation" (*Proceedings of the Royal Society of Medicine,* July 1973). Dr. Parks, who has given bran to a number of his patients with diverticular disease, says that this kind of stool is precisely what might be expected to prevent formation of high-pressure segments of the bowels from which diverticula can explode.

Some of the other advantages of bran are that it is easy to regulate the dose, is extremely inexpensive, has very little taste, and can be kept sealed in the refrigerator for a long time.

## Bran . . . Better Than Surgery?

An interesting perspective on the potential of bran in dealing with bowel disease was offered by Dr. Adam N. Smith, consultant surgeon at the University of Edinburgh in Scotland, to doctors attending the Fifteenth Biennial Congress of the International Society of Colon and Rectal Surgery in 1974. Dr. Smith reported on the results of a long study designed to determine how much good bowel surgery did, and if a dietary change could influence the outcome.

Dr. Smith explained that "if high intraluminal pressure [inside the segments of the colon] is one of the predisposing factors in the genesis of diverticular disease, it follows that operations for this condition may be judged effectively in terms of colonic motility [pressure-creating contractions]."

The operations Dr. Smith is talking about are performed on diverticular patients who have a very severe condition which causes extreme pain and inflammation. The worst eventuality is a break in the mucous membrane lining the colon, which allows fecal bacteria to migrate into the bloodstream, where they can cause life-threatening infections.

There are two kinds of operations given and patients receiving each kind were followed and tested regularly for five subsequent years.

It was found that patients who had a portion of their tracts removed in an operation known as a colon resection had no reduction at all in motility or pressure following surgery. Although the sigmoid colon portion of the bowel had been removed in these patients, the problems had simply moved higher up in the bowel.

In the patients who had had a longitudinal myotomy, a relatively new operation in which some of the muscles which create the contracting effect are surgically cut, there was at first a considerable reduction in motility following surgery. However, the doctors found this only lasted for about a year. After that, the pressure began climbing again, so that in three years, it was very nearly back to what it was before surgery.

The Scottish surgeons then set out to see what the course of improvement would be if bran was added to the postoperative diet. Five patients from each group were put on a daily dose of 20 grams of unprocessed bran in addition to their normal diet. (That works out to about four tablespoons of bran a day.) The patients were monitored for five years, during which time they were repeatedly subjected to tests to measure intraluminal pressure. And here is what the doctors found:

Among the myotomy patients, who with surgery alone typically experience only a one-year improvement, the bran diet kept the pressure down during all five years of observation. In fact, said Dr. Smith, "The colonic activity fell even lower than it did with myotomy alone and has been well maintained."

In patients who had undergone a colonic resection, and who with surgery alone do not even achieve a temporary drop in pressure, the added bran resulted in a significant pressure reduction which was maintained throughout the five years. "In light of our findings we advise giving patients bran after either a resection or myotomy," Dr. Smith concluded.

There is no doubt that in some instances the bowel has become so damaged or infected that it must be surgically redesigned to prevent waste matters of the intestines from polluting the bloodstream. However, there is good indication that—at least in some cases—a bran regimen given to diverticulitis patients can actually make surgery unnecessary.

That was one of the conclusions of the previously cited study by Dr. Painter. And here we quote this well-known surgeon: "Twelve patients who suffered from painful diverticular disease had recurrent attacks of severe colic and *might well have come to surgery. . . .* In four, the colic was relieved and in seven it was abolished by the bran diet. None came to surgery despite the fact that formerly they had had attacks of severe pain. One woman of 50 had had three attacks of left renal colic . . . she was placed on a bran diet and had no further pain for two years. Occasionally she experienced mild cramp. . . . This disappeared when she doubled her intake of bran for a few days. *Thus even severe pain which might have lead to surgery will respond to a high-residue diet*" (emphasis added).

Dr. Painter adds that he is frequently asked if bran irritates the bowel. Here is his answer: "In not one of the 62 patients was the appetite made worse by bran. This suggests that the widely held view that so-called 'roughage' irritates the gut is not founded on fact; bran when moist becomes 'softage.' "

Dr. Goldstein, whom we mentioned earlier in this discussion, points out that physicians should also check to see if their patients are unable to properly digest milk because of a lactase deficiency. When people with this deficiency drink milk, especially relatively large amounts of milk or dairy products, they can develop diarrhea and crampy abdominal pains. This condition may exist simultaneously with a diverticular problem or ulcerative colitis. Dr. Goldstein notes that some patients complaining of bowel irritability are occasionally placed on dairy-rich ulcer diets which can aggravate all their symptoms.

Dr. Goldstein also points out that there *are* some indications for a low-residue diet, and these are during the acute phases of diverticulitis, ulcerative colitis, or any other condition in which the bowel is markedly inflamed. Once the crisis is past, he says, it appears that the addition of bulk agents to the diet is beneficial to patients who have bowel irritability or diverticulosis—and to some, but not all patients with ulcerative colitis. Dietary changes in ulcerative colitis and other relatively serious conditions should always be discussed with your physician, preferably a specialist who is up-to-date on the latest work in the field.

# Doctor: When To See One

**by Alan S. Bricklin, M.D.***

There can be no simple, straightforward answer to the question of when it's advisable to see your doctor. We all know from experience that doctors have individual criteria for when they want to talk to their patients on the telephone, and when they want them to come to the office or hospital. Beyond this, these criteria will vary greatly depending on the age and health status of the patient. A cold may be a mere nuisance to most of us, but to an older person with a long history of smoking and emphysema, for instance, a cold may be very dangerous.

What follow, therefore, are general guidelines that apply to *normally healthy adults,* but not those who are so old or weak that they cannot get around by themselves.

*Fever* is one of the more common indicators of infectious disease and every household should have a fever thermometer. Suppose you're home with a cold; your nose is stuffed up, you have laryngitis, you feel achy, and you have a temperature of 100.6° F. Do you call a doctor? Well, the temperature is not unduly high for an upper respiratory infection and in itself is not threatening. A fever of over 101° F. probably warrants a call to your doctor, although that degree of fever is also not particularly threatening in itself.

Let's take another situation where you haven't had any noticeable symptoms, but for the past week or so your temperature has been 99.6° to 100° F. In this case, with no explanation for the fever, you should consult your doctor. Generally, in adults, the fever secondary to an infectious process is seldom of itself a cause for alarm, while in a fever of unknown origin it is the underlying cause which is of concern.

*Pain* is a symptom, and once again it is the reason for the symptom, rather than the symptom itself which is of prime importance. Pain in the chest, particularly if it spreads to the left shoulder or arm, or is accompanied by sweating, nausea, or vomiting is reason

---

*Alan S. Bricklin earned his M.D. degree at Thomas Jefferson University School of Medicine and completed his residency in anatomical pathology at the Hospital of the University of Pennsylvania. He currently practices in the Los Angeles area.*

for immediately contacting a physician, since these are the classic symptoms of a heart attack. Chest pain which is made worse by breathing may have its origin in the lungs, and when shortness of breath is associated with chest pain, it is usually the heart or lungs that are responsible. Muscular or skeletal pain is generally worsened by direct pressure, while the pain of indigestion is most often beneath the lower portion of the breastbone and may respond to milk or antacids.

Because the pain involved in a heart attack may be rather mild (although it usually is severe) and the symptoms quite varied, it is probably wise to be very careful where chest pain is concerned and not to hesitate to contact your doctor.

*Pain in the head,* experienced as a headache, is one of the most common forms of pain. Recurrent headaches, ones that are particularly severe, and the sudden onset of headaches in a person who generally does not get them, warrant a medical consultation since they may signify a tumor within the substance of the brain. However, far and away the commonest cause of headaches is tension, and this can be relieved by body relaxing techniques. In general, head pain (except for headaches) is not very common. Many serious lesions involving the brain first produce symptoms other than pain.

*Pain of a sore throat* is something almost all of us have experienced at one time or another and is most often due to a viral infection. There is really nothing presently known to cure such an infection, although there are many methods for treating the pain, including saltwater gargles, medicinal gargles, honey and lemon, and usually a favorite grandmother's special formula. The main concern in throat pain is to determine whether or not you are dealing with a sore throat due to a particular type of streptococcal bacteria, since these infections can cause serious complications (such as rheumatic fever and kidney damage), which may be prevented by proper antibiotic therapy.

In viral sore throats the onset is generally gradual and may be associated with other signs and symptoms of a cold. The fever tends to be mild, usually below 101° F. (orally). A "strep throat" usually has a more sudden onset with fever of 102° F. or greater, and the person affected tends to appear "sicker" than one would expect for a routine cold. Although an experienced physician can make a good judgment as to whether a sore throat is viral or bacterial, the only way to be sure is by taking a throat culture. Physicians often disagree on the necessity of taking a culture, some maintaining that it should be done more routinely while others feel that clinical judgment is sufficiently accurate for the large majority of cases.

Because not all physicians agree on how to manage sore throats, it is somewhat difficult to offer practical advice to all readers. Probably the best advice is to ask your own physician (presumably someone in whom you have confidence) how he thinks you should deal with a sore throat and at what point he would like to be notified. My own personal opinion is that mild throat pain occurring in the setting of a typical cold and with little or no fever is most likely a viral infection. Where the pain is severe, the fever high, or the symptoms unusual in any way, it is best to consult a physician.

Pain in the throat not associated with signs and symptoms of an infection is an indication for a medical consultation.

*Pain and/or difficulty in swallowing* (dysphagia) may occur as part of a sore throat or cold but may indicate other, more serious disorders. If dysphagia lasts more than a few days or occurs for no apparent reason, a physician should be consulted.

*Hoarseness* (or a deepening and rough quality to the voice) may be due to upper respiratory viral infections (colds), excessive use of the voice, tumors (benign or malignant) on the vocal cords, damage to the nerves of the vocal cords, endocrine disturbances, and other more unusual causes. The first two reasons account for the large majority of cases. Hoarseness, sometimes called laryngitis, may progress to a temporary inability to speak. When one's voice becomes hoarse during a cold or after shouting all afternoon at a football game, it will usually return to normal in a day or so, if given the proper rest. If hoarseness develops for no apparent reason or if it lasts more than a few days, it would be wise to consult a doctor.

*Abdominal pain* is commonly associated with viral gastroenteritis and is experienced as a diffuse "crampy" type of pain. When pain localizes in one particular area, it often is a signal that something more serious has occurred and it is time to call a doctor. Pain that is relieved by eating is characteristic of a duodenal ulcer, while the pain of a stomach ulcer is often worsened following a meal. In women, pain sometimes occurs during the middle of the menstrual cycle at the time of ovulation and is presumed to be due to rupture of an egg from the surface of the ovary (a normal process). This pain, known as mittelschmerz (middle pain), occurs low down in the abdomen, on either side, depending on which ovary is ovulating at the time.

*Pain arising from skeletal structures* (muscle, bone, or connective tissue) in the torso or extremities due to exercise or physical exertion is usually recognizable as such because of the circumstances in which it occurs. It usually subsides in several days to a week. When this type of pain is associated with redness or a mass in the area involved it usually indicates a significant amount of tissue damage and may require medical attention. Other types of pain probably warrant a medical consultation.

*Coughing* is often part of the symptom complex known as an upper respiratory infection (URI) and may last for one to two weeks. If coughing persists longer than this, it is advisable to consult a physician. Smokers may have a chronic cough which is easily cleared up in a few days simply by stopping smoking.

*Coughing up blood* (hemoptysis) is an indication to see your doctor. Occasionally this may be due to bleeding from the gums, mouth, or nose; more often it is an indication of a serious disorder of the lungs. Among the diseases causing hemoptysis are pneumonia, tuberculosis, and tumors both benign and malignant.

*Shortness of breath* (dyspnea) may be an early symptom of either heart or lung disease. The shortness of breath is due to a lack of oxygen and may occur when inflammation or other damage to the lungs such as emphysema prevents the proper oxygenation of the blood or when the heart is not able to pump a sufficient amount of blood to supply oxygen to the various parts of the body. After varying amounts of physical exertion, we all experience dyspnea, but when we become short of breath after only nominal physical activity or when our tolerance to exertion suddenly decreases, it is time to see a doctor.

*Difficulty breathing when lying in a horizontal position* (orthopnea) usually indicates heart disease and is due to an accumulation of fluid in the lungs. This is often associated with exertional dyspnea and also warrants medical consultation.

*Vomiting* (emesis) occurs as a symptom of numerous varied disorders, many not directly associated with the digestive system. Vomiting following a blow to the head may indicate swelling of the brain or bleeding within the skull. Heart attacks often present with chest pain and vomiting. These conditions, of course, require prompt medical attention. An episode or two of vomiting may occur as part of many viral disorders or infections in general. In these situations, it is the nature of the primary disorder that determines if medical attention is needed. Anxiety or other emotional states may cause vomiting. Excessive coughing, particularly in children, may also cause vomiting.

Presumed viral infections of the gastrointestinal tract (known by some people as the "24-hour virus") are usually accompanied by vomiting and tend to follow a fairly typical course. Nausea and more or less diffuse abdominal pain or discomfort are followed by vomiting. This usually brings some relief for a while (minutes to hours) to be followed by renewed discomfort. By 12 to 24 hours the vomiting has usually stopped, although vague, mild abdominal discomfort may persist for a day or so. If the pain ever becomes localized to one specific part of the abdomen, especially the right lower quadrant, a physician or hospital should be contacted immediately, since this may indicate appendicitis or some other serious disorder.

If vomiting persists for more than a day, a physician should be contacted, since the loss of fluids may lead to significant dehydration.

*Vomiting of blood* (hematemesis) is serious and requires immediate medical consultation. After violent or extensive vomiting, there may be a few tiny streaks of blood in the vomitus from minute tears in the lining of the stomach or esophagus. The presence of these tiny flecks of blood is, by itself, not a cause for alarm.

*Diarrhea* often accompanies vomiting as part of a viral gastroenteritis and usually subsides within a day. Episodic diarrhea such as this is usually of little consequence, although the loss of water may lead to mild dehydration. It is therefore important to keep up your fluid intake when you have diarrhea. A large variety of foods and drinks may cause diarrhea in different people (this is usually a matter of personal idiosyncrasy), but this will subside after one to several episodes. When diarrhea is so severe as to be incapacitating, when it is associated with the passage of blood, or when it lasts longer than a day or two without improving, it is time to call your doctor.

*Constipation* almost defies definition, since bowel habits show such wide normal variation from person to person, and since there is so much psychological overlay associated with bowel functions. Some people have several bowel movements each day, while others have only one bowel movement every several days. What is important, however, is a persistent change in *your* usual bowel habits, or in the nature of your stools. What we eat and drink and to a certain extent, our activity, can alter the color or nature of the stools, but this is only transient. Changes in the stool that are of significance include narrowing of the caliber, greasiness, presence of mucus or blood, or pain on defecation.

*Passage of blood in the stool* (melena) may occur in several forms—as bright red blood; as black or tarry stools from bleeding in the upper portion of the gastrointestinal tract; and as microscopic melena, detectable only by laboratory tests. In any form, melena is reason for a medical evaluation.

Most cases of rectal bleeding are due to hemorrhoids but even if hemorrhoids are present, bleeding requires a medical workup since the presence of hemorrhoids does not mean that one cannot also have a tumor.

*Changes in weight* of a mild degree may occur in a short period of time—one or several days—due to dehydration from vomiting or diarrhea. Losses of 10 or more pounds (when not part of a planned diet) occurring over longer periods of time, often but not always associated with a decreased appetite, may signify a serious underlying disorder and should prompt a visit to your physician. Fluid retention, often due to heart disease, kidney disease, or as a side effect of certain drugs, may cause a significant increase in weight and is often manifested as swelling of the ankles. This may be the first sign of the underlying disease and a medical workup is indicated.

*Fatigue* is a very common complaint and has many varied etiologies, including poor nutrition, boredom, and various disease states. If you are sure that you are receiving an adequate amount of vitamins, minerals, iron, and other foodstuffs, persistent fatigue then requires investigation by your doctor.

*Palpitations* (or an awareness of your heart beating) may be of no significance, but also may indicate heart disease. Following strenuous physical activity, or when scared, you may be aware of your heartbeat or hear your heart "pounding in your ears," but usually the beating of your heart goes unnoticed. When palpitations occur at other times, or when associated with any type of distress, a medical consultation is in order.

*Swelling of the lymph nodes* (lymphadenopathy) may occur as a reaction to infection, either generalized or localized. When infection is the cause of the lymphadenopathy, the nodes are often tender. Lymphadenopathy may also be caused by cancer, and if there is no obvious cause for the swelling (such as a nearby infection), consult a doctor.

*When a skin wound becomes infected* there is usually a discharge of pus. Sometimes, however, the area merely becomes hot, tender, and red because the infected area is too far beneath the skin. Red streaks leading away from a wound are a sure sign of an infection of the lymphatic vessels (lymphangitis) and are an indication for immediate medical care.

*Pain on urination* (dysuria) is usually due to an infection and requires medical care.

*Blood in the urine* (hematuria) may be visible to the naked eye (tea-colored urine) or may be detected only by laboratory tests. In either case medical care is indicated.

*Waking up at night to urinate* (nocturia) is often an indication of disease, either genitourinary or cardiac. Persons who drink coffee or alcohol before retiring or who drink large quantities of other liquids shortly before bedtime may have to void during the night.

*Frequency of urination* may be due to anxiety but is often a sign of infection or other disorders of the bladder. Unless it is of short duration, at a time when nervous tension is high, it should be investigated.

*Vaginal bleeding* except during menses is reason to consult a physician. Although most cases eventually prove to be due to a benign disorder, bleeding may be the first sign of several types of cancer involving the female genital tract. Postmenopausal women who bleed should consult a physician immediately, since there is a greater likelihood that this type of bleeding is due to a malignant or premalignant disorder.

*A yellowing of the skin and whites of the eyes* (jaundice) may be due to a variety of diseases, all of them serious, and requires immediate medical consultation.

*Personality changes* are often subtle and difficult to detect. They may represent a "normal" change or a stage in our development. However, certain disorders and tumors of the brain can present with personality changes and because of this, if we recognize what appears to be an inappropriate change in ourselves or someone close to us, it would be wise to investigate it further.

Let me emphasize that whenever you think there may be something seriously wrong, but you aren't sure, do not hesitate to call your doctor, even in the middle of the night. Being awakened in the middle of the night is part of being a doctor; we all knew that before going to medical school. Doctors who don't want their sleep interrupted will have someone covering their night calls. Hospital emergency rooms are generally staffed 24 hours a day and you shouldn't hesitate to call one of these if you can't reach your own physician.

# Eczema

Here we are using the term "eczema" to mean chronic dermatitis—a rash that won't go away. If the eczema is distressing, or spreading, or appears on a child, consultation with a skin specialist is of course advisable.

No one who has or has had eczema would be surprised to learn that natural therapies do not work for everyone: they know the same is true with drugs, which in this case typically mean cortisone ointments. In my experience, cortisone ointments are often helpful in "knocking down" a rash which has flared up, but all too frequently the condition returns when the ointment is stopped. Sometimes the ointment doesn't help at all. So although natural therapies are not 100 percent effective, it may be that they are equally or even more effective than medicated salves. They're also a lot cheaper.

The first thing to keep in mind is that it is horrendously difficult to look at any given rash and determine what's causing it. Although a dermatologist has even more labels than he has ointments to apply to your skin condition, those labels do not in themselves constitute an understanding of the underlying cause. Even rashes which have been identified with a specific vitamin deficiency may not respond to that vitamin at all unless other nutrients are also given. The practical approach then, from a nutritional point of view, is to insure that your intake of *all* necessary vitamins and minerals is adequate.

With skin rashes, the B complex is crucially important. An appropriate supplement would include every factor in the B complex in amounts several times higher than the Recommended Dietary Allowance. For such therapeutic purposes, my personal view is that the B-complex supplement should contain at least: $B_1$—10 mg.; $B_2$—10 mg.; niacin—25-50 mg.; pantothenic acid—100 mg.; $B_6$—10 mg.; $B_{12}$—25-50 mcg.; folic acid—400 mcg.; PABA—100 mg.; biotin—300 mcg.; plus several hundred milligrams each of choline and inositol.

Vitamin E is also important in skin conditions, and an appropriate therapeutic figure is between 400 and 800 units a day. Almost any of the other vitamins or minerals can be involved in a skin condition, so that's why we recommended across-the-board supplementation, or the shotgun approach, rather than trying only one nutrient.

This approach, for one thing, will take care of any skin condition which is a direct result of an absolute deficiency of a certain vitamin or mineral, and so we will not have to spend time discussing the various skin lesions associated with scurvy, pellagra, and so on.

With a few exceptions, the therapies which follow should be considered folk remedies more than anything else, because there do not seem to be any convincing medical studies showing that they are uniformly effective. The exceptions to these are in the case of the absolute deficiencies, which of course do respond uniformly to supplements.

## Try Vitamin E

A woman from New York reports that after her dermatologist explained that there was no treatment for the eczema on her hands except periodic cortisone injections, she began taking 300 units daily of vitamin E. Her hands then healed satisfactorily, except that from time to time the condition would again flare up, at which time she would increase the dose of vitamin E and it would subside again.

Another reader was bothered with a skin rash that caused itching for five years. He tried all the other remedies, but nothing helped until he began taking vitamin E. In short order, the rash began to clear and the itching stopped.

A chemist told us he went to a skin specialist at one of the leading medical clinics in California and was given a salve to put on a skin rash he had on both sides of his nose. It worked beautifully, he said, but whenever he stopped using it, the rash came back.

At that point, he began taking 600 units of vitamin E and 50,000 units of vitamin A every day. "No more skin problems and no more chemicals," this chemist said. Let me add that 50,000 units of vitamin A is a bit much to be taking on a long-term basis. It is an appropriate amount for an adult who believes he is deficient in vitamin A, for a week or so. After that, a maintenance amount of 10,000 to 20,000 units daily should be more than sufficient.

Sometimes vitamin E works better when it is applied directly to the rash. A woman who had been taking an unspecified amount of vitamin E for five years said she developed a rash on her face that wouldn't go away. "It made my face feel like sandpaper. I tried everything on it, even went to the skin doctor, but nothing I put on it would make it go away. Then I decided to try vitamin E on it. Every night I broke 100 I.U. of E and put it on my face. Within three days the rash was gone. Now the skin on my face is as smooth as a rose petal."

We know of one case, where, ironically, vitamin E was able to reverse the ill effects of herbal therapy. A California woman, apparently of Chinese background, hurt her leg when she fell into a gopher hole and went to an old Chinese doctor who wrapped her leg in a mixture of Chinese herbs. "This potent poultice was just too strong for my sensitive skin and it broke out into blisters—almost killing me with itching all night long," she said. "Washing with baking soda always stopped itching before, but this time nothing helped. By sheer luck I opened up a few vitamin E capsules and smeared my inflamed skin with vitamin E. Relief came instantly!"

## Brewer's Yeast Can Do Wonders

In our entry on DERMATITIS, we noted that contact dermatitis can hang around for years even after the irritating agent has been removed. That was the experience of a reader who developed an itching rash under one of her rings. Naturally, she took the ring off, but instead of getting better, the itching became worse, even though she went to several dermatologists. At that point, she said, the rash, "diagnosed as eczema, covered my whole hand and none of the expensive prescribed ointments worked. Not only would the intense itching keep me from sleeping some nights, but I was also embarrassed by the way it looked." Finally, she went to an M.D. who was interested in nutrition, and was put on what she called "an incredible diet," which after three months stopped the itching completely and almost entirely cleared up the rash.

"His diet for me included brewer's yeast, desiccated liver and lecithin granules dissolved in prune juice, as well as blackstrap molasses mixed with large quantities of lemon juice."

The brewer's yeast and desiccated liver prescribed by that doctor are rich not only in B vitamins, but in trace elements and other nutrients which the body may need more of. Whatever is in brewer's yeast seemed to be exactly what one reader who had a very bad case of eczema for four years needed. She told us her hands looked like those of an "old, old lady; scales, red bumps, cracks, itching, etc., and very swollen all the time." (She was 26 years old.) She then began taking six brewer's yeast tablets a day and the results amazed her. She put it this way: "I can't believe it, it's gone, all gone, not even a trace, really. My hands were clear, not swollen, smooth, not itching, small and beautiful like they used to be, for the first time in at least four years."

It's interesting that she goes on to say that when she forgets to take at least four tablets a day of the brewer's yeast, her hands break out again in a few days. This indicates either that her diet is in general very deficient in B vitamins, or that she has a special need for more B vitamins or the other factors which occur in brewer's yeast. She added that although she had been to a doctor, his treatments did not help very much. We might well ask if that doctor was wrong in not prescribing B-complex vitamins or foods such as brewer's yeast. From a medical point of view, the answer is that he was *not* wrong, because the symptoms described do not exactly fit any particular deficiency. Were she deficient in niacin, for example, the rash *should*—theoretically—have appeared around her neck as well as her hands, and there would have been other symptoms, too. But that's from a *medical* point of view. The commonsense, practical point of view which should complement the strictly medical view, is something else. And from this perspective, we recognize that the B vitamins are so important to the skin that it pays to at least try them in almost any skin condition, particularly rashes.

Brewer's yeast was used externally by a woman whose face frequently broke out in allergic reactions to her food. On one occasion, she related, her face broke out worse than it ever had before and she was desperate. Nothing she did, including applying a prescribed medicine, helped very much. She then tried applying a brewer's yeast facial mask, left it on for about 10 minutes, and then washed her face. "The next day my skin had healed considerably, and by the next day, with another facial mask, my face was almost cleared up." For directions on how to make a brewer's yeast facial mask, see SKIN, OILY.

## Herbal Remedies for Eczema

The fact that the herbal world offers innumerable remedies for eczema and other skin conditions is good evidence that mankind has been plagued with skin problems for many years. After reading a great deal of herbal literature and talking with many people who have used herbs for chronic skin conditions, it seems that the most valuable or trustworthy are burdock, slippery elm, comfrey, and goldenseal. Luckily, these herbs are not at all difficult to get. Any botanical supply house will have them and so will some health food stores.

Grieve, whose opinion is always to be valued, says this of burdock (a common broad-leaved weed with prickly heads or burrs which you may find sticking to your clothing after you've walked through some underbrush): "In all skin diseases, it is a certain remedy and has effected a cure in many cases of eczema, either taken alone or combined with other remedies such as yellow dock and sarsaparilla. The root is principally employed, but the leaves and seeds are equally valuable." She adds that the oily seeds are especially valued for chronic skin conditions.

To use burdock, steep the seeds and/or the other parts in hot water, let cool, and then apply to the skin, perhaps with a dressing to make a poultice. Generally speaking, a slight handful of herbal material is used with one cup of water which has been brought to a boil. This may be too strong for a tea, but a poultice should have a greater concentration of herbs than a tea.

Herbalists usually combine several plant substances for treatment in order to get a better balance of healing elements, just as we recommend a well-balanced B-complex supplement instead of a single vitamin. Therefore, you could reduce the amount of burdock in the brew and make up the difference with some chopped up roots and/or leaves of comfrey, along with a generous pinch of powdered goldenseal root. When the brew has steeped for a good 20 minutes in a covered vessel, soak a clean dressing in it and apply to the skin. A poultice should be warm, not hot.

As an alternative to a poultice, you might do well to take the above brew and mix enough of it with some coarse powdered bark of slippery elm to make a paste. Dab a little olive oil on the skin first, to make sure the paste doesn't adhere too tightly to the skin. If this proves a bit messy, there's nothing wrong with putting the paste on a clean dressing and then applying that to the skin. In any case, slippery elm is highly valued for all conditions where the skin is irritated.

One reader passed along to us a Gypsy remedy which made use of slippery elm. It seems that some years ago, a band of Gypsies was traveling west and stopped at the family house to ask for some eggs and milk. When one of the women saw eczema all over the arms of a young girl (she had suffered from it for years and hundreds of dollars had been spent on various treatments), she promised to fix it. An hour later, she returned with some boiled jimsonweed and slippery elm bark. She put some cloth in this "goo" and wrapped it around the girl's arms. Then she wrapped more cloth around that and left the fluid with the family so that they could continue to moisten the dressing.

The itching stopped almost immediately, and five days later, "the arms were cleared, all but the redness of the new skin, which developed to its natural color. The girl had no more eczema after that."

Two herbs that may very well be growing on your lawn also have a certain amount of herbal tradition behind them for skin conditions. They are the common dandelion and plantain, the round, broad-leaved weed. A wash brewed from the root of the dandelion is said to be good for skin conditions, as are the mashed-up fresh leaves of plantain. Do you have any strawberries, wild or domesticated, growing around your house? If you do, you can make a strong wash from them and try that as well.

See also DERMATITIS and ITCHING.

# Emotional Problems

Some of the more clear-cut emotional problems are discussed elsewhere in this volume under the headings of PSYCHOTHERAPY, SCHIZOPHRENIA, DEPRESSION, and HYPERACTIVITY. Here we'll discuss such less sharply defined symptoms as anxiety, nervousness, irritability, poor memory, fearfulness, and confusion. The individual bothered by such problems may be labeled as neurotic, or senile, but such labels are often meaningless or downright misleading.

Nutrition may play a key role in a surprisingly large number of these problems. That was the conclusion of a group of investigators at the Institute of Medicine and Pharmacy in Bucharest, Rumania, who compared 65 patients with neurotic symptoms to 49 healthy individuals (*Nutrition Reports International,* September 1975). The Rumanian researchers found that the neurotics excreted only half as much thiamine, or vitamin $B_1$, in their urine as the controls. This normally indicates a thiamine deficiency. In addition, blood tests revealed an excess of pyruvate in the neurotic patient. Pyruvate is an intermediate breakdown product which accumulates in the blood when dietary thiamine intake is insufficient.

"These differences suggest that patients with neurosis exhibited biochemical evidences of thiamine deficiency," the authors point out. "When the intake of thiamine is reduced, mental symptoms appear resembling those of neurasthenia—intolerance of noise, inability to concentrate, memory defects, irritability, depression, and other neurological manifestations. . . . Such a biochemical lesion could diminish the individual's ability to adapt to the multitude and rapidity of stimuli of modern lifestyles."

The Rumanians, like most Americans, had a high sugar intake as a result of their dependence on refined, processed foods. According to the authors, this aggravated their mental symptoms, because additional thiamine is used up as the body metabolizes sugar. "A consideration of the changes in food habits prevailing in many countries raises the question as to whether the increasing occurrence of neurosis may not arise from a thiamine-glucose imbalance," the researchers conclude.

## Brain Cells Are Also Body Cells

The report from Bucharest is part of a growing trend among scientists and health practitioners to recognize the role food can play in affecting the psyche.

"Psychiatrists continue to think of emotions as separate from the human body, unconnected with the chemistry of the brain cells," writes H. L. Newbold, M.D., in *Mega-Nutrients for Your Nerves* (Peter H. Wyden, New York, 1975). "Freud, misinterpreted, has so captured our imaginations that even physicians forget that the brain is an organ in the body.

"The idea of treating emotional illness with nutritional supplements is still new," says Dr. Newbold, "but is rapidly unfolding into a fascinating psychiatric subspecialty. I say subspecialty, but it should really be a part of every psychiatrists' knowledge, for the enzyme defects demonstrated in the emotionally ill are so widespread that I feel every patient with an emotional disorder deserves a trial at this form of therapy."

Dr. Newbold calls thiamine "the granddaddy of the 'nerve' vitamins. It is essential for the proper functioning of the central nervous system, and its lack can result in almost any nervous manifestation you can name: depression, difficulty in concentration, fatigue, tension, hyperactivity, confusion, disorientation, hallucinations, numbness in the arms or legs, and many more." Unlike a drug, thiamine works as an emotional "normalizer." Dr. Newbold says that thiamine "can have a lifting effect on tired or depressed people and a tranquilizing effect on excited people."

## Thiamine Deficiency Sets Moods Swinging

A classic study of thiamine and its effect on behavior was described by Josef Brozek, Ph.D., at a Symposium on Nutrition and Behavior held at the University of Minnesota, April 27, 1956. Dr. Brozek, a professor in that university's School of Public Health, reported that large swings in mood and attitude were observed among 10 healthy male volunteers deprived of thiamine.

Each man received a diet carefully balanced in every respect save one: thiamine was partially restricted for a period of 168 days, then totally removed for a period of from 15 to 27 days, depending on the individual. Without thiamine, the subjects became more depressed. They lost their ability to concentrate, their mental alertness, and feeling of well-being. They became more apprehensive, irritable, forgetful, and nervous. Some complained of dizziness and headaches. The men began to lose patience with each other and with staff members conducting the study. Tempers flared. Those whose diets had contained the least thiamine during the 168-day period of partial restriction went downhill fastest and farthest during the days of total $B_1$ deprivation.

Oral $B_1$ supplements (five mg. per day) were then added to the men's diets, said Dr. Brozek, "when it appeared that the deficiency had progressed as far as we considered safe." Within a few short days, he continued, "thiamine supplements restored appetite and brought about a dramatic change in the attitudes of the subjects . . . the effects of supplementation were dramatic both in the speed and degree of recovery."

Where can you find thiamine? Whole grain cereals, sunflower and sesame seeds, pork, organ meats like heart and liver, are all good sources. Brewer's yeast, wheat germ, and desiccated liver are especially concentrated natural sources of thiamine as well as all the other members of the B complex. That's especially significant, because there's much evidence that other B vitamins are also important for emotional stability.

## Niacin and Riboflavin Also Important

For example, a deficiency of niacin or vitamin $B_3$ can produce nervousness, suspiciousness, apprehensiveness, irritability, memory loss, and other "mild" symptoms long before it leads to the outright dementia or insecurity of pellagra. "To date, no method has been devised to determine precise niacin levels in the blood or brain cells," report E. Cheraskin, M.D., D.M.D., and W. M. Ringsdorf, Jr., D.M.D., in their book *Psychodietetics* (Stein and Day, New York, 1974). However, they point out, "The late Dr. Tom Spies, an internationally famous nutritionist, developed his method of detecting vitamin $B_3$ deficiencies. Whenever he saw patients who were short tempered and 'swimmy-headed', he told them a funny story. If he couldn't get a laugh, he suspected a niacin deficiency. After hundreds of trials he learned that one of the early signs of niacin depletion is the loss of a sense of humor."

Riboflavin, or vitamin $B_2$, is one member of the B complex whose role in mental health was not pinpointed with any degree of certainty until fairly recently. Two research psychologists attached to the U.S. Army's Medical Research and Nutrition Laboratory at Fitzsimons General Hospital, Denver, Colorado, subjected six male volunteers to a 56-day regimen of near total riboflavin restriction. The results are reported in the February 1973 issue of *American Journal of Clinical Nutrition*. Psychological testing showed that riboflavin deficiency significantly affected the subjects' personalities in a number of cases. Depression scores increased, along with levels of hysteria. Some of the volunteers became lethargic; others complained of varied symptoms of illness.

Researchers have found similar ties between "steady nerves" and adequate amounts of various other components of the B complex. For example, many women taking oral contraceptives develop mental depression that responds favorably to vitamin $B_6$ administration.

Deficiency of vitamin $B_{12}$ can lead to nervous system degeneration, characterized in its earlier stages by mental changes and behavioral disturbances.

Lack of pantothenic acid, another B vitamin, can affect the personality, cause profound depression, and lower resistance to stress.

Deficiency of biotin, also part of the B complex, can result in lassitude, hallucinations, and panic, says Dr. Roger Williams. "When biotin was administered," he writes, "all these symptoms disappeared. Biotin is something that we expect to get as a matter of course, and usually we do, but there may be exceptions. It is clear, however, that if we do not get enough biotin, mental disease results."

## Hypoglycemia Sometimes the Culprit

Faulty diet can affect our brain in other ways than by depriving us of B vitamins. Skipping breakfast or eating a diet too high in carbohydrates and low in protein can cause hypoglycemia, or low blood sugar, in susceptible individuals. If blood levels drop too low, mental confusion, anxiety, depression, and personality change can result.

"A typical hypoglycemia victim," say Drs. Cheraskin and Ringsdorf, "is, in fact, an emotional yo-yo, strung out on a chemical reaction he cannot control, with reactions so severe they frequently resemble insanity.

Dr. Newbold points out that dramatic behavior shifts can occur while an individual is in the throes of a hypoglycemia attack: "Once a patient consulted me because of a depression. I did a glucose tolerance test, and between the third and fourth hour she became paranoid and suspicious of the laboratory technicians, believing that they were going to harm her. Checking back, we found that during this period there had been a rapid fall in her blood sugar level. This was the first and only time this woman had ever had paranoid symptoms."

Unfortunately, many times victims never suspect that they may have hypoglycemia, and their doctors never think to look for it.

"I know of one Texas physician," continues Dr. Newbold, "who came home from the office one afternoon, had a cocktail, and spent the next hour mowing the grass. Then he showered and went to a cocktail party, where he had one more drink and passed out. At the hospital emergency room they tested his blood sugar level, found it to be very low, administered some intravenous glucose, and within an hour he was back at the party. That's one way to discover hypoglycemia."

Frazzled nerves and undue anxiety or depression don't necessarily mean that you have hypoglycemia. But if you are suspicious, ask your doctor to administer a six-hour glucose tolerance test. This is the only way to determine for sure if low blood sugar is behind your symptoms. Confirmed cases of hypoglycemia can usually be treated by adapting a more sensible pattern of eating, including the avoidance of sugar, alcohol, and other empty-calorie foods.

## Minerals and Moods

In addition to B vitamin deficiencies and hypoglycemia, below-optimum levels of certain *mineral* nutrients in our diets also can affect our nerves. Writing in the June 25, 1973, issue of the *Journal of the American Medical Association,* Dr. Richard C. W. Hall of the U.S. Naval Hospital in Orlando, Florida, and Joy R. Joffe, M.D., of the Johns Hopkins University College of Medicine in Baltimore list the following psychiatric and neurological signs and symptoms of magnesium deficiency: depression, marked agitation, disorientation, confusion, irritability, restlessness, vertigo, and pronounced startle response.

Drs. Cheraskin and Ringsdorf, in their book *Psychodietetics,* describe a study carried out a number of years ago at the University of Iowa by Willard A. Krehl, M.D. Analyzing a group of patients with *mild* magnesium deficiencies, Dr. Krehl found that 78 percent experienced mental confusion, 83 percent were so disoriented they couldn't remember where they were or what day it was, and 100 percent were easily startled by unexpected movement or loud noises.

Calcium is another important mineral which, when present in our diets in sufficient amounts, acts to calm the nerves. This was demonstrated by two Washington University School of Medicine psychiatrists, Ferris Pitts, Jr., and James McClure, Jr., in a study involving nine patients suffering from anxiety neurosis and nine normal controls. The patients displayed a variety of symptoms: feelings of impending doom, fears of insanity, fears of heart attacks, fears of smothering or choking to death, etc. The researchers found that by infusing lactate, a normal chemical product of glucose metabolism, anxiety symptoms could be provoked in all nine patients, as well as in two of the normal controls. But when calcium was administered along with the lactate in subsequent tests, the anxiety symptoms generally did not occur (*New England Journal of Medicine,* December 21, 1967).

There may even be an as yet unidentified link between zinc and personality. Eight of eighteen emotionally disturbed youngsters hospitalized in Detroit's Lafayette Clinic were recently found to be suffering from zinc deficiency (*Family Practice News,* April 1, 1975). Researchers made this discovery by analyzing samples of the children's hair for trace mineral content.

Even if your particular nervous upset or emotional problem isn't tied to a vitamin-mineral deficiency or dependency, you may still be better off taking a natural nutritional supplement regularly rather than commonly prescribed tranquilizers or other medication.

That fact was brought to light in a study conducted at Harvard Medical School and the Massachusetts Mental Health Center in Boston. Forty male volunteers over the age of 60 took either a daily dose of diazepam (a popular tranquilizer sold under the trade name of Valium) or a placebo pill containing nothing of therapeutic significance. The patients, considered normal for their age group, suffered mild anxiety and depression but their mental health was rated adequate. What the four researchers discovered and reported in the October 1975 issue of the *Journal of the American Geriatrics Society* is that while Valium had a modest antidepressant effect, it actually produced memory loss and sedative side effect in many subjects. The placebo, on the other hand, had a significant anxiety-reducing effect, especially in the older subjects, and also *improved* memory and motor function, as well as decreasing fatigue!

When we consider that Valium, like so many mind-altering drugs, can trigger side effects such as venous thrombosis, phlebitis, tremor, vertigo, constipation, and jaundice, the desirability of a natural nutritional approach to better mental health seems even more obvious.

### Herbs for Nerves

A number of herbs are valued for their reported ability to produce a calming effect. Chief among these are skullcap, lady's slipper, valerian, linden, camomile, basil, catnip, hops, and rosemary.

Skullcap, lady's slipper, and valerian are herbs which must be used in small amounts. Herbalists would ordinarily make a tea combining small portions of several of these herbs.

While herb tea is a substitute for neither better nutrition nor psychological counseling, it does have its legitimate uses. Simply taking the time to brew a cup and sitting down to enjoy it will help calm you. After drinking the tea, you might want to clear your mind and relax for 20 minutes, perhaps enjoying some meditation.

# Emphysema

For the emphysema victim who really wants to be able to breathe again, there is considerable hope. And that hope depends not on any miracle drug or miracle vitamin but the patient's own determination.

Harry Bass, M.D., formerly head of the Pulmonary Division of the Peter Bent Brigham Hospital in Boston, has shown in studies extending over many years that daily exercise on a stationary bicycle, increasing gradually in intensity, can not only largely arrest the progress of emphysema and chronic bronchitis but even bring about enormous improvement in these chronic conditions.

Dr. Bass told us that in his latest series of tests, one group of patients was followed fully for five years. Some men and women who were barely able to walk from one end of their house to another were, after five years, working every day, enjoying vigorous hobbies such as gardening, and enjoying world travel. At the biochemical level, they were also using oxygen much more efficiently. Before the long exercise program, a great part of what little oxygen they were able to get into their systems was consumed merely in the process of reaching the body cells.

For those who may be interested, it is necessary first to have a medical evaluation to make sure that your health is good enough to begin an exercise program. In the beginning, of course, the exercise is very light, but the distance pedaled each day—measured by an odometer attached to the bike—should increase gradually until the equivalent of a considerable distance is being pedaled each day. Draw breaths deep down into your lungs by expanding your lower belly—*not* your chest.

The determination to return to a more active life is essential for this kind of therapy to succeed, but according to Dr. Bass's work, the result is much greater vigor, fewer crises requiring hospitalization, and in all likelihood, increased life expectancy.

A specialist in lung diseases or rehabilitation medicine would be the one to talk to about getting started on such a program.

# Enterostomal Healing Problems

Enterostomal therapy is a specialized medical and nursing field which deals with the problems encountered by people who have undergone surgery to create substitute routes for elimination of body wastes. Well over one million people in North America have had such operations as colostomies, ileostomies, and urinary diversions. And over 100,000 people join the ranks of the "ostomates" every year.

One of the problems faced by ostomates is that the opening or stoma in their body is very susceptible to infection, often resistant to healing, and sometimes causes more trouble than the surgery or condition which made the creation of the stoma necessary.

In 1975, we learned that a major breakthrough in preventing and curing these problems had been made at the Pottsville Hospital and Warne Clinic in Pottsville, Pennsylvania. There, nurse Dorothy Fisher is the chief enterostomal therapist. In studying the literature on skin healing, Fisher was excited by reports coming from the Shute

Institute in Canada about quick healing of difficult wounds when vitamin E is used.

With the full cooperation of doctors and administrators at Pottsville, Fisher went to London, Ontario, where she met with Dr. Evan Shute.

"Dr. Shute was most generous with his time and counsel and opened up his records to demonstrate the best uses of vitamin E— orally, by spray, ointment, or cream."

Dr. Shute suggested using only the natural vitamin E (results with the synthetic are not the same), so Fisher's first hurdle was to get the hospital pharmacy to stock the natural.

It turned out that the hospital pharmacist not only stocked the clinic with natural vitamin E products, but also made them available in his community pharmacy so that patients could continue their therapy after discharge.

Fisher told us that there are seven surgeons on the staff of the Pottsville Hospital prescribing vitamin E. "And we don't waste time using small amounts anymore. Twelve hundred I.U. is the minimum we start with. Some surgeons order four hundred I.U. to be given four times a day. And we get marvelous results!"

## Some Case Histories

In one case, a badly ulcerated colostomy was completely healed in seven days—which is phenomenal considering the deficiencies of the patient, who was in a very poor state of nutrition.

Three days after surgery was performed for carcinoma of the rectum, with a resultant sigmoid colostomy stoma, the area of the stoma was ulcerating. The surgeon was dismayed and considered reopening the wound. "Why don't we see first what we can do with vitamin E," Fisher urged. "Give us three days." Then she set to work. She treated the stoma and the area around it every day with vitamin E oil (60 I.U. of vitamin E in every gram of oil). "We practically drowned it in vitamin E oil. And we gave the patient 400 I.U. natural vitamin E orally four times a day. The patient made a fantastic recovery in a week and no further surgery was necessary."

They use vitamin E therapy at Pottsville Hospital not only on ostomates but for recalcitrant hard-to-heal wounds like gangrene, diabetic ulcers, and decubitus ulcers (bedsores) which are the bane of every hospital in the country and a torment to every bedfast patient.

A diabetic patient whose right foot was severely ulcerated was given 800 units of vitamin E daily. (Such low dosages are seldom ordered anymore.) The denuded areas of her foot were treated with the vitamin E oil. Cotton balls were saturated with this oil and spread over the affected areas and a light dressing was applied. There was complete healing in less than two months.

Another patient who had been bedfast at home due to a stroke was admitted to the hospital with a bowel obstruction and a huge bedsore in the sacrolumbar area. The bedsore was treated topically with daily applications of vitamin E oil and the patient received 800 I.U. of natural vitamin E per day. In less than six months there was total healing and the area involved has remained well healed. In fact, it now looks very healthy.

## No Adverse Reactions

Bedsores are very hard to heal and six months for this kind of a sore is a very good outcome. But Fisher feels the cure time would have been even better if they hadn't been so timid. "When we first started using vitamin E, we were not courageous enough to use high dosages. Now we don't fool around with anything less than 1,200 or 1,600 I.U. daily and it hasn't disturbed anything. There has been no adverse reaction, not even in hypertensive patients."

When a patient is anemic, he gets all his prescribed iron in the morning and all his vitamin E in the evening. That's because inorganic iron, the kind usually used in hospitals, destroys vitamin E. Organic iron, which is enclosed in a carbon-containing molecule, does not have this effect, but organic iron is seldom stocked in a hospital pharmacy.

Fisher knows the importance of treating the whole patient and starts out by improving his or her diet with fresh vegetables, fruits, salad, and bran. She recommends multivitamins and, where needed, megavitamins. Many patients are given vitamin C, up to 1,000 mg. daily.

# Exercise Therapy

If there is one supreme natural therapy for chronic and degenerative disorders, it is exercise. And if there is one natural therapy that is *more* natural than any others, that too is exercise.

You don't need a degree in anthropology or physiology to realize that human beings were literally designed to be highly active organisms. Our leg muscles, particularly, seem shaped by a need to walk or run for great distances. It's said, in fact, that thanks in no small part to the relatively large size of our buttock muscles (which are much larger than those of other primates), there is no other mammal that can keep up with man over the long haul. An antelope, of course, can leave us behind in a burst of speed, but if a man sets out in the morning to stalk an antelope on foot, he will, if he is able to follow the trail, overtake the exhausted animal that same day. Some anthropologists believe that before the days of spears and bows and arrows, men got most of their meat by running game to the ground on a long march.

So when we say that exercise is therapy, we are also saying that returning to a more natural mode of activity is therapeutic.

Throughout this book, you will read how exercise can be used to improve, arrest, and even reverse a number of serious debilitating illnesses.

You will read that in most cases of low back pain, for instance, the very best therapy is gradually progressive exercises that stretch the hamstring muscles of the thighs. These same exercises will also stretch the calf and will eliminate many cases of cramps and even knee problems that runners get.

You will read that gradually progressive long walks will do wonders not only for circulatory problems of the legs but for the entire vascular system.

You will read that the pulmonary exercise involved in playing a wind instrument will benefit many asthmatic children.

That adults with emphysema are helped by stationary cycling.

That progressive exercise which moves limbs through the full range of motion will prevent joints afflicted with bursitis or arthritis from freezing up.

That exercises which stretch the pelvic area will make life easier for women troubled with menstrual cramps.

That exercise helps you lose or maintain your weight by burning off fat and normalizing the appetite.

That exercise helps you relax and get a better night's sleep.

That exercise will even help relieve the symptoms of hay fever.

When you look at this range of benefits, you get some idea of how basic exercise is to health. Yet, even though people today are more health conscious than ever before, the average person probably gets less exercise than any of his ancestors did all through the history of the human race.

First we got desk jobs. Then we drove to them in cars. Then the cars got power steering and power brakes. Then the buildings where we work got elevators and intercoms. For recreation, we watch athletic events on television or go to a concert or a movie. We got rid of our handmowers and bought self-propelled gas mowers, and then threw them away and bought lawn tractors.

The effect on our health has been profound. One doctor has given this mode of living a name, *hypokinesis,* meaning an abnormally low amount of movement. Hypokinesis is not itself a disease, but rather a condition which promotes the emergence of a host of debilities, and it is a condition that most of us have.

When we escape from hypokinesis into the world of regular vigorous exercises, we are causing surprisingly profound changes in our physiology. The act of walking, for instance, combining both the exercise and the actual striking of the feet on a hard surface, promotes the addition of minerals to bones. That is apparently why astronauts, whose feet do not bump on any surfaces because of the absence of gravity, lose bone minerals despite dietary supplementation and exercise. Regular long walks should be a part of the program of anyone hoping to prevent or arrest the progress of osteoporosis.

Exercise also burns up cholesterol and other fats. It improves circulation to the point that areas which are stressed with regular exercise will actually develop additional tiny blood vessels to deliver oxygen and remove wastes. Muscles trained by exercise develop greater stores of ready energy in the form of glycogen. The muscles themselves grow larger and stronger. Lung function improves, and the heart rate becomes lower.

The secret, I believe, to the effective use of exercise as a therapy is to develop an avid interest not so much in exercise itself, but in some hobby which requires vigorous movements of all kinds. Some of the best are swimming, folk dancing, yoga, Tai-Chi, karate, tennis, gardening, and hiking.

# Fasting

Fasting has been recommended both as a general health measure and a therapy for specific disorders. Much of the literature on fasting is based on personal anecdotes by people lacking a medical or biological education. That in itself is not necessarily bad, but it does, perhaps, explain why many popular books on fasting contain emphatic statements about metabolism and health that are pathetically inaccurate. One popular book, for instance, published as late as 1964, recommends prolonged fasting for, among other things, gonorrhea and the nausea of pregnancy.

Whatever physiological events may occur during fasting, some people simply enjoy it and report that it makes them feel and think better. It's also been said that it's natural for people to fast, since many of our early ancestors probably had to go without food for days or weeks at a time.

If fasting gives you pleasure, enjoy it. Be aware, though, that in middle age and beyond the body does not respond to fasting as it does during youth. For some reason, the ability to burn up fat in response to fasting diminishes, and energy is largely produced by burning up protein. That means your body is losing some of the basic structural material of its muscles, connective tissue, and even skin.

As for fasting being natural, that may or may not be true. It seems to me much more likely that it's natural for people to sometimes be *hungry,* which is quite different from fasting. In fasting, no food at all is consumed. Most likely, our early ancestors did not fast during the lean weeks and months but ate what they could find of roots and small animals. In semistarvation, the body is ordinarily able to extract considerably more nourishment from food than it does when it is well fed, so the importance of a small amount of the food cannot be underestimated.

## Fasting and Sanity

If there is one area in which controlled fasting seems to hold the greatest promise, it is in the treatment of certain forms of schizophrenia, where the individual has not responded to other modalities. The use of fasting to treat schizophrenia has been used most extensively in the Soviet Union, notably by Dr. Yuri Nikolayev, Director of the Fasting Treatment Unit of the Moscow Research Institute of Psychiatry. New York psychiatrist Dr. Alan Cott spent two weeks observing the fasting treatment conducted by Dr. Nikolayev in 1970 and reported on his observations in the journal *Schizophrenia* (First Quarter, 1971). A later report, in which he described his own results using fasting for schizophrenics, appeared in *Applied Nutrition in Clinical Practice* (Walczak and Huemer, eds., Symposia Specialists, Miami, 1973).

Dr. Cott first explains that there is an important distinction between fasting and starvation. In fasting, there is no sense of hunger, at least after the first day or two. All food is excluded, while fluids are given plentifully. In starvation, on the other hand, food is eaten, but not enough, and there is a great sensation of hunger. He further notes that "fasting patients never appear ill or emaciated. Their skin color becomes healthy and ruddy. Muscle tone improves remarkably, especially in those patients who are normally sedentary, since three hours of exercise daily is a prerequisite throughout the period of fasting."

Further describing the regimen which has been used for some 25 years by Dr. Nikolayev in his 80-bed unit in Moscow, Dr. Cott says that breathing exercises, stimulating baths or showers, daily enemas, and massage are also given. Typically, that period of the fast consisting of total abstinence from food lasts 25 to 30 days. However, once he has begun to eat again, the patient must remain hospitalized and under close observation for the same length of time as the period of his fast. Food is reintroduced slowly, beginning with salt-free fruits, vegetables, and fermented milk products. Slowly, other foods are returned, although meat should not be eaten again for at least six months after ending the fast.

Professor Nikolayev says that such a fasting regimen is effective in more than 70 percent of all cases of schizophrenia of long duration, with nearly half of these cases maintaining improvement for a period of at least six years.

It is important to emphasize that the patient undergoing such a fast goes through a series of profound biochemical changes. According to Dr. Nikolayev, somewhere between the second or third to the seventh or fifteenth day of fasting, a state of acidosis of the blood sets in, along with other abnormalities, such as hypoglycemia and physical and emotional depression. Acute exhaustion may follow.

Eventually, most of these symptoms vanish, but other ones may appear. During the time the patient is slowly beginning to eat again, there may be irritability, anxiety, and other problems, particularly if too much food is eaten too quickly.

Significantly, those patients who do *not* show marked biochemical changes as a result of fasting are least likely to improve. Apparently, these changes are intimately connected to a disease process in schizophrenia.

## A New York Study

Dr. Cott began an experimental controlled fasting program as part of the research project at the Gracie Square Hospital in New York. The patients he used were all schizophrenic for at least five years and had failed to improve under previous forms of treatment. After treating some 28 individuals, Dr. Cott reported, 60 percent of those who completed the fast remained well. This, of course, would seem to be a very gratifying rate of success, although it is not clear how many patients were *unable* to complete the fast.

In this regard, it is worth noting that Dr. Cott states that if the patient does not drink at least a quart of water a day, the fast must be broken. Severe hunger is another sign that the fast should not continue for the usual 25 or 30 days. If a patient who smokes cannot give up the habit during the first few days, that is another indication to take him off the fast.

Dr. Cott also points out that the patient must be given a thorough physical examination, and his medical history taken before he is put on a fast. If there is a tendency or a history of thrombosis, that is a definite contraindication, because there seems to be a high danger of thrombosis in "predisposed patients" both during certain parts of the fast and even at a certain stage of the recovery period.

It is likely that if further research such as that described by Dr. Cott is carried out under controlled circumstances, we will learn a lot more about the usefulness of fasting. Eventually, we may even learn whether or not fasting is of any real use for the dozens of conditions which its proponents say it is. At present, though, it seems that fasting is of the most *practical* use in cases of schizophrenia, where other treatments have not worked. It is always possible, of course, that further work will show that if fasting is given as the primary treatment rather than the treatment of last resort, it will be found to be extremely useful.

The only other medical use of fasting I have found is during the acute stages of pain in ulcerative colitis and similar inflammatory diseases of the intestinal tract. Here, it is used for a few days only, to rest the inflamed tissue.

# Fever

A very high fever, which I will define as anything over 102°F., deserves swift medical attention or at least advice. Another indication for medical attention is when a fever persists in the absence of an obvious cause, like the flu or some other infectious disease.

A mild fever in itself is not necessarily dangerous, and there is some evidence to indicate that elevated temperature is part of the body's defensive reaction to invading germs. The defensive value of fever, however, does not seem to be very great, and it usually causes more harm than good. A prolonged fever may be very debilitating, rapidly dehydrate the person, and bring about malnutrition as well, which can only weaken resistance.

A simple, logical, and effective means of reducing fevers is to apply cold wet compresses. In cases of serious fever, general sponging of the body or wrapping the patient in a wet sheet for short periods of time will help.

Plenty of fluids should be given and as much food as can be comfortably eaten. If the fever persists, make certain that salt is also eaten.

There are a number of alternatives to aspirin, although in an acute fever, I would not scorn the judicious use of this drug. American Indians specifically used willow bark to reduce fevers. Willow bark contains salicin, which apparently decomposes in the human system into salicylic acid—just about the same thing as aspirin. Indians boiled the inner bark and drank the tea in strong doses. The same remedy was also used by Greeks living 2,000 years ago.

Herbal teas have long been used to reduce fever and they offer the bonus of providing badly needed fluids.

Cayenne, or common red pepper (the *hot* kind), is one of the most highly regarded herbs for treating fevers. You can add small amounts to warm water, milk, or tea, or if you happen to have some gelatin capsules, fill one or two with cayenne and then follow with a glass of water. Boneset is another old Indian remedy which all herbalists agree is a specific for reducing fevers. Why is it called boneset? Not, as some people believe, because it helps bones to set, but because of its use in olden days for what was known as break-bone fever. Use boneset moderately in your cup of tea, or it may make you nauseous.

Yarrow is valued in fevers because it causes the pores of the skin to dilate and produces copious sweating. Vervain is also highly regarded in treating fevers. The berries of the barberry, a perennial shrub that grows very tall and has sharp spines, have been used to make a brew taken for fever.

Whatever kind of tea you may drink, add a lot of fresh lemon juice to it and some extra vitamin C as well.

# Gout

People who suffer with the sharp pains of gout would do well to educate themselves about the drugs they may be taking. On one hand, medications for gout can cause some very unpleasant side effects. Conversely, drugs taken for other conditions, such as high blood pressure, can cause gout as a side effect.

When gout begins at a young age, or the attacks become more and more frequent, treatment is necessary to prevent permanent damage caused by the precipitation of uric acid crystals. Although uric acid formation in the blood is encouraged by foods containing substances known as purines, the problem with most gout victims is not that they are eating too many rich foods, but that their bodies are *synthesizing* uric acid too aggressively. Therefore, although elimination from the diet of high-purine food such as bouillon, meat extracts, organ meats, yeast, anchovies, herring, and sardines may help a little, it will probably not control a severe case.

Is there an alternative to gout medication in less severe cases? It seems that there may well be, and that alternative is to eat cherries.

Yes, plain cherries—sour or sweet. They can all do the trick, and it doesn't matter much if they're fresh, canned, or frozen.

The cherries-for-gout story seems to start with Ludwig W. Blau, Ph.D., whose big toe at one time gave him so much torment that he was confined to a wheelchair. One day, quite by accident, he polished off a whole bowl of cherries and the next morning the pain in his foot was practically gone. This sudden relief was almost unbelievable, and since the only thing he had done was to eat the cherries, he continued to eat at least six cherries every day and was soon out of the wheelchair and free of pain. If he forgot to take the cherries, while traveling, it only took a few days for the stabbing pain in his big toe to return with a vengeance. More than 20 years after Dr. Blau wrote up his experiences in a medical journal (his research at that time revealed that there were 12 other case histories of people whose gout or arthritis had been helped by eating cherries or drinking cherry juice), he told us that he was still eating six to eight cherries every day and was still in good health.

Letters from readers received after the publication of this information in PREVENTION magazine indicate that cherries can indeed bring relief to at least some gout victims. A typical response came from a woman who had an "aching, throbbing knee for almost two years. After going to several doctors, chiropractors and having X-rays and taking bottles of aspirin, I was about to give up," she wrote. After reading that article about cherries for gout, she bought several cans and ate them for about a week "and all the swelling and stiffness disappeared! It was a miracle!" She added that "As long as I eat cherries, there is no pain. Exercise, walking, bicycling, and no pain." But when she forgets to take the cherries, the swelling and pain return to her knees.

A chiropractor reported that when the "cherry therapy" was tried by one of his patients for two months, "the results have been nothing less than spectacular." Another man, who had suffered with gout for many years, ate about 15 cherries every day for two years. "During this period of time the gout would flare up slightly but not so much as to be uncomfortable or to immobilize me. About December of 1973 I gave up eating cherries to see if anything would happen. In May of 1974 I suffered a painful and immobilizing attack of gout. I had to revert to the old medication and pain pills I used to use before discovering the benefits of cherries."

We mentioned before that medication may cause or aggravate gout, and one woman told us that because she had gout and high blood pressure simultaneously, her doctor put her on drugs for both conditions. The condition only became worse, and consultation with other doctors did not bring any improvement. Finally, she read in a magazine (PREVENTION) that one of the side effects of high blood pressure medicine can be gout. She checked this in a medical library, confirmed it, and then went back to her doctor. At first, he thought that it couldn't be true but when he checked his own books, he found that the woman was right. He changed her hypertension medication to one which does not eliminate body fluids and the woman immediately began to improve, being able to walk with less pain and feeling much better. At the same time, her blood pressure actually decreased.

The famous botanist Linnaeus was reportedly cured of gout by eating almost nothing but large quantities of strawberries morning and evening, which led him to call these berries a "blessing of the gods." The French herbalist Mességué also recommends that a "strawberry cure" of several days' duration "will bring great relief to people with gout or kidney stones."

A tea made from the flowers of the broom plant is another traditional folk remedy for gout.

The *Merck Manual* advises that the tendency to form kidney stones in gout may be diminished by drinking at least three quarts of fluids a day. Those fluids should definitely *not* be alcoholic. Slimming down if you're overweight is another sensible step to take. However, don't go on a crash diet or try to lose weight while you're having an active attack, because the sudden loss of weight increases the concentration of uric acid in the body.

# Hay Fever

Here is my basic remedy for hay fever. Three times a day—morning, noon, and night—take 500 mg. of vitamin C. Morning and evening, take 50 mg. of pantothenic acid and a teaspoon of grated orange or lemon peel sweetened with some honey.

Chances are it will help you considerably. You may well be amazed at the results. It won't help everyone uniformly, but neither does anything else when it comes to hay fever.

Granville F. Knight, M.D., of Santa Monica, California, told us that in his own experience B-complex vitamins often hold the key to solving allergy problems. It seems, though, that pantothenic acid, one of the B vitamins, is especially important. Nutritionist Adelle

Davis recognized this and related it to the fact that allergies are "stress diseases" and pantothenic acid is crucial in building resistance to stress. "Allergies have been repeatedly produced in animals by injections of numerous foreign substances, and invariably the allergic reaction is particularly severe or fatal when pantothenic acid is deficient; the lack of no other nutrient has a comparable effect," she wrote in her classic *Let's Get Well* (Harcourt Brace Jovanovich, New York, 1965).

One person who has tried pantothenic acid for an allergy is Sandra M. Stewart, M.D., of the Children's Hospital in Columbus, Ohio. We learned of her experience in a book by pediatrician-allergist William Grant Crook, M.D., *Can Your Child Read? Is He Hyperactive?* (Pedicenter Press, Jackson, Tenn., 1975), and we confirmed in a conversation with her what she told Dr. Crook.

Plagued with an allergy problem and with "unfavorable response to the usual antihistamine decongestants, I decided to experiment and try pantothenic acid," she told Dr. Crook. "I took a 100 mg. tablet at night. And I found my nasal stuffiness would clear in less than 15 minutes. I could breathe. And, rather than waking up at four or five in the morning with cough and mucous secretion, I wouldn't have it. The pantothenic acid appeared to have an antimucous-secreting effect on me personally."

Equally pleased with pantothenic acid was a California reader who related that she had been a longtime victim of sinus attacks brought on by her allergies. "For five months I had one solid sinus attack that never completely cleared up," she wrote.

She said she was entering a particularly bad attack when she decided to take two 100 mg. tablets of pantothenic acid every day, along with a B-complex supplement. "I was startled (and thought it surely must be my imagination) to begin feeling better in about four hours! I couldn't believe how quickly my trouble began to disappear. Within 10 days I had such complete relief I began to 'walk on eggs', fearing any minute I would have a relapse."

## Vitamin C Important

Vitamin C also plays a very important role in the allergy and hay fever picture. A report in the *Eye, Ear, Nose and Throat Monthly* (July 1968) indicated that allergy victims show low plasma and urine levels of vitamin C during the active stages of allergy. There is a positive side to this study: "Heavy medication with vitamin C produced a rise in the blood and urinary ascorbic acid levels which coincided with subjective and objective improvement of the allergic disorder."

Inhibiting the release of histamine seems to be one of the chief characteristics of vitamin C as an allergy agent. This was demonstrated by Arend Bouhuys, M.D., Ph.D., of the Yale University Lung Research Center, and two colleagues. As reported in the *Journal of Allergy and Clinical Immunology* (April 1973), the doctors had 17 healthy people inhale a histamine mixture. Then they measured their ability to breathe immediately afterwards, at three hours, and finally six hours after each person had been given 500 mg. of vitamin C. Several days later each person's breathing ability was again measured after taking a placebo or dummy pill.

They reported finding a "significant" increase in the ease of breathing after receiving vitamin C. Specifically, they said that "a single oral dose of 500 mg. of ascorbic acid inhibits the constrictor effect of histamine on airways of human subjects," an inhibition lasting at least six hours.

There are several other studies that show the same thing. But when small doses are used, results are negative. Use *at least* 500 mg. several times a day.

Bioflavonoids, the natural substances usually found with vitamin C in nature, and particularly abundant in the white pulpy portion and rind of oranges and lemons (and the juice of tangerines), seem to make vitamin C "work better" and this is especially true when it comes to hay fever. Although you can buy tablets of bioflavonoids such as rutin, and some vitamin C tablets contain them, you can't do better than go directly to nature. One woman told us that "I have found orange peel to be the best antihistamine I have ever tried. I have been a victim of allergy all my life. I keep the peels in the refrigerator for several days until there is enough to work up, and I cut them in small strips and soak them in apple cider vinegar solution for several hours, drain off well, place in a pan with honey, and cook down but not to the candy stage. Then I put them in the refrigerator and eat as I need them. I place some pieces in my mouth when I go to bed at night. No more stuffiness and clogged passages to keep waking me from sleep."

A strong cup of comfrey leaf tea sweetened with honey is said by some to do wonders for respiratory allergies complicated by constant coughing. It's also said that eating some tender young comfrey leaves from your garden every day will stop hay fever.

The most dramatic anecdote we received about nutritional therapy for allergies came from a woman in the Pacific Northwest who said that for 16 years she suffered with allergies, asthma, and nasal polyps. She had an incredible amount of medical work done, including seven operations for the removal of a total of 130 polyps. For the last two years, though, she said that she has become a completely new person and has even managed to keep away new polyps. What did she do? Nothing more—or less—than take just about every vitamin and mineral supplement in the book, as well as brewer's yeast, lecithin, and even garlic. Her regimen was especially heavy in vitamin C (1500 mg. a day) and included extra bioflavonoids and rutin.

Diet is not the only thing you can do for your runny nose. At home, you can run your air conditioner with the vent closed. Most air conditioners won't keep out pollen, but with the vent closed, at least you aren't getting more than is already in the house. There are also special air filters you can get which remove nearly all particulate matter from the air.

And, strange as it may sound, there is good evidence that getting exercise can actually help. It seems that when you exercise, a kind of constricting effect is produced in the small blood vessels and symptoms improve in a matter of three to five minutes. Try some vigorous yoga or rope skipping or stationary bike riding.

## An Unsuspected Cause of Respiratory Allergy

Finally, I want to mention an extremely instructive case which came to us from a reader in New Jersey. He said he had been the "victim of a severe allergy condition which has cost me over $1,000 in medical expenses." The usual shots did nothing for him. After months of cortisone and antibiotics, he began to improve, but his sore throat "never did go away completely."

He lived with this miserable condition for three years. Luckily, he found the answer in an article in PREVENTION magazine and cured himself in three days.

The article was on dry winter air and methods for normalizing the humidity inside your home. But it also cautioned that mold can grow in a home humidifier unless it is regularly and thoroughly cleaned out. And these molds can cause all sorts of respiratory problems.

The reader said "I remembered that when I cleaned the lime deposits from the humidifier, it always had a greenish slimy growth in the float chamber. I never expected that this growth could cause airborne spores which could circulate about the house by the action of the blower. The very minute I read the article, I jumped up and pulled the unit out to give it a thorough cleaning. In about two to three days, all traces of sore throat were gone. It has been nearly two months now, and I have not had a single allergy symptom."

# Headaches

Occasional headaches which are not terribly severe are one thing, while migraine attacks are something else again. Let's talk about the former first.

It's been said that at least 90 percent of occasional headaches are a result of nervous tension. While that may be true, it is also misleading and possibly dangerous, because a surprising number of environmental factors entirely unrelated to the state of your nerves may be the real culprit.

One such environmental cause of headaches which is easily corrected without aspirin *or* psychotherapy is what Dr. Gordon J. Gilbert of St. Petersburg, Florida, has dubbed the "turtle headache." In a letter published in the *Journal of the American Medical Association* in 1972, Dr. Gilbert said that several of his patients ceased having headaches immediately after they quit sleeping with their heads under the covers. He explained that sleeping in this manner can create a shortage of oxygen and build up the concentration of carbon dioxide, which in turn can make you wake up in the morning with a nasty headache.

If you are habituated to drinking one or more cups of coffee first thing in the morning before going to work, you may get a headache on weekends if you stay in bed an extra hour or two. It seems that your body can become addicted to the caffeine in coffee or tea, which tends to constrict blood vessels. Apparently, without the daily jolt of caffeine, the blood vessels in the head of some people may dilate, which can produce a headache.

If you *are* addicted to coffee, you have an option at this point. You can either maintain your addiction, making certain to hop out of bed even on a Sunday and get your morning caffeine, or you can gradually wean yourself off this artificial stimulation. One man wrote to us and said that he suffered from headaches for many years until he quit drinking coffee. He added, though, that after a while, he found he was able to have his one cup of coffee in the morning without suffering for it. It seems that in his case, and possibly many others, the repeated bombardment of the blood vessels with caffeine throughout the day made them dependent on this chemical.

## Eating Habits Important

Remaining in bed longer than usual in the morning can cause a headache for an entirely different reason: low blood sugar. It's likely that many people who have mild functional hypoglycemia *do* suffer when they delay having breakfast. That tendency could be greatly aggravated if the last thing consumed before retiring was a sweet snack or alcoholic beverage. The system of a hypoglycemic can overreact to this flood of sugars and drop the blood sugar level so low that the brain is deprived of the glucose it requires, and the result is a morning headache. Low blood sugar can also cause wicked and recurrent migraine headaches (see HYPOGLYCEMIA). So eat a good breakfast at the regular hour.

Occasional headaches can also be caused by a great variety of food allergies and by allergies or reactions to industrial or household chemicals, including strong detergents, polishes, waxes, paint, and pesticides of all kinds. In such cases, you have to be your own detective. If you keep a diary of everything that you eat and every exposure to a chemical and every activity—such as walking through the garage or doing the laundry or talking to your father-in-law on the phone—you may be very satisfied when you can pinpoint the cause of your headaches.

Once a headache has hit you, there are several things you can do besides taking aspirin. One is to brew yourself a stiff cup of peppermint tea, drink it, and lie down for 20 minutes. Rosemary, catnip, and sage are other herbs traditionally valued for their effectiveness against headaches. The favorite of the American Indians for a headache was a tea brewed from the bark of the willow tree. This bark is now known to contain a substance called salicin, which may well change in the human system to salicylic acid, the active ingredient in common aspirin tablets. Last but not least, try a cup of coffee.

A good neck massage can also do a lot for some headaches. First, let your head droop forward as far as it will go, and then slowly roll it around in the widest possible circle. Repeat several times, and then reverse directions. Then let your head slump forward again and begin massaging the back of the head and the neck.

A naturopath suggests treating a headache by taking a hot footbath and at the same time applying a cold towel to the head. That may sound arcane, but it might prove to be very effective in drawing blood away from the head.

## Migraine and Food

Migraine headaches, like simple headaches, are also believed by some doctors to be caused largely by nervous tension. And again, while that may be the case, it would be foolish not to make some careful checks on the diet and environment.

Hypoglycemia may cause migraines, and in our entry on that subject, we describe the case of an individual who suffered for years from an apparently classic migraine headache, which eventually proved to be the result of reactive hypoglycemia and disappeared when the appropriate dietary changes were made.

There are a large number of individual food substances which doctors have associated with migraine attacks, including milk and other dairy products, chocolate, cola drinks, corn, onion, garlic, pork, eggs, citrus fruits, wheat, coffee, alcohol in all forms (especially red wines and champagne), cheese (particularly aged or cheddar), chicken liver, pickled herring, canned figs, and the pods of broad beans.

In addition, two extremely common food additives are known to cause headaches in sensitive individuals. They are monosodium glutamate (MSG) and nitrates. MSG may be present in almost any processed food. Read the label very carefully. Nitrates and nitrites are found in hot dogs, bacon, ham, and salami.

I mentioned before that anyone with headaches should keep a careful diary of everything she or he eats and does. Such a diary will be very helpful in producing prime suspects of a dietary nature, which can then be eliminated one or two at a time.

Curiously, though, studies conducted both in the United States and Britain in which migraine victims were fed either dummy pills or pills containing the foods they believed were causing their migraines, revealed that there was no difference at all in the number of headaches produced by the placebo pills vs. the foods. In one study, pills containing tyramine, a substance found in many "suspect" foods and believed to cause migraine attacks in sensitive individuals, were found to cause *fewer* migraine attacks than placebo pills.

There are two conclusions that may be drawn from these studies. One is that laboratory or hospital conditions do not truly duplicate actual eating conditions. The other is that psychological factors play a greater role in producing migraines than food per se.

## Estrogen Can Cause Migraine

Any woman who suffers from migraine and is taking either oral contraceptives or supplemental estrogen should immediately suspect those hormones as a possible cause of her headaches. Lee Kudrow, M.D., of Encino, California, reported in the journal *Headache* (April 1975), that he found a definite association between the hormones and migraines in 239 patients.

He reported that 70 percent of the women with migraines who were taking estrogen-containing oral contraceptives benefited "in terms of a marked reduction of headache frequency, following the discontinuation of birth control pills," although it often took a month for the effect of the hormones to wear off. Among women taking supplemental estrogen, 58 percent were "improved following the reduction and decycling of their hormone therapy."

Another unsuspected cause of chronic headaches is sinusitis. From the medical reports we have seen, it appears that some physicians may not be able to diagnose a sinusitis headache accurately, or simply do not think of it. One ear, nose, and throat specialist indicates that people who have suffered for years with headaches, and have been to many physicians, can sometimes find swift relief after an abnormality in the sinuses is surgically corrected.

One simple folk remedy that seems almost ridiculous was suggested by Dr. Charles Adler, of Denver, at the 1974 Annual Meeting of the American Association for the Study of Headache. Dr. Adler said that Kirk Peffer, a doctoral candidate working at Dr. Adler's clinic, found an obscure reference to the treatment of migraine with a hair dryer and decided to try it on some of his "tougher" patients. The patients were instructed to use a bonnet-type hair dryer applied to their heads at the first signs of a migraine. At the time of his report, he said that eight patients had used the treatment, and all had found it successful. Although, as he put it, "it seems too pat, too simple," he added that if the results continue to be positive, "someone will have to make up a complex theory to explain it."

### Acupuncture Worthwhile

For the person with recurrent migraine attacks which have not responded to other therapies, acupuncture offers an excellent opportunity for relief. A great many studies have reported extremely gratifying success, and usually, the patients were those who had not been helped by any other form of treatment.

A fairly typical report appeared in the *American Journal of Chinese Medicine* in 1974 (vol. 2, no. 4), written by K. C. Kim, M.D., Ph.D., and R. A. Yount, of the Departments of Anesthesiology and Biophysics at the Indiana University School of Medicine. They worked with twenty-one women and four men who had been referred to them by other physicians. The patients were instructed to come to the acupuncture clinic whenever they had pain. Over a period of six months most of the patients required only from one to five treatments. The results were that "Frequency of headaches and duration were reduced 68 percent and 60 percent, respectively. Sixty-eight percent of patients were improved enough to stop their use of medication after the treatment. Twelve of the twenty-five patients were completely well . . . five patients got no significant relief from the treatment." Those helped least were those who before treatment had suffered from migraine attacks on a daily basis. Other experiences with acupuncture for migraine are discussed under ACUPUNCTURE.

# Hearing Problems

Old-time remedy and herb books are full of advice on what to do for ear problems. Most of it is bad advice and I wouldn't trust *any* of it.

Modern medical findings, though, show that there are a number of natural and good things you can do for your ears and hearing problems with perfect safety.

The first thing worth knowing about is that excessive buildup of earwax—called ceruminosis—is, in the words of one physician, "a condition which is all too commonly overlooked." Normally, earwax is a blessing, rather than a curse, serving to lubricate the ear canal and trap bacteria, dust, and other foreign substances which may enter the ear. Entirely without intervention, earwax has a way of working itself out of the ear and taking with it these foreign substances.

Sometimes, though, earwax accumulates in such amounts that it seriously interferes with hearing.

Dr. Harold J. Harris of Plattsburgh, New York, described a case of a young boy in *Consultant* (May 1973). When the 10-year-old youth came to Dr. Harris, he had a history of hearing problems going back to the time when he was only two years old. Since then, he had been treated for a speech defect and fitted with two hearing aids which didn't help very much. Although he had been examined by several specialists, apparently not one physician had checked for the presence of earwax. "I discovered that both ear canals were occluded with wax that had been pressed against the drums, probably by the ear pieces [of the hearing aids]. Its removal resulted in greatly improved hearing, with and without the hearing aids."

Some years ago, a random examination of about 1,000 people found that roughly one out of five had enough earwax to totally obscure the eardrum. Although these people were not considered deaf, they certainly suffered from some degree of hearing loss. A study published in the *Journal of the American Medical Association* in 1970 reported that 42 percent of the population of a mental hospital failed a hearing test, while in the general population only 10 percent fail such tests. "The majority of those who failed had impacted cerumen in both ears . . . ," the article said, adding that in some cases, "cerumen was impacted to an extent that general anesthesia was necessary to remove it."

Following wax removal, 50 of about 1,700 patients were rehabilitated to the extent that they were actually dismissed from the hospital. Here is dramatic evidence that at least in some cases, the "confused" or "indifferent" attitude which might be taken for mental illness or senility may merely reflect the fact that the person cannot hear what others are saying and becomes confused and depressed.

What do you do about excess earwax? First of all, don't use an ear swab. After studying 27 patients who were treated at two hospitals for ear injuries, one doctor wrote in 1973 that "The most common object causing damage to the tympanic membrane and ossicular chain was a cotton-tipped applicator (13 cases)." Not only is the risk of permanent ear damage high in using the swabs—they aren't even effective. Any wax that can be dislocated by them is on its way to falling out of the ear of its own accord anyway. And wax that is not removed is only packed in more tightly by the swab.

Glycerol is one of the few substances which can soften earwax without causing it to swell. Some preparations available without prescription are little more than a form of glycerol and some antiseptic. If this does not accomplish what is desired, an examination by an ear specialist is in order. Some people, in fact, apparently because of the shape of their ear canal, need to have a doctor remove the wax periodically.

## A Nutritional Approach to Inner Ear Disease

Excessive earwax is a problem of the external ear, and as such, is much easier to treat than inner ear problems. Nevertheless, many cases of inner ear disease can be successfully treated by putting patients on a high-nutrition, low-fat diet similar to that prescribed for heart patients, a West Virginia ear, nose, and throat specialist has reported. In fact, James T. Spencer, Jr., M.D., believes that hearing loss and other inner ear symptoms may actually be early forerunners of heart and artery disease.

Dr. Spencer, assistant clinical professor of otolaryngology at West Virginia University School of Medicine's Charleston Clinical Division, examined 444 patients with hearing loss, ringing or fullness in the ears, vertigo, and other symptoms of inner ear problems. Staggering, nausea, vomiting, and headaches were also present in some cases. Laboratory analyses revealed that 46.6 percent of the subjects were suffering from hyperlipoproteinemia, or elevated levels of cholesterol, triglycerides, or similar fats in the blood. Abnormal glucose tolerance indicative of diabetes or a prediabetic condition was evident in 87 percent of the patients. And 80 percent of the subjects were overweight to the point of obesity.

Putting the emphasis on what he calls "good basic nutrition," Dr. Spencer altered the patients' diet to restrict saturated fats, refined sugars and starches, and concentrated sweets. He also urged all overweight patients to reduce their weight to an ideal level.

Among those who conscientiously followed his instructions, the majority reported significant improvement. "Phenomenal gain in hearing has resulted with as much as a 30 decibel improvement in an affected ear," Dr. Spencer reported (*West Virginia Medical Journal,* September 1974). Ear discomfort, vertigo, headaches, and other symptoms were also relieved as blood lipid levels fell.

There was an added bonus. "In addition to these improvements," Dr. Spencer wrote, "these patients generally improve in appearance from weight loss, exhibt or admit to having more energy, and feel more youthful. They are very grateful patients."

Any diet that corrects hyperlipoproteinemia must also be assumed to be beneficial for the heart and arteries: "While treating the patients' inner ear disorder," Dr. Spencer noted, "simultaneous improvement in their general health and increased longevity can be expected to follow."

## Airplane Earache

Did you ever take a relatively long trip on a jet and discover, as the plane began to descend, that your ears hurt like the devil?

I did. Short flights have never bothered me, but the first time I flew directly from Philadelphia to Chicago, my ears began to ache as the plane descended. For several hours after landing, I had a very difficult time understanding what people were saying. Even worse, I could hardly hear what I was saying and somehow wound up shouting, quite unnecessarily, to try to make myself heard.

But that was nothing compared to what happened on the flight back. This time, my ears not only felt funny—they hurt; *really* hurt! I was chewing gum, sipping drinks, and swallowing constantly, but nothing did *anything* to relieve the pressure. And this time, instead of going away after a few hours, the pain lingered for about three days.

Several years after that, I was planning another jet trip—this time from the East Coast to Los Angeles. I had some important meetings scheduled in Los Angeles and I had this nagging fear that an earache would ruin my trip and prevent me from hearing clearly what people were saying. That was a good time, I thought, for PREVENTION magazine to do some research into how to prevent airplane earache!

The first thing we did was to call up several major airlines and ask their medical people what should be done. Surprisingly, all we got was the usual business about chewing gum and swallowing.

Someone asked a friend who was a stewardess, thinking that surely she would know the answer, and was told only to sip water and keep swallowing. But I knew this didn't work—at least in my case.

Finally, we asked Robert D. Strauss, M.D., an otolaryngologist in Allentown, Pennsylvania, and got an answer—and an explanation —that seemed to make sense.

When the plane is gaining altitude, the surrounding air pressure decreases swiftly, causing pressure to build up inside the middle ear cavity, which pushes the eardrum outward as the plane climbs. Normally, and sometimes with the help of swallowing or yawning, the eustachian tube takes some of the air we breathe into this cavity and serves to equalize pressure. But the pressure changes that take place during air travel are too swift for some people to adjust to.

Usually, though, going *up* is no big problem. Air earache most often hits passengers as the plane descends and the heavier pressure outside pushes the eardrum inward, creating a sense of blockage or outright pain. That's because the eustachian tube is more resistant to opening under the conditions of descent; the low pressure in the middle ear cavity creates a vacuumlike effect, which tends to "suck" the flexible tube walls together, like a flattened drinking straw.

If swallowing doesn't do the trick for you, Dr. Strauss had two suggestions. First, if you have a problem with swollen tissue in your respiratory tract, probably because of an allergy, the physician said he often recommends an oral drug, to be taken an hour or so before landing, which combines an antihistamine and a decongestant. There are also sprays and inhalants that shrink the mucous membrane, and these can be applied shortly before and again during descent. This is not, obviously, a recommendation to use such drugs routinely. But for the short period of flight descent it is certainly sensible to take advantage of such help if you really need it.

Then there's a technique known as the "Valsalva maneuver," for venting the middle ear, which Dr. Strauss described for us. "Close your mouth and pinch your nose tight shut. Then blow out your cheeks and that will force air into the middle ear," he explained. Be sure to summon up every bit of air you've got to make those cheeks bulge, he advised, and don't be worried if you hear a click— that's the sound that tells you your "maneuver" has been successful.

Well, it so happened that when I was ready to take my flight, it was just that time of year when I sometimes suffer mildly from some sort of pollen. I have found that with vitamin C, bioflavonoids, and pantothenic acid, I don't need antihistamines, so I skipped that part of the program. The particular flight that I was on stopped at Pittsburgh and Chicago before heading out for Los Angeles. So each time the plane began to descend, I glanced quickly around me to make sure no one was looking and went through a couple of Valsalva maneuvers.

It worked like a charm. There was no blockage, no fullness, and no pain. The trip back was just as delightful. Subsequent flights have been just as comfortable.

# Heart Disease

This is a book about the healing of illness rather than its prevention. But the evidence shows that it is safe—even necessary—to assume that nearly all of us Westerners have some degree of heart or circulatory illness. So when we talk about "preventing" heart disease, what we are really talking about is halting or reversing the progress of an already existing pathology.

It is an important reflection on the state of our knowledge about the epidemiology of chronic disease that we do not know with any kind of real certainty what causes the disease which takes more American lives than any other. Because chronic heart disease and atherosclerosis occur far less frequently in "primitive" societies, it's assumed that there is *something* about civilization that sets off a series of developments resulting in a heart attack. Exactly *which* factors are involved, or which are most important, is presently unknown.

The need to discover and evaluate these factors, and just as important, develop ways of motivating people to modify their diets and lives accordingly, is particularly urgent because of the failure of the pharmaceutical approach to control chronic heart disease.

Although heart patients are routinely given a number of drugs intended to perform such mechanical functions as reducing coagulation, lowering blood pressure, and lowering cholesterol, when mortality figures are examined, the net result of all these drugs is far from impressive. Recently, a major study conducted at a number of medical centers around the United States found that while commonly given drugs meant to lower cholesterol did in fact lower it, the heart patients who took these drugs tended to survive for *less* time than patients who did *not* receive them.

After spending several years reading hundreds of articles in medical journals about the supposed causes of chronic heart disease, it seems to me that the most reasonable personal approach to arresting the progress of this disease is to imitate—to the greatest practical extent—the lifestyle of "primitive" people among whom the disease is so rare. In doing that, we beg the question of whether the villain is cholesterol, lack of exercise, stress, too many calories, too much fat, or insufficient vitamins or minerals, and take the attitude that by modifying our lifestyle we can simultaneously reduce the effect of *all* these factors.

We might say that what we are doing is returning to a more *natural* way of life, the habits and foods that man survived on for a million or more years before things began to change radically in the last few thousand years for the very wealthy, and for nearly all of us in the last half century.

From this historical perspective, the question, for instance, of whether or not eating a low-fat, high-fiber diet is good for the heart is overshadowed by the undeniable fact that for well over 99 percent of man's time on earth, he has survived on just such a diet. And if you look today at the habits and diets of groups of people who are notably free of degenerative heart disease (and many other chronic diseases which plague Westerners), you will find that they, too, thrive on a diet containing a low level of fat, a relatively modest intake of protein, and great amounts of unrefined carbohydrates in the form of fruits, nuts, grains, leaves, and roots.

Apparently, it is not necessary to follow every last facet of a "natural" or "primitive" lifestyle in order to enjoy relative freedom from heart disease. There are some fairly remote and primitive peoples whose circulatory systems are in beautiful condition, who indulge moderately in smoking or drinking, who do not get much exercise, or whose food supply seems relatively lacking in one or more important nutrients. Nonetheless, because the overall *pattern* of natural living is followed, their hearts seem able to accept some moderate insults without suffering much in the process.

With us moderns, the story is just the reverse. Beginning with an *un*natural lifestyle, in which virtually everything is out of tune with our biological heritage, each added insult challenges the integrity of the entire system. In this situation, removing just one additional burden, such as excessive fat intake or insufficient vitamins, may not be enough to pacify the physiological hurricane of smoking, unrelieved stress, too many calories, and not enough exercise. That's why the best approach seems to be one which changes total behavior, rather than one or two habits.

## Simpler Diet and Long Walks

Late in 1975, news came from the Longevity Research Institute of Santa Barbara, California, that a relatively conservative approach to this kind of modified lifestyle may be the best answer yet found to actually *reversing* heart disease.

The people in the experimental program, according to Dr. Stewart Gorney, were put on a diet that calls for a total fat intake of only 10 percent—compared to an average American diet of 42 percent. A typical menu for patients consists of rolled oats, skim milk, whole wheat bread, and fresh fruits for breakfast; for lunch, fresh and cooked vegetables along with two or three ounces of lean meat, preferably poultry or fish; and a modification of the luncheon diet for dinner.

To this diet, which is clearly a more *natural* diet for man, was added a controlled exercise routine.

While it may sound rather too simple to accomplish much, this combined diet and exercise program, Dr. Gorney says, "produces changes within a few weeks which increase the blood flow and raise the oxygen content of the blood. The improved circulation quickly betters the patient's condition and permits the body to start the healing process that is the key to permanent recovery."

Some of the elderly people in the study who had heart disease and who could walk only a few hundred feet when first seen, were able to increase their walking distance to *at least* six miles and as much as ten miles a day at the conclusion of the six-month study.

Angina pains were greatly relieved—completely in some patients —and high blood pressure dropped precipitously without drugs.

"The rapid return to normal health occurred in patients with symptoms of coronary insufficiency, with angina, hypertension, leg pain, diabetes, arthritis, gout, and other symptoms of degenerative vascular disease. In 30 days many patients had improved to the point where drugs were no longer needed," Dr. Gorney and his colleagues declared.

That is what can be accomplished by returning to a more natural style of eating and living. How many people will be able to adopt these new habits is another question, unfortunately. If you have the motivation, though, to follow such a program—or a reasonable facsimile thereof—there is no question in my mind that you are on the most reliable road to a healthier heart.

Some people take an approach to heart disease which is almost entirely nutritional in character. While such an approach is not particularly holistic, it must be said that realistically, this approach is the only one that many people are willing to take. And to the extent that it is a positive program, emphasizing the addition of certain nutrients to the diet, rather than largely negative, stressing complete avoidance of eggs, whole milk, and the like, it is even more acceptable.

But let's at least take a rounded and well-balanced view of nutrition and the heart, rather than zeroing in only on one particular nutrient as the answer to heart problems. A number of food elements, some minerals, some vitamins, other bulky substances containing unknown compounds, have been shown to be of possible use in maintaining the health of the circulatory system.

## Vitamin E and the Heart

Vitamin E is easily the best known nutrient that has been recommended for the heart. Whatever its worth, however, it is not easily proved by common tests. It does not have any reliable effect on cholesterol levels, and although it does seem to have some retarding influence on blood clotting, this influence seems to be rather weak. It's more likely that the beneficial effect of vitamin E will be found to be in its reputed ability to permit tissues to survive and thrive with less oxygen, or its protective effect on artery walls and muscular tissue, particularly the heart muscle.

Wilfrid E. Shute, M.D., and his brother Evan Shute, M.D., are the great pioneers in the field of vitamin E therapy for the heart. For over a period of many years, they administered vitamin E to thousands of patients at the Shute Institute for Clinical and Laboratory Medicine in London, Ontario. Innumerable case histories have been reported which seem to demonstrate excellent results from the administration of vitamin E, typically in amounts ranging from 800 to 1,600 I.U. a day for heart patients.

Dr. Wilfrid Shute cautions that patients with chronic rheumatic heart disease should be started on no more than 90 units a day for a month, then 120 units a day for a month, then 150 units. He also cautions that patients who have serious elevations of blood pressure first have that elevation brought under control by the appropriate medication before receiving vitamin E therapy.

Although acceptance by the medical profession of vitamin E therapy for the heart has been limited and slow, there is little question that thousands upon thousands of people are convinced that it has done them a world of good. Statistically, this means nothing; to the heart, which has a difficult time understanding statistics, it may mean everything.

In 1974, PREVENTION magazine invited readers to fill out a questionnaire relating their experiences with vitamin E. Nearly 20,000 responses were received, and it took many months to organize the information. Designed and analyzed by Richard Passwater, a biochemist, the survey did not pretend to be scientifically conclusive; such an approach would have meant retrieving the medical records of thousands of people, interviewing and examining them, and determining exactly how much vitamin E they had taken for how long. Like I said, impossible. What Passwater did instead was to simply ask each respondent for this information, including subjective changes in the state of well-being and freedom from pain.

There emerged an overwhelming picture of vitamin E's ability to bring about gradual but very significant improvement in angina, irregular heartbeat, leg pain, and a number of other circulatory conditions. Many people volunteered extended descriptions of their progress and these were highly supportive of the idea that vitamin E can make a real difference in health.

Passwater commented that in looking at the final figures, which he submitted to a statistician for analysis, the trend emerged that the maximum degree of protection came from taking 400 I.U. of vitamin E over a period of ten years, or from taking 1,200 I.U. or more a day for four years.

Recently, a branch of the National Institutes of Health examined a group of people who had been taking relatively large amounts of vitamin E for some time, with the specific purpose of trying to find undesirable side effects. They found no such side effects that were clinically significant but *did* find that half of those taking vitamin E said they "felt better."

## Vitamin C and the Arteries

Vitamin C is another nutrient which may play a most important role in protecting and possibly even reversing heart disease. The available evidence points to the fact that its action is directed at the interface of the arterial lining and cholesterol, somehow protecting the artery from becoming clogged with fatty deposits.

An important review of evidence suggesting a beneficial role for vitamin C (and for lecithin) was published in August 1974 in the *American Journal of Clinical Nutrition* by Charles E. Butterworth, Jr., M.D., former chairman of the Food and Nutrition Council of the American Medical Association, and Carlos Krumdieck, M.D., Ph.D. The two physicians cite one study showing that when patients with atherosclerotic fatty plaques in their arteries were given vitamin C supplements, six out of ten experienced partial regression of these deposits. There was no improvement at all in patients who did not receive vitamin C.

Dr. E. G. Knox has reported in *Lancet* (June 30, 1973) that when the intake of various nutrients is correlated with the causes of death in a very large number of people, it becomes evident that the more vitamin C there is in a diet, the less chance there is of suffering a fatal heart attack or stroke.

In 1975, we interviewed Dr. Constance Leslie (nee Spittle), a British pathologist who has published extensively on the role of vitamin C in preventing thrombosis, and she told us that in her hospital, those wards which routinely give patients vitamin C before and after surgery have experienced no problem at all with dangerous blood clots.

Late in 1975, we spoke with Anthony Verlangieri, Ph.D., of Rutgers University, a young biochemist who believes he may have found the underlying reason why vitamin C can protect the heart. First, he explained, his research showed that when rabbits are fed cholesterol, they are protected from developing atherosclerosis when vitamin C is added to the diet. That in itself was no great surprise. The important finding was that vitamin C apparently accomplishes this feat by encouraging the synthesis in the arterial lining of substances known as mucopolysaccharides. While a number of these substances increased during vitamin C supplementation, the most dramatic increase was discovered in one known as chondroitin-4-sulfate.

**Chondroitin-4-Sulfate** ● That in itself is interesting, but what made it truly exciting was that this same substance, chondroitin-4-sulfate (formerly known as chondroitin sulfate A or CSA for short), has been tested clinically by Dr. Lester Morrison of Los Angeles, who reported dramatic success when he gave this substance to 60 cardiovascular patients.

While chondroitin-4-sulfate sounds like a pure chemical, it is actually a purified extract of the throat cartilage of cattle. That particular tissue is used only because it occurs there very abundantly; the same substance is found as a naturally occurring and vital component in a great number of human tissues. In this sense, it might be compared to one of those vitamins which the body can synthesize itself, but which—apparently—pays big dividends when taken in supplemental form. ·

Dr. Morrison and his colleague Norbert L. Enrick, Ph.D., wrote in *Angiology* (May 1973) that over a period of six years, 50 patients given CSA fared much better than another 60 heart patients who were given only conventional therapy over the same period of time. The latter group suffered a total of 42 coronary incidents, while the CSA group had only 6. And while 14 died in the control group, only 4 patients taking CSA died.

There is a great deal more we could say about chondroitin-4-sulfate or CSA, but since—as of this writing—the product is not available to the public in the United States, it may be premature to dwell at length on this seemingly miraculous substance. If it does in fact become available, it would be well to insure that the product has been thoroughly tested for biological activity (this is done by measuring its ability to prevent experimental arterial thrombosis) and that it has been prepared in such a way as to negate the possibility of an allergic reaction. The form of CSA which Dr. Morrison has used, we should add, has proven to be quite safe, and the most recent report we've seen—from a large hospital in South America—indicates that this natural substance has enormous therapeutic potentials for a wide variety of circulatory ailments.

**How Much Vitamin C?** ● Meanwhile, we have Dr. Verlangieri's evidence that supplemental vitamin C causes the body to synthesize more of the substance by itself. Whether or not the "bottom line" on vitamin C will turn out to be as dramatic as the CSA story, we cannot say. Dr. Verlangieri says he *knows* it works in rabbits and that he feels 99 percent certain that this vitamin would have a similar protective effect in humans.

Drs. Krumdieck and Butterworth, whose article was mentioned earlier, seem favorable to the idea that somewhere between one and two full grams (1,000 to 2,000 mg.) of vitamin C daily may be the ideal intake. At least, they write, they are not aware of any reliable reports of ill effects resulting from high intakes of vitamin C. They make a point of shooting down the vague threat that a lot of vitamin C can cause oxalate stone formation in kidneys by citing medical evidence that even on 3,000 mg. a day of vitamin C, there is no noticeable increase in oxalates in the urine.

There is some rather weak evidence that if a person takes very large amounts of vitamin C with every meal and continues to do so for a year or more, vitamin $B_{12}$ absorption may suffer. The answer to this problem is either not to take vitamin C along with your meals, or to take a supplemental $B_{12}$ tablet at some time other than when you are ingesting vitamin C.

## Lecithin and Cholesterol

Lecithin, an oily substance derived from soybeans, is another nutrient which has been rather extensively investigated in relation to heart disease. Lecithin's action seems to be directed solely at combining with cholesterol in such a way as to prevent its deposit in arteries.

Drs. Krumdieck and Butterworth relate that it's been shown in rabbits that putting more lecithin into the system results in deposits of cholesterol being broken up and carried away. However, in order to do this effectively, the lecithin must be a polyunsaturated lecithin. In the rabbit experiment it was this kind of polyunsaturated lecithin, derived from soybeans, that proved effective. When lecithin from egg yolks, which is a saturated lecithin, was used, it was not nearly as effective as the soybean lecithin.

In this particular experiment, the lecithin was injected into the animals, but Drs. Krumdieck and Butterworth cite other research which shows that a substantial amount of lecithin which is eaten is actually absorbed intact through the wall of the intestines.

And in fact, there is evidence going back many years which shows quite clearly that lecithin consumed in the same manner as food is a potent weapon against excessive cholesterol. Back in 1943, two doctors at Mt. Sinai Hospital in New York City reported on five cases of high cholesterol associated with various clinical conditions in which "a striking decrease of the serum cholesterol level was achieved by addition of commercial lecithin to the diet." One woman, 41, had a cholesterol count of 620 when she began taking 12 grams of soybean lecithin a day. Two months later, it was down to 420 and a month after that, down to 300. Probably the most striking case was that of a 38-year-old woman who had multiple health problems, including fatty plaques on her skin, who dropped her cholesterol from an extremely high 1,370 all the way down to 445 during the three months in which she took 15 grams of lecithin a day.

One of the important figures in lecithin research is Lester M. Morrison, M.D., the same Los Angeles physician who has worked for many years with chondroitin-4-sulfate. Dr. Morrison reported in *Geriatrics* (January 1958) that 12 out of 15 patients experienced an average fall of serum cholesterol of 156 mg., or 41 percent, after three months of taking soybean lecithin supplements daily. It should be mentioned that these particular patients had all been on a low-fat diet as well as the full medical treatment for some time but had failed to respond until lecithin was added to the low-fat regimen.

Lecithin, I should mention, comes in several forms, including liquid, granules, and the encapsulated oil. The liquid is quite tasteless but very viscous and needs to be washed down with some fluids. The granules are best taken mixed with some liquid or food. The capsules are quite convenient, but about 10 or 12 of the larger variety (1,200 mg.) must be taken to equal the dose used in most research.

## Magnesium and Heart Disease

At least two minerals are suspected of having important beneficial effects on the circulatory system. They are magnesium and calcium.

A great deal has been written in medical literature about these minerals, particularly in relation to their occurrence in hard water, and the apparent protective effect that hard water has against heart attacks. Here, we will limit ourselves to discussing the most recent findings.

A team of five Canadian scientists headed by Dr. T. W. Anderson of the University of Toronto's Department of Preventive Medicine and Biostatistics, collected samples of heart tissue at autopsy in

83 cases of accidental death and analyzed them for mineral content. Samples were specifically collected from various cities in Ontario, where the water hardness, a measure of the dissolved minerals in the public water supply, is known to vary from extremely high to extremely low. Of seven minerals analyzed, only one element, magnesium, varied significantly between hard- and soft-water areas. Those who lived in soft-water regions had seven percent less magnesium in the myocardium, the middle and thickest layer of the heart wall, composed of cardiac muscle (*Canadian Medical Association Journal,* August 9, 1975).

Dr. Anderson and his colleagues also collected and analyzed myocardial tissue from 40 people who died as a direct consequence of severe and irreversible heart disease. *Regardless* of whether those subjects had lived in hard- or soft-water communities, the average concentration of magnesium in their hearts was 22 percent lower than among all those who died accidentally. Combined with the overall findings, "these results are compatible with the belief that the higher cardiac death rate in the soft-water areas of Ontario is due to the relative lack of magnesium in the water supply," the authors conclude.

They suggest—but do not recommend, since such recommendations are scarcely ever made—that it might make a lot of sense if oral magnesium supplements were taken to insure adequacy of this mineral.

Such a supplement might be in the form of magnesium oxide, commonly available in tablet form, some containing 250 mg. of magnesium, which is an appropriate daily supplementary amount.

## Why Calcium Is Important

Like magnesium, calcium has long been suspected of being the mysterious factor in hard water that provides a measure of protection against heart and artery disease. After analyzing mortality statistics and sampling the tap water from 48 communities in South Wales, three Welsh scientists reported a strong negative association between the amount of calcium and the incidence of fatal heart disease in each area (*Lancet,* December 21, 1974). In fact, the more calcium in the tap water, the fewer the deaths from *any* cause.

A similar statistical study, conducted by E. G. Knox of the University of Birmingham, England, found that when dietary intake of 13 nutrients was matched against deaths from six natural causes (including heart disease), the strongest single relationship was between calcium and heart disease, and it was a negative one. That is, the more calcium in the diet, the less the chance of dying of heart disease. In second place as a protector was vitamin C, which we discussed earlier.

Both magnesium and calcium are important for normal contraction and relaxation of muscles, and it is possible that their protective effect lies in this area. Calcium, however, also has a very specific ability to lower serum cholesterol.

It does not seem to do this as dramatically as lecithin, but the effect is still there.

Anthony A. Albanese, Ph.D., and five colleagues related in *Nutrition Reports International,* August 1973, that women between the ages of 53 and 88 experienced a general reduction of cholesterol levels while taking 750 mg. of calcium daily, along with vitamin D to enhance absorption. A control group taking a placebo experienced no such benefit. The doctors suggest that calcium's ability to lower cholesterol "may prove to be a meaningful therapeutic and prophylactic action in the management of cardiovascular diseases."

Earlier, Alan I. Fleischman, Ph.D., and M. L. Bierenbaum, M.D., of the Atherosclerosis Research Group at St. Vincent's Hospital in Montclair, New Jersey, reported similar results feeding supplemental calcium to ten men and women between the ages of 26 and 61. All had high levels of cholesterol and other fats circulating in their blood. Three of the subjects had previously suffered heart attacks; three others were plagued by angina pain.

After taking two grams (2,000 mg.) of calcium in four divided doses daily for one year, their serum cholesterol fell an average of 24 percent, the two researchers told a convention of experimental biologists in 1969. Blood and urine analyses indicated no harmful side effects at that high dosage, they added.

The nice thing about calcium's effect on cholesterol levels is that, unlike a drug, it appears to act as a normalizer. In an earlier study in which the St. Vincent's researchers participated, calcium lowered serum cholesterol readings *most* in people with especially high initial readings. Those who had only moderately elevated readings experienced moderate reductions. And among those whose serum cholesterol levels were normal, there was no decrease after taking calcium (*British Medical Journal,* June 1965).

For mature people, an appropriate supplemental amount of

calcium seems to be about 1,000 mg. a day. This may be conveniently obtained in a number of forms, including calcium lactate, calcium gluconate, or bone meal. It is advisable either to use a powdered form or to chew the tablets to insure maximum absorption. Personally, I prefer chewable bone meal tablets because bone meal is the most natural form of calcium and it contains a number of trace elements that are valuable for developing strong bones. It used to be believed that phosphorus inhibited calcium absorption and for this reason, some people questioned the use of bone meal, which contains phosphorus as well as calcium. Recently, though, it's been shown by Dr. Herta Spencer, one of the nation's leading mineral researchers, that even very large amounts of phosphorus have no effect on calcium absorption in human beings.

## Use Unsaturated Oil

Although there is still considerable controversy over the importance of fats and oils in relation to heart disease, it does seem fairly clear that cutting out saturated fats and substituting polyunsaturates is a step in the right direction. For one thing, polyunsaturates tend to lower cholesterol. More than that, it's now been shown that changing from saturates to unsaturates has a very beneficial effect on the clotting properties of the blood. Dr. Fleischman and colleagues reported in the *Journal of Nutrition* (October 1975) that when residents of a geriatrics center were switched from using butter to a "highly unsaturated margarine," the average aggregation time of their blood platelets doubled.

That could be very important in preventing an abnormal blood clot or thrombosis, because the tendency of the platelets to aggregate (i.e., clot) is abnormally high in many people. Medication is commonly given to reduce platelet aggregation time but it appears that simply using polyunsaturated oils is also very beneficial. The key substance is linoleic acid, or linoleate, which is found abundantly in safflower oil, sunflower oil, and corn oil. Check labels if you are uncertain.

## Alfalfa and Pectin

I do not believe in making a fetish out of cholesterol reduction, but it is worth mentioning that at least two natural substances other than lecithin and calcium have a definite ability to do the job. They are alfalfa and pectin, the latter being the substance found in many fruits and berries and which is added to jellies to make them thick. Both alfalfa and pectin do their work in the intestinal tract, apparently binding up cholesterol and carrying it right through the system, so it cannot be absorbed (or reabsorbed). Relatively large amounts of each are needed to do the job. With alfalfa, for instance, you will probably need to chew up a dozen or more tablets a day, preferably before a meal so that it would have a chance to combine with dietary cholesterol. A daily salad of alfalfa sprouts would also be worthwhile.

Pectin is found abundantly in apples, and a good way to get a lot of pectin is to eat a large amount of fresh raw applesauce every day, because when apples are grated, they have a greater cholesterol-inhibiting effect. While one or two apples a day are good for you, the full effect on cholesterol is not achieved until about two pounds of apples are eaten daily. When pectin is extracted from apples, it is measured in terms of grams and an appropriate amount is 10 grams of pectin a day, equivalent to about 20 pectin tablets (assuming you aren't eating any apples). This was the amount used in research by Dr. Hans Fisher, Chairman of the Department of Nutrition at Rutgers University in New Brunswick, New Jersey, in his tests. Dr. Fisher tested college students who were eating at least two eggs daily and found that after three weeks, those who took pectin had an average cholesterol count of 157, while those who did not take the pectin had a count of 191—more than 25 percent higher. "It is clear," Dr. Fisher and his colleagues have written, "that pectin offers partial protection against the problem which may arise from cholesterol ingestion." Dr. Fisher told us that his research indicates that when there is no "overload" of cholesterol in the diet, pectin may not be necessary to limit its absorption. But when the typically fat-rich American diet is eaten, pectin does have a definite regulatory role to play.

Finally, I have recently come across reports in scientific literature indicating that both the fruit and leaves of the common eggplant have the same kind of effect on cholesterol absorption as alfalfa and pectin. So far, the work has only been done on rabbits, but like all the other work we've discussed here, it's been carried out by scientists with gold-plated credentials.

## Garlic and the Heart

There is at least one herb that has a proven effect on parameters involving the health of the heart, and that is garlic. R. C. Jain, M.D., of the University of Benghazi (Libya) Pathology Department, has written extensively on the subject of garlic and health. In *Lancet* (May 31, 1975) he describes a study with rabbits which showed that when these animals were fed a high-cholesterol diet, their serum cholesterol zoomed over 2,100 and postmortem examination revealed they were well along the road to artery disease. Rabbits fed the same diet but which also were fed garlic juice had an average serum cholesterol level of just 419. That is still much higher than normal, but the protective effect is obvious. Dr. Jain also found that fatty plaque formation inside the arteries of those rabbits fed garlic juice was less severe than in the other animals.

Does it work for human beings? No one is about to do a biopsy on the human arteries following garlic ingestion, but doctors in India have demonstrated that when healthy subjects were fed about two ounces of garlic or an equivalent amount of garlic extract, serum cholesterol decreased from an average of 229 to 213 within three hours after a quarter pound of butter was eaten. With the same subjects who were fed the butter without the garlic, serum cholesterol *rose* about 15 points.

Perhaps more important, among those who took the garlic, blood coagulation time, a measure of blood platelet stickiness, became longer. Since most Westerners have a tendency to form clots too fast, that is a good healthy sign. Dr. Arun Bordia and H. C. Bansal concluded their communication to *Lancet* (December 29, 1973) with the suggestion that for patients predisposed to cardiovascular disease, garlic "could be recommended for long-term use without danger of toxicity."

In addition, there are anecdotal reasons to believe that eating garlic also tends to lower blood pressure somewhat.

## Rinse Breakfast Mash

We said at the beginning of this journey through natural remedies for heart disease that the best approach is to cover as many bets as possible. Such an approach has been worked out by Jacobus Rinse, Ph.D., a chemist who has published a number of articles on how he cured his own angina. Using his knowledge of chemistry and a careful reading of a great deal of research, he came up with a mixture of nutrients which can be eaten for breakfast. Dr. Rinse has told us that a great many people who have tried this mixture have enjoyed gratifying relief of symptoms of circulatory problems, including some very severe ones. Here are his instructions for what has come to be known as the Rinse Breakfast Mash:

> A mixture is made of one tablespoon each of soybean lecithin granules, debittered yeast, and raw wheat germ, with one teaspoon of bone meal powder. A larger quantity can be prepared for storage.
>
> Then, says Dr. Rinse, mix in a bowl: two tablespoons of the above mixture, one tablespoon of dark brown sugar (if you wish), and one tablespoon of safflower oil or some other linoleate oil such as sunflower or soybean oil. Add milk to dissolve sugar and yeast and then add some yogurt to increase consistency. Then add some cold or hot cereal such as oatmeal and if you wish, some raisins or other fruits. Some bran flakes may also be added to increase fiber.

For severe cases of atherosclerosis, Dr. Rinse says, the quantity of lecithin should be doubled.

Finally, he recommends taking daily 500 mg. of vitamin C, 100 to 200 I.U. of vitamin E, and one multivitamin-mineral tablet.

## Exercise Is Important

As a final note, let me urge anyone who takes a nutritional approach to cardiac health to try to begin a regular exercise program as well, working *gradually* up to the equivalent of walking several miles a day. In the successful research conducted at the Longevity Research Institute, which we mentioned at the beginning of this discussion, even "elderly" people were walking at least six miles a day, and some even more. When you eat right, quit smoking, and walk that far, every day, your heart seems to realize that you mean business and have no intention of closing shop at any time in the near future.

# Heartburn

As common as heartburn is, it isn't easy to treat. The truth is that much remains to be learned about the basic causes of this condition, in which stomach acid is regurgitated up onto the delicate lining of the esophagus.

A carefully controlled study conducted in Great Britain revealed several interesting facts about heartburn "remedies." One is that placebo tablets (dummy pills) had no significant effect on heartburn pain, indicating that the condition apparently does not respond well to simple "suggestion."

More surprising was that antacid tablets containing the usual aluminum hydroxide, magnesium, and sodium bicarbonate also failed to cause any significant reduction of suffering.

What *did* work, at least for some patients, was a tablet containing the usual antacid ingredients plus algin in the form of alginic acid, a natural substance derived from seaweeds.

The doctors explained in *Lancet* (January 26, 1974) that algin apparently forms a soothing, gel-like solution inside the stomach "which will float on the surface of the gastric contents as a thick surface layer or 'raft'."

Let me hasten to add, however, that even this preparation was not a resounding success in all patients; only a little more than half described their symptoms as definitely improved. If you want to try the algin therapy, thoroughly chew up one or two sodium alginate tablets (do not swallow them whole) and wash them down with a glass of milk. This is a tasteless concoction but somewhat messy, because the algin tends to stick to your teeth. You might also try adding some magnesium oxide or crushed dolomite to the milk, as the British results show that the effectiveness of algin is enhanced when combined with antacid.

If you do take antacids containing aluminum compounds, with or without algin, note well this warning: long-term consumption of these preparations may seriously deplete you of calcium, resulting in thinning of the bones and possible bone pain. This has been demonstrated by Herta Spencer, M.D. In laboratory experiments, she found that even relatively small amounts of one widely sold antacid preparation caused a loss of about 130 mg. of calcium a day. The second product caused *twice* this level of calcium loss. Adding weight to these findings was the case of a 48-year-old man who had "marked demineralization of the skeleton, probably a mixture of osteoporosis and osteomalacia," but who had "none of the usual causes of osteoporosis." What he did have was a history of having taken aluminum-containing antacids for 10 to 12 years.

So much for antacids. Now let's mention a number of other simple steps heartburn sufferers can take to quell the fire down below. Just losing weight can sometimes be a big help. That's because persistent heartburn is occasionally caused by hiatal hernia, a condition in which either the stomach or esophagus is squeezed out of proper position. The pressure of extra weight or a flabby diaphragm may be responsible. Shedding excess pounds and toning up the muscles with regular, moderate exercise can relieve hiatal hernia distress in many cases. You should avoid tight-fitting clothes and belts for the same reason.

Heartburn victims should eat smaller meals, especially in the evening, and avoid lying down after meals. Lying down only invites the contents of the stomach to slosh into the esophagus.

Avoid alcohol, chocolate, caffeine, and fried, fatty, or spicy foods. In addition to stimulating your stomach to produce extra acid, some of these foods have been found to lower sphincter pressure at the stomach-esophagus junction. This opening of the "gate" permits stomach acid to move upwards.

Cigarette smoking is one of the worst offenders in this regard, because nicotine can have a dramatic effect on sphincter pressure, causing it to drop and permitting the reflux of acid. In fact, if you are a heavy cigarette smoker and have heartburn, the chances that you can get rid of your condition by getting rid of your nicotine habit are very great.

# Heel Spurs

As an alternative to surgery, great relief from the pain of a heel spur may be obtained by inserting a properly fitted pad of foam rubber into the bottoms of your shoes. There should be a hole cut in the foam rubber where the spur projects, so that when you walk, it is spared from bearing the incredible amount of pressure which results when a tiny portion of your foot must absorb the pressure of your entire body with each step.

A podiatrist will be able to help you build such a cushion, or make one for you.

# Hemorrhoids

According to conservative estimates, half the adults in this country over the age of 40 are sitting on a case of hemorrhoids. Some put the incidence among mature people as high as four out of five.

Architectural structure has something to do with the fact that these pesty lesions bedevil so many of us. Gravity imposes a constant load on the delicate veins which supply the anus. While most veins have check valves to prevent backflow of blood and keep it moving toward the heart, for some reason nature neglected to install check valves in the column of blood which extends through the veins down the abdomen to the hemorrhoidal area. Therefore, the entire weight of this column of blood bears on these tiny blood vessels.

Gravity alone imposes a constant burden; abdominal pressure of any kind makes matters worse. These veins are not meant for hard use. They exist as an auxiliary pathway only. But when pressure causes an excessive flow of blood to the rectal area, the normal channels are unable to handle it all.

While straining at stool is the prime cause preventing the blood from getting through the larger veins, straining applies to conditions other than a difficult bowel movement. When you lift a heavy object, and even when you cough, you tighten your abdominal muscles, thus squeezing on these veins. The pressure builds up in the rectal area and blood piles up above. Avoid such actions and you can keep the hemorrhoids away from your backdoor or retard their development if they are already knocking.

## Learn to Lift Properly

Learn to lift objects in the proper way—by stooping instead of bending—so you can push with your legs instead of with your stomach and back muscles. While lifting, breathe freely to minimize abdominal pressure on the hemorrhoidal veins. Inhale and exhale constantly. The idea, while lifting or during bowel movements, is not to hold your breath—a common practice among those who strain at stool. Learn this breathing technique which is based on the same principle as that taught for natural childbirth, and you will vastly improve traffic conditions in your internal superhighway.

Avoid constipation in the first place and straining will be unnecessary. Drink lots of liquids—water and fruit juices. Avoid sugar and refined foods made of white flour. Among people who live on unrefined foods, such as the Zulus in Africa, hemorrhoids and varicose veins are virtually unknown. Eat high-residue foods like fresh fruits and vegetables and especially bran. Use the unprocessed or coarse bran; the greater water-holding capacity of coarse bran makes it preferable.

In our country there is a strong emphasis on "being regular" and it's nice to be regular, but don't force the issue. The important thing is that when you do have a strong urge to go, do so immediately. You should also avoid the popular custom of making a library out of your bathroom. Getting engrossed in an article may cause you to spend too much time on the commode. Prolonged periods of sitting invites engorgement and varicosities of those delicate veins.

## Try the Bioflavonoids

Your veins might be less likely to become varicosed if your diet were rich in rutin, one of the family of bioflavonoids which combats capillary fragility. A doctor in Switzerland reported he cured thousands of patients suffering various types of hemorrhoids with orally administered trioxyethylrutin, a bioflavonoid sometimes referred to as $P_4$ (*Current Therapeutic Research*, August 1963).

In 1974, Dr. P. Muller and colleagues of the Hospices Civils in Strasbourg, France, reported that when they administered flavone or bioflavonoid compounds to women who had varicose veins in their legs and rectum, most enjoyed marked relief from pain.

Clinical research using bioflavonoid compounds for hemorrhoids is almost completely lacking in American medical literature, we have to admit. So for what they are worth, here are some anecdotes sent to us by readers of PREVENTION.

"I have been to my doctor and he said I had hemorrhoids," a reader in Union, New Jersey, told us. "I saw the article on citrus bioflavonoids. After taking three tablets per day, my hemorrhoids have disappeared after three months. I take the multivitamins and minerals, vitamin E, citrus bioflavonoids, and acerola (vitamin C) every day."

A pleasant surprise was experienced by a reader in Pennsylvania, practically on the way to the operating room. "I found this complete cure quite by accident," she wrote. "I was ready to tell the doctor I would have the operation because I couldn't stand the pain any more, when they [the hemorrhoids] completely disappeared. I was having some internal trouble besides and I went to the doctor. He said I was having capillary breakdown and prescribed vitamin P . . . he told me to take one a day. I knew that wasn't enough so I started to take six a day. I still wasn't getting the relief that I thought this vitamin should bring and began to take twelve a day. Within 48 hours, the hemorrhoids disappeared, and not one bit of pain. I couldn't believe it. I had been in terrible pain constantly for two and a half months. Here is . . . what [in the vitamin P tablet] I took: citrus bioflavonoid complex, vitamin C (and rose hips), hesperidin complex, and rutin. This has been like a miracle for me," she wrote.

"In the summer of 1968," a reader in Washington told us, "I was having a great deal of trouble with hemorrhoids. The swelling was bad and the pain was terrible. I tried various remedies and nothing seemed to help. Then in August of that summer, a special report appeared in PREVENTION on how rutin was used to help this problem. I started to use it and got relief within just a few days. A friend of mine a couple of years after this was having the same trouble and I recommended rutin to him, and he also used it and got help immediately. I have continued to take rutin since that time as it is very cheap and it will help prevent a recurrence."

Rutin is chiefly contained in buckwheat. But rutin and other flavonoid substances also occur in rose hips, grapes, plums, black currants, apricots, cherries, blackberries, and all citrus fruits. Of these, rose hips is extremely rich in flavonoid activity and gives you the added benefit of large amounts of vitamin C, which scientists say is essential to the proper use of the flavonoids.

Wilfrid E. Shute, M.D., of Canada tells of his successful treatment of many cases of varicose veins in his book *Vitamin E for Ailing and Healthy Hearts* (Pyramid House, New York, 1969). Since hemorrhoids are, in fact, varicose veins of the anal canal, it would certainly make sense to increase your intake of this versatile vitamin which can be very helpful to you in yet another area.

## More Natural Aids

Do not overlook the importance of regular exercise. Take brisk walks, join a yoga class or calisthenics class, a class in modern dance, go square dancing or folk dancing. Do shoulder stands frequently to reverse the pull of gravity. Never ride when you can walk. If you avoid the sedentary life, you have a much better chance of avoiding constipation and consequently hemorrhoids.

For relief of pain and for lubrication, try A and D ointment, vitamin E ointment, or better yet a vitamin E suppository which contains no drugs.

Recently, two readers described to us what they said was near-miraculous success in ending itching by scrupulously washing with warm water after each bowel movement and then applying wheat germ oil. No matter what else you try, do practice meticulous cleanliness of the anal area. But be gentle.

All of these measures—improved diet, more exercise, and cleanliness—comprise a self-help program which will help prevent and in some cases even cure a case of hemorrhoids.

If, however, you have rectal bleeding, with or without pain and with or without any sign of hemorrhoids, don't let any false sense of modesty or embarrassment keep you from seeking medical advice. It may be nothing at all to worry about, in which case you will be greatly relieved. But, do have it checked out. "As far as I'm concerned," one doctor has written, "rectal bleeding means cancer until proven otherwise." Chances are it isn't. Only one of 50 complaining of hemorrhoids actually has a tumor. If you are the one in 50, catching it early may save your life. The exam will free you of the nagging worry that bothers you almost as much as the discomfort.

# Herbal Medicine

The specific use of herbs as aids in healing is discussed in many of the entries in this book. Here, I want to present a broader view of herbal medicine as well as some details that may not appear in other sections.

Included here are:

- Dr. George Zofchak: 45 Years of Healing With Herbs
- A Pharmacist's Experiences With 'Yesterday's Miracle Drugs'
- The Ten Most Practical Medicinal Herbs: How To Grow and Use Them
- Dangerous Herbs

- 'Quack' Salad and Cancer
- Pharmacognosy, The Scientific Approach to Medicinal Herbs
- Herbal Formulations For Mind and Body
- A Critical Review of Correspondence Courses in Herbalism
- An Annotated Bibliography of Herbal Medicine and Folk Remedy Books

I have attempted to avoid completely all the herbal jargon and technical terminology which makes some herb books difficult to understand. Perhaps the only two terms which need explanation are "infusion" and "decoction."

An infusion is simply a tea made from an herb. Ordinarily, about a teaspoon of the leaves or flowers are put in a pot and a cup of boiling water is poured over them. The vessel—which is not heated—is then covered and the tea allowed to steep for five or ten minutes. It may be necessary to reheat the tea. You may also want to use more or less than a teaspoon of herbal material, depending upon how powerful or unpleasant the taste is. Goldenseal, for instance, tastes awful, and it is usually used in the ground root form, which is quite potent. So rather than use a teaspoon, you would be using only a scant *half* teaspoon of the powder. By way of contrast, a teaspoon of peppermint leaves may not give you the strength you want in your tea, but because it tastes so good, you can simply add more leaves.

A decoction is also an herbal tea but differs from an infusion in that the herbal material is actually boiled or at least simmered. Typically, seeds, pieces of root or bark, or branches which would not easily release their essence when steeped are prepared in this way. Begin with cold water, bring to a boil, and keep on the heat for as long as necessary to extract the virtues of the plant material. Keep the pot covered while cooking, and cool before using.

When preparing herbs to be applied in a poultice or ointment, greater strength is usually desired, so more herbs should be added to either the infusion or decoction.

To make an ointment, add approximately one part of a strong brew of the herb you want to use to about four parts of something like Vaseline or lanolin anhydrous. Technically, a poultice includes not only a warm brew of herbs into which some cloth is dipped, but something like bread to keep the herbal material in contact with the skin. You may find it simpler to saturate a clean piece of cloth in a strong warm herbal brew, apply to the skin, and cover with a clean, dry cloth.

When you purchase herbs for medicinal purposes, it's always best to get them in a tightly sealed container. I have found that when herbs are bought in tea-bag form, they have generally lost much of their potency by the time they are used.

## Dr. George Zofchak: 45 Years of Healing With Herbs

"We had our first son, George Jr., 27 years ago. A few years went by, and we decided we wanted more children. But my wife Irene had trouble carrying, and there were several miscarriages. Finally, in restudying herbal literature, I learned that red raspberry leaves can help a woman in many ways throughout her pregnancy, strengthening the attachment of the fetus and even easing delivery at the time of birth. Although I had been selling herbs and herbal teas for some years before this, I had somehow overlooked the usefulness of raspberry leaves in our own situation. So Irene began drinking a few cups of raspberry leaf tea when she next became pregnant. Everything went beautifully, even though 10 years had passed since the birth of our first son. The following year, Irene had another very easy and successful pregnancy. Now, besides George, we have Thomas, who is 17, and Janet, 16."

Dr. George Zofchak, herbalist, chiropractor, and naturopath, was talking to us in his office at the Tatra Herb Co., a business he has conducted for 45 years. During most of that time, his establishment has been located in the small, bustling town of Morrisville in Bucks County, Pennsylvania. Although he is actively licensed as a chiropractor, Dr. Zofchak today devotes most of his time to his herb business, headquartered in a small frame building on a quiet residential street, just a healthy stone's throw from the Delaware River.

Here, Dr. Zofchak stores and sells—mostly by mail order—hundreds of different kinds of herbs to customers all over the United States, and even Europe. Inside the building, as we talked with him for several hours, we somehow never stopped being aware of the lovely, unique fragrances emanating from all those herbs—even though most of them are in tightly sealed containers.

"I went into the herb business all the way back in 1929, when I was a student at the American School of Naturopathy and Chiropractic, the school then operated by Benedict Lust in New York. I needed money to help me get through school, and since my folks had done some trading in herbs back in Czechoslovakia—I can still remember roaming through the fields there picking herbs at the right time of year—I decided to try going into the business myself. I called my company the Tatra Herb Company after the Tatra Mountains in Czechoslovakia," Dr. Zofchak explained.

Today, nearly half a century after beginning his active interest in herbs, Dr. Zofchak is more convinced than ever that many people would be better off if they knew more about herbs. "Herbs, of course, are not looked upon as a substitute for medicine, not even by naturopaths. In my practice, I used herbs as an adjunct to other forms of treatment such as manipulation, massage, exercises, dietary guidance, and other natural techniques," the herbalist explained. "But very often, herbs are useful as a preventive measure and are also better to use, I think, than aspirin, tranquilizers, and all the other patent medicines that so many people use so heavily. And when you get into the habit of drinking herb tea instead of coffee, Coke, or a cocktail, you're not only avoiding the caffeine and sugar and alcohol, but helping to keep yourself healthy with herbs at the same time."

It is easy to believe Dr. Zofchak when he talks about the part that herbs can play in a healthier life. Now in his late 60s, Dr. Zofchak looks at least 10 years younger. Tall and powerfully built, he speaks in a calm and quiet voice as he moves swiftly around his immaculate offices locating various herbs. And lately, he's found that his vigor comes in handy, because his business has increased dramatically with the recent rebirth of interest in herbs.

## Experiences of an Herbalist

We asked Dr. Zofchak to tell us about a few cases he recalls where herbs seem to have an especially dramatic effect.

"Yes, sometimes there are real surprises, where the effect is especially outstanding," he said. "For example, there was a woman who had a badly infected toe. She came hobbling in here on crutches with other members of her family who said that doctors told her that they would have to amputate. The woman had diabetes, and her toe was becoming gangrenous.

"Now, in diabetes, I've found that in some advanced cases, the cells of the pancreas seem to be dead. Then there is nothing to do except provide the body with sufficient insulin. In other cases, you can help the body normalize itself. Well, this woman began drinking a tea made mostly from blueberry and huckleberry leaves and followed strict dietary advice. At the same time, she began soaking her foot in a decoction of comfrey root. The condition began to improve —not overnight—but gradually. In a few months, she came back to see me, this time with no crutches. Her toe was completely healed."

This particular case is rather illustrative in that it demonstrates that herbalists always work with a combination of herbs and other treatments, rather than one herb or treatment by itself. But when it comes to healing epithelial tissue, whether externally or internally, Dr. Zofchak has the highest praise for comfrey as a key ingredient in the healing formula.

"One of the best examples I can think of showing what comfrey can do happened to me personally," he told us. "Once I had a terrible case of poison ivy. I had it all over my face. In a couple of days, my skin was actually cracking and plasma oozing out. I applied repeated poultices of comfrey herb and the skin immediately began to heal. The cracks closed up and the swelling subsided and I was soon back to normal."

Powdered goldenseal root is another highly effective herb in healing skin lesions, Dr. Zofchak believes. For ulcers, which represent lesions of the "skin" of the stomach, he recommends an herbal mixture of goldenseal, comfrey, angelica, and valerian. The valerian is in the mixture because it helps to relax the nerves, and nervous agitation aggravates ulcers, the herbalist explained.

Eczema and psoriasis are two skin conditions which are notoriously difficult to heal. Dr. Zofchak admits that relieving these conditions may be as difficult for the herbalist as it is for the doctor. He believes that in cases of eczema, for example, the rash may be only a symptom of an underlying condition, such as a fungus, a reaction to a medicine, or some other environmental pollutant. As a practicing doctor he says he always inquired about the general health of the individual before making any recommendations for these skin conditions. For eczema, he says, he's found that in general, the most effective treatment is a decoction of comfrey root, witch hazel bark, and white oak bark, with a little goldenseal added.

For psoriasis, he recommends external application of a strong comfrey root decoction and goldenseal.

## How to Use Herbs on Your Skin

In applying herbs to the skin in this way, he said, the usual method is the poultice. A strong tea is brewed, cooled somewhat, and then the mixture is used to soak a clean piece of white cloth. Some of the herbs may actually be placed in the cloth, which is then wrapped around the herbs, and applied to the skin. The liquid and the vapor of the herbs soak through the cloth to the skin, while the herbs themselves are separated from the skin by the cloth. This technique is somewhat neater than applying crushed herbs directly to the skin and also reduces the chances of skin irritation.

If it is more convenient, the warm or cool tea can be applied directly to the skin as a wash. In treating the hands or the feet, a simple soak is often the most convenient method.

A wash is also a convenient method of application when dealing with animals who won't abide a poultice wrapped around them. Asked if he had much experience with animals, Dr. Zofchak said that pets frequently respond just as well or even better to herbs than humans. "Goldenseal, especially, seems to be very helpful for skin conditions. There was a woman who came in here with her poodle, whose hair had all come out. The tail looked like a big rat tail. She got some goldenseal, made a weak solution out of it, and applied it as a wash wherever the dog's hair had fallen out. As soon as she put it on, the dog would lick it off, but this didn't hurt matters because this meant the dog was getting goldenseal internally as well as externally. The funny thing was, she put some goldenseal in his food and even in his water, and the dog lapped it up, even though goldenseal is very bitter and bad tasting. This is a very common occurrence—many people find that dogs almost instinctively know when they need herbs and will eat them if given the chance. Anyway, the poodle's hair came back quickly, and the woman returned to show me how the herbs had helped her pet after all the veterinarians had failed."

## A Severe Sinus Headache

Sinus congestion is one of those hard-to-handle chronic problems, and we asked Dr. Zofchak if he had any experiences with sinusitis. "Yes, I had a really fascinating experience with a sinus problem. A man came in who works outdoors with heavy equipment. He had these terrific headaches and was taking aspirin and Darvon, but even the Darvon was of no help. He had been going to a doctor but had not been able to get relief. The man told me that his doctor informed him that if he didn't get relief soon he would have to operate —I presume he had a nerve block in mind.

"Well, I could tell just from listening to this man's voice that he had congestion of his sinus nodes. I suggested that he take a tea mixture which we call the pectoral tea, because it's designed mainly to clear up congestion in the chest, although it also helps congestion in any part of the respiratory tract.

"The man took the tea for about a week. Then he came back. 'God', he told me, 'my headaches are gone!' He said that blobs and blobs of phlegm and mucus had come up. He was one of the most grateful customers I ever had. If his headaches hadn't stopped, he would have had to quit his job or have that operation."

We told Dr. Zofchak that by coincidence, we had just read a medical journal article by a surgeon who reported on over a dozen cases of "migraine headache" that turned out to be nothing but cases of obstructed sinuses. In every case, the initial doctors treating the "headaches" had failed to make a careful check of the sinuses. Dr. Zofchak smiled at this but was clearly less than overwhelmed, as he has learned through the years that incorrect diagnoses by doctors are hardly unusual. It is worth noting that in this case, Dr. Zofchak's training as a naturopath may have played an important role, because naturopaths are trained to pick up subtle clues about a patient, such as the tone of his voice, the appearance of his eyes, the color of his skin, even his breath and body odor, which many M.D.'s simply ignore. Here, it was the tone of the laborer's voice that revealed he had a sinus problem. This by itself was no guarantee that his sinuses were causing his intractable headaches, but it did suggest that clearing up the sinus congestion was the first therapeutic target.

The herbal mixture which this man took consisted of horehound, coltsfoot leaves, wild cherry bark, eucalyptus, and mullein as the active ingredients, with a few other herbs added to improve the taste. Mullein and coltsfoot are probably the two most effective ingredients, Dr. Zofchak said, adding that to get the maximum effect against congestion, the brew should not only be taken as a tea, but the vapors of the simmering herb inhaled. If you want to, he says, you can put some of the tea into a vaporizer, or else stand over the hot herbs as they steam on the stove with a towel over your head as a hood, breathing in the aromatic and curative vapors.

## The Relaxing Herb

Valerian is another herb which Dr. Zofchak has found extremely helpful. When we asked him about high blood pressure, he recalled a case of one man who was getting "jittery and woozy" on his blood pressure medicine and asked for some tea. "He didn't tell me he was going to stop taking his medicine, but a few weeks later, he said that he had been to his doctor, and his blood pressure was down to normal. But he said he didn't have the nerve to tell the doctor that he had stopped taking the medicine and was drinking a tea composed mostly of valerian and hawthorn. Valerian, Dr. Zofchak explained, has a powerful relaxing effect on the parasympathetic nervous system. This herb was also of help to a retired Army captain with a long-standing heart condition who had taken all kinds of medication. After taking valerian he reported that "nothing has helped me more than this."

As a calmative, nervine, and antispasmodic, valerian also plays an important role in treating headaches. It should be combined with wood betony and camomile, Dr. Zofchak said, adding that if the headache is due to an upset stomach, peppermint should also be taken.

For insomnia, valerian again is indicated, this time along with lady's slipper, skullcap, passionflower, and hops. Because valerian, lady's slipper, and skullcap are all powerful relaxants, these herbs should only be taken in small amounts, Dr. Zofchak emphasized. In using valerian root, for example, only half a teaspoon is added to a cup of boiling water. When it cools, only one cup should be consumed a day, a large mouthful at a time. If lady's slipper or skullcap are also being used, proportionately less valerian should be employed, so that the total amount of all three herbs does not exceed more than one-half teaspoon a day. By drinking this tea a large mouthful at a time, any danger of overreaction is minimized, as the size of your mouth automatically tailors the dose to your size.

## Urinary Problems

Kidney and urinary problems are a common complaint with advancing age, and Dr. Zofchak recommends a tea brewed from buchu leaves, bearberry (*Arctostaphylos uva-ursi*), cubeb berries, and althea or marshmallow root as the active ingredients, with other herbs added for balance and taste, including anise, licorice, hydrangea leaves, and others.

"Many people come in after a prostate operation," Dr. Zofchak said. "The three major herbs indicated to ease prostate distress are buchu leaves, uva-ursi, and saw palmetto. Buchu leaves are especially valued for soothing irritation to the bladder. If there is a problem with incontinence of urine, St.-John's-wort is indicated at least for a trial. Remember," Dr. Zofchak stressed, "these conditions must not be oversimplified. Pain or irritation in any part of the body may stem from a number of causes. Just as the physician wants to find out exactly what the source of the trouble is, the herbalist, in attempting to cooperate with the program and help ease the person's pain, must also try to find out the underlying nature of the problem before he recommends a particular herb. Urinary incontinence, just as one example, may stem from a failure of muscle control, but may also be involved with structural damage, inflammation, irritation, allergy, or psychological problems. You can't—or shouldn't—approach herbalism with the idea that there's one herb for every symptom and expect to get very favorable results."

Kelp is not usually regarded as an herb, but to Dr. Zofchak, kelp is an herb from the sea. "Kelp contains organic iodine and trace elements such as gold, silver, and many others which act as catalysts, sparking vital enzyme reactions. Specifically, kelp increases thyroid metabolism and can help some people to reduce excess weight."

What about the old-fashioned mustard plaster? Does it really work, and what is it good for? "For sore, stiff muscles or a sore back, the mustard plaster really helps," Dr. Zofchak says. "It acts as a rubefacient—drawing blood to the area. This loosens up the muscles and carries away the toxins that cause the muscles to tighten up. Linseed oil also makes a good poultice for muscles that are in a spastic state. It's also good for softening boils."

Asked for a few examples of "home remedies" or folk medicine which he's personally found useful, Dr. Zofchak said, "My wife has an interesting one. When she gets an insect bite, such as a mosquito bite, she puts a little dab of toothpaste on it. She says it really takes the itch out fast.

"When one of the children gets a sore throat, they gargle with sage tea. This is a very fine gargle. In our house, we've also had occasion to use myrrh for gum irritation. My son had some dental work and developed gum irritation. The dentist gave him glycol to put on it, but that only made it worse. I made a mouthwash out of myrrh and the irritation quickly went away. You use one-quarter teaspoon of myrrh in one-third glass of water and wash your mouth with it. Or you can apply the wet powder to the gums directly at night and by morning you will notice that bleeding gums will be noticeably better."

## Herbs and Sex

Any discussion of herbs must get around to ginseng sooner or later. In the Orient, ginseng has long been regarded as the supreme herb, good for everything from sex problems to terminal diseases. We asked Dr. Zofchak what he honestly thought of ginseng.

"First of all, I think that American ginseng is definitely superior —if you can get it. Here, it grows wild in virgin soil, because it needs certain elements to grow and thrive. Korean ginseng is cultivated in the same soil year after year, and the reason why I think it isn't as good as American ginseng is that it is not getting the elements that it needs.

"Does it work? Many people tell me that they find it a good *tonic*, better than caffeine or even amphetamines. It has a sustained energy-building effect. Some like to chew on the root. In fact, I do this myself when I have to work very hard, and I find that it refreshes me."

And the sexual effect of ginseng? "Ginseng *does* have aphrodisiac power, because it works through the glands. I regard it as a normalizer of many functions. Now ginseng is not going to perform miracles. Many men have problems with their sex lives, and there can be many reasons for this, including, of course, psychological problems. A cup of ginseng tea is not going to abolish a problem that stems from a deep psychological cause. But I will say, though, that taken over a period of time, ginseng can have a general stimulating and normalizing effect, which may also help with the sexual problem."

And damiana? Is it truly the aphrodisiac it is reputed to be? "Yes, damiana is a powerful aphrodisiac," Dr. Zofchak declared. "If you are taking it, you should take it along with juniper berries and saw palmetto at the same time, which work to give strength and allay irritation of the sexual and urinary tract."

When the problem is menopause, he added, life root (female regulator) and motherwort are the herbs of choice.

Dr. Zofchak says he has often thought about a profound philosophical question that arises whenever herbs as healing agents are studied. "How is it," he asks, "that nature has provided us with herbs from the jungle, the ocean, the deserts, the high mountains, even the Arctic, that have so many different effects on us, and yet can safely be mixed together?" He has no easy answer to the question, if indeed there is one. In a purely practical vein, Dr. Zofchak advises that herbs can be mixed just like vegetables. "Your body will take what it needs from them and throw off the rest."

# A Pharmacist's Experiences With 'Yesterday's Miracle Drugs'
by Richard Lee Lindner, B.Sc., R.Ph.*

My childhood memories of "home remedies" are rather vivid, because both my mother and maternal grandmother were recognized in their small farm community as having quite some knowledge of herbs and their curative powers. In fact, in our neighborhood they were often referred to as "herb doctors," and as such, treated many complaints of their family and friends. As though it were yesterday, I remember a panic-stricken mother running through our front door, an infant in her arms, yelling for my mother. Mother took one look at the child, exclaimed "Seizure!" and grabbed the black mustard, ran some hot water into the bathtub and dunked the child in the mixture. What was happening, I do not exactly know, but I do know that the infant snapped out of her seizure. It must have been the shock of the mustard and hot water that brought her back to normal.

I can still see and smell our old smokehouse and attic, hanging full with drying herbs: sassafras root, often used as a blood tonic; elder and dandelion flowers for fevers; white elm and white birch barks for coughs and colds; pumpkin and raspberry seeds for "liver

*Richard Lee Lindner received his pharmacy degree from Philadelphia College of Pharmacy and Science in 1950 and currently operates his own small family pharmacy in Allentown, Pennsylvania.*

tonics"; and other leaves too numerous to mention, each having a specific function in the herb doctor's formulas.

What impressed me most was that my mother and grandmother knew exactly which plant or part of which plant was to be used alone or in combination with other plants for the treatment of a specific ailment.

The entire family was subject each spring to a week's course of spigelia-compound worm syrup, the theory being that every species of "animal" should be wormed at least once a year. A combination of boneset, catnip, and comfrey was administered for colds, fevers, and minor stomach complaints.

The "girls," as my mother and grandmother were referred to by my father, always had a cure for whatever ailed the human body and did not hesitate to use it. Although many of the medicines and mixtures were not very tasty, they must have done their job. My father, although critical, did not waste time when his stomach kicked up to have my mother mix up some camomile, catnip, and fennel, a mixture he used for many years. I must confess the whole family was disgustingly healthy; I believe we owed this entirely to the energy of the "girls."

Since I was the only member of the family not openly critical of some of their concoctions—perhaps because I was the youngest—I was more or less taken into the confidence of my mother and grandmother. Thanks to them, I have inherited many of these old family secrets and remedies. I have in turn used them in the treatment of some childhood maladies in my own children and can offer no complaints as to their efficacy.

## A Close Fight With Dysentery

My oldest daughter, at the age of nine weeks, contracted amoebic dysentery. The physician had never seen a similar case and referred us to a specialist, who treated her in the prescribed manner of the time—to no avail. She continued to lose weight, run a high fever, and was rapidly becoming dehydrated. After one week of treatment there was no response and she was slipping very close to the edge. The attending physicians advised hospitalization, although admitting they were not sure what could be done except retard dehydration.

The advice of my mother was to take the bull by the horns and treat my child as she had treated me and many others. We gave her boiled skim milk and a mixture of herbs and chemicals in miniature doses. In 24 hours the diarrhea stopped, the fever was lower, and a great general improvement was noticed. The specialist could not believe the improvement and when I told him what I had done, he remarked that his grandfather had used just such a treatment, but he was not aware that it was still available. I am proud to report that he has since used this mixture on some of the most stubborn cases with a very high percentage of success. The active ingredients in this remedy are bismuth subsalicylate, salol, fennel, catnip, and paregoric camphorata. But this is not something that I advise making yourself. It should, and in fact must be made by an experienced pharmacist (paregoric, which is tincture of opium, is a prescription item in most areas).

I have studied herbs from the academic point of view as well. As a registered retail pharmacist for the past 25 years, I have constantly been reminded of the practical application of crude plants and their active principles. During my college years I seemed to take naturally to my class in pharmacognosy, where a minimum of 154 crude plants and their potent constituents were separated and microscopically examined in order to identify them by their American name, Latin name, value, and the active ingredients of leaves, roots, seeds, flowers, and whole plants. Today, an in-depth study like this is not considered essential, as the use of these plants is restricted to a minority of people in this country. However, I cannot help but feel that some of us are missing a great deal by not using the knowledge passed down through time for the alleviation of some of man's ills.

I was very fortunate to have served my apprenticeship under a preceptor who was well versed in the collection, curing, and use of what were called "crude drugs" (crude in the sense that after drying, they are used in their original form). He encouraged my interest in herbs. His many years in a small "corner drugstore" only proved to him that there are many things to be said for "crude" plants and their value. He had many concrete examples in his old stockroom of the advantages of crude drugs. His tapeworm remedy was at that time over a hundred years old and just as effective then as now. He used an emulsion of male fern oleoresin (*Aspidium oleoresin*) which, to my knowledge, never failed to expel the worm, witnessed by numerous expelled worms housed in formaldehyde jugs that lined his shelves.

When he found I was interested and had some background in plant study, he opened up many avenues for study and confided some of his old remedies to me, a gift for which I shall be eternally grateful.

When I compare that time period with today, it isn't difficult to notice that most health professionals tend to focus their attention on the many man-made drugs, such as the growing family of anti-biotics. But these started from the study of mold growths and soil samples. So even here, we went to Mother Nature's bounty and then tried to improve on it.

Recently, though, it has been very pleasant to witness the inevitable return of interest in crude drugs. The general public is asking questions and looking for more definitive information on the use of plants and their extracts. I find this to be true in my own shop each day, and I share with others some of the knowledge I've gained.

## Slippery Elm's Many Uses

Elm bark, or slippery elm, as it is sometimes called, is generally used as the whole dried bark of the elm tree (*Ulmus fulva*). A poultice is made with equal parts of cornstarch and powdered elm along with black mustard as an external heat-producing decongestant for chest colds. The mixture is spread on white muslin or flannel and applied to the chest. Don't use more than 10 percent mustard at the very most. Slippery elm is also used in the form of a tea, often in combination with other herbs to coat the throat and stop coughing.

An old miner put elm bark to the most unique use I have ever seen. He bought the elm bark in its whole form (before it was powdered), consisting of long sticks looking just like the inner bark of a tree. He then broke the sticks into one-inch by one-inch pieces. To these pieces he added 10 drops of kerosene and then sucked on the bark during the day in the mine pits to keep the coal dust from adhering to his throat and make it easier to spit out the black dust. He explained this was an old miner's remedy used by his father in the Polish coal fields before he came to this country. Although sucking on kerosene is definitely a bad idea, on analysis this remedy makes a kind of sense: the kerosene would act as an irritant, causing him to cough, and the elm, because of its moistening nature, made the coughing easier, producing the desired effect.

Elm bark can be purchased in most drugstores either in the stick, chipped, or powdered form. By steeping it in boiled water, the characteristic mucilaginous matter is released. When cooled to a proper temperature it can be used whenever a soothing effect is desired, internally or externally. Medical science cannot agree on the precise value of elm in its many forms but this by no means indicates that it has no use!

## More Herbal Friends

Eucalyptus is a very interesting herb which comes chiefly from Australia. Its use in this country is so extensive that we import it by the ton. Most cough lozenges and cough preparations contain eucalyptus. Many nasal sprays also use some eucalyptus because of its cooling and soothing effect on the lining of the nasal passages: Dristan, Vapex, and Sinex are just a few of the many such products. An herbalist would generally use the pure expressed oil of eucalyptus in making liniments and creams. It has a peculiar effect in that it seems to cool at the same time that its mild irritant effect produces heat in the area to which it is applied. When eucalyptus, or any other herb, is used in the pure oil form, it is very concentrated, and a much smaller amount is needed than when you're using a simple infusion made from the whole herb.

In my opinion, one of our most useful herbs is fennel seed, which comes to us from the *Foeniculum vulcare*, as a dried, ripe fruit. Our greatest problem is getting enough pure fennel from Asia Minor, where it is commercially cultivated for export. Although it still comes to us in sufficiently large amounts, this herb is often adulterated with fruits of other similar plants, and when people in the trade buy it, we must know whom we are dealing with if we are to get the expected results.

I have used fennel seed by itself and in combination with other herbs as a carminative for mild stomach upset, especially for colic in infants. I am happy to say that all of our four children were raised on an old family mixture of fennel, catnip, and other dried herbs made into a rather tasty substance, which never failed to relieve their minor stomachaches. Fennel is also present in the preparation known as Official Catnip and Fennel Elixir (National Formulary) and is available in many pharmacies. Perhaps I should qualify this by saying it is available in most *older* pharmacies. I suppose that dates me, but the younger pharmacists feel, as they have been taught, that the use of "crude drugs" is outdated and passé. However, herbal remedies have had their critics for thousands of years, if we can believe our historical writers. I feel that in most instances, the herbs which survive do so because of their success, and often outlive their staunchest foes.

It is difficult for me to separate fennel from common catnip, since many of the old formulations call for a mixture of the two. With catnip (*Nepeta cataria*), we use the dried leaves and flowering tops. These leaves and flowers are still important enough in commerce to be raised and cultivated as a money crop. Catnip formulated as a tea is used for colic in infants and mixed with fennel and many other herbs as a tonic and stomachic (sour stomach sweetener). In my own experience, catnip (and catnip mixtures) is most effective and should not be passed over as another worthless weed.

Speaking again from my personal experience, one of the most impressive herbs is the common elder flower and its berries. I vividly recall walking down the old railroad tracks at high noon looking for elder flowers, because according to my mother and grandmother, the active constituents were more concentrated then, as the plant reached towards the sun. As a child this seemed to me rather ridiculous, but I learned in the years to come that each herb has an appropriate time to be harvested. I was only allowed to cut the uppermost berries in bunches, being careful not to disturb them or crush them. It was many years before I was allowed to remove the berries from the slim twigs, for as my mother explained, my hands were not yet well-enough educated to extract the berries in their whole state for the drying process.

Elder is of great value and is used with many other herbs in combination and by itself. It is fine when used as a tea to reduce fever and promote perspiration. It is also a mild stimulant. When allowed to ferment with dandelion, sugar, and other makings, a delicious sweet wine is produced which is both relaxing and healthful when properly imbibed. In the old days it was not considered ladylike to drink alcoholic beverages, but a glass of elder and dandelion wine was considered acceptable because of its therapeutic effect. Even when I was a child it was considered harmless for me to have a small wine glass of the nectar. Perhaps because of the many nostalgic memories connected with elder, I find it one of my favorites.

A long-time favored herb of my mother was feverwort or boneset. Once again, the leaves and flowering tops of the weedlike plant (*Eupatorium perfoliatum*) are used to make a steeped tea or decoction. As a fever-reducer, it has been my experience that it lives up to its name of feverwort ("wort" means herb). Although its taste leaves much to be desired, its effectiveness more than makes up for that. I believe my mother favored this herb because of a mixture she made with tansy. She used this combination for many illnesses, usually combined with still other herbs. On a visit to our home, the simple statement that you were not feeling up to par called for boneset tea or the boneset and tansy mixture. Although I know today many people did not care for the taste, I cannot remember anyone refusing the cup, even our old country doctor, who always made our house his last stop. I think he really wanted the elder wine but knew none would be forthcoming without the boneset first. So he suffered in silence.

Another of the older "drugs" that may prove interesting is tansy (*Tanacetum*). The dried leaves and flowering tops are used. After being dried they are made into a tea and used as an aromatic bitter to sweeten the stomach and increase the appetite. Another use, still in vogue, is for "female complaints." There are properties in tansy that when properly used, relieve the cramps of painful menstruation and delayed menses. Asiatic midwives have used tansy oil extract applied alone or in a clay pack to the abdomen of women with similar problems, and the herb is believed to bring on an easy childbirth. But let me hasten to point out that tansy can be toxic if taken in more than very small amounts. Used excessively, it can cause abortion. Herbalists who are aware of its good points as well as its dangers have long used tansy safely. But it must not be abused.

Licorice root, or sweet root as it is sometimes called, has been used in the past as a flavoring agent for the tobacco industry, in candy, and in many cough drops, because of its ability to cover or add to the taste of the drug contained therein. As a youth, I remember going to the drugstore for five cents' worth of sweet wood, which meant a handful of wooden roots that when slowly chewed gave up their delightful flavor and served as a real "candy" treat. The reference books tell me that licorice has been cultivated as a money crop since the early 13th century. The part used is the dried feeler roots.

Licorice, in the form of compound licorice powder, is a powerful laxative and is incorporated today in some of our most sophisticated medicines. Where constipation is due to "normal" systemic faults, I have never seen compound licorice powder fail to work as a complete bowel evacuant.

Licorice is found both wild and cultivated by peoples in all parts of the world, where it serves many small communities as their sole money crop. So we see that all herbs are not obscure and none are as obscure as some authorities would have us believe.

## How a Pharmacist Can Help

While the pharmacist usually serves his clients by filling a doctor's prescription or dispensing nonprescription medications, he can also admirably serve the person who is interested in using herbal preparations—providing he has the interest. Often, he can provide materials that are hard to come by in health food stores that carry herbs. Essential oils, which are very highly concentrated herbal extracts, are available in many pharmacies. Clove, wintergreen, sassafras, eucalyptus, and others are widely available. Other essential oils may be ordered for you. Such oils are ordinarily used in very small quantities, mixed with other materials. A small dab of oil of clove on a swab is an old but quite reliable way to numb the pain of a toothache.

The pharmacist can also be of great help in providing ointments and salves to act as the base or vehicle for herbs you want to apply topically. If you talk to your pharmacist and tell him what you want to do, he will be able to make a number of useful suggestions. He might recommend a cream, such as hydrophilic base, Vaseline, or lanoline anhydrous. If you want the product to be purely "natural," or as close to natural as possible, explain this to the pharmacist. Many ointments today contain synthetics, although it must be said that many of them are quite effective. If the pharmacist does compound something himself from scratch, it is naturally going to cost you more than a prepackaged item that contains more synthetics. For example, cold cream, or rose water ointment, has the following formula:

| | |
|---|---|
| Spermaceti | 125.0 gm. |
| White Wax | 120.0 gm. |
| Almond Oil | 560.0 gm. |
| Sodium Borate | 5.0 gm. |
| Stronger Rose Water | 25.0 ml. |
| Purified Water | 165.0 ml. |
| Rose Oil | 0.2 ml. |

If you are on good terms with your pharmacist, you can even benefit if he doesn't make up the formula for you. Just by learning what's *in* something like cold cream (notice the large amount of almond oil, which is so soothing to the skin), you can learn things which you can use at home.

The witch hazel that you buy from your pharmacist is a pure water of witch hazel with enough alcohol added to preserve it. However, if you buy oil of wintergreen, you'll have to pay 10 to 20 times as much for the natural oil as you will for the synthetic. The wintergreen alcohol you buy probably contains methyl salicylate.

The active ingredients of most herbs are more soluble in alcohol than water, especially when the water is not very hot. For this reason, our forefathers frequently mixed herbs with whiskey—usually adding about two to four ounces of the herb to a pint of whiskey. If you want to be more medicinal about it, you can get pure ethyl alcohol from a liquor store, but this is usually 90 percent alcohol or 180 proof and must be diluted by adding anywhere from an equal amount to four times as much water. A mixture of the active ingredient and alcohol, or alcohol and water, is known as a tincture. (Since it was frowned upon to drink alcoholic beverages in the past, some of the old-time herbalists used to say they made a nonalcoholic tincture, which by definition cannot be so. At best, they used a homemade wine such as elderberry or dandelion. Such beverages were considered to be "tonics" rather than true alcoholic beverages—a simple aid to salve one's conscience.)

An elixir is similar to a tincture in that it contains alcohol, but it is also aromatic and sweetened.

Let me say again that your average chain-store-type pharmacist is not apt to have the facilities or interest to help you much along these lines. But if you try a private pharmacy, you may find that the pharmacist has a great interest in herbs and has just been waiting for someone like you to walk in and ask him a question. He may feel, as I do, that we today are much too quick to buy any prepackaged "cure" advertised by Madison Avenue. In my own case, my 25 years of practicing pharmacy have only reinforced my childhood beliefs that the art of using and mixing herbs is well worth learning.

Let us all take another look at Mother Nature's gifts and enjoy the good health meant to be ours through them.

# The Ten Most Practical Medicinal Herbs: How to Grow and Use Them

Luckily for those who enjoy gardening but don't like to water their plants with perspiration, cultivating herbs in your backyard (or front lawn) is relatively easy. In general, herbs tend not to be very fussy about soil, don't require optimal fertilization, and are seldom bothered to any extent by bugs.

When we talk about growing and using the "most practical" herbs, we're referring to those which are not only famed for their medicinal properties (and often, good taste) but are also used frequently enough throughout the year to make it worthwhile cultivating them yourself. Goldenseal, for instance, is certainly a most useful herb, but its successful cultivation is no easy trick, and most people use it in rather small quantities. So it is probably more practical to buy your goldenseal root powder than to grow it yourself. Needless to say, the same goes for the bark of slippery elm and wild cherry. Comfrey, on the other hand, is definitely worth growing yourself, not just because it's easy, but because you will be able to use the fresh leaves as well as the dried, and harvest the roots in the early spring, when you can be sure that their content of allantoin is highest.

The herbs discussed below are mentioned frequently throughout the text of this book (along with dozens of other herbs) in relation to specific ailments and applications. Here, we are summing up some of what is known about how to use and grow them, and in some cases, giving additional information not mentioned elsewhere.

## Comfrey

Three thousand years ago, the Greeks in their wisdom were using comfrey, and it wasn't long before it was entered into the very earliest catalogs of medicinal herbs.

Three *hundred* years ago, the great Elizabethan herbalist Nicholas Culpeper listed comfrey among the most effective natural healing agents.

About *three* years ago, a woman in Veneta, Oregon, decided to apply a comfrey dressing to painful varicose veins that had troubled her for 13 years, threatening to immobilize her. Where countless doctors and remedies had failed, the herb succeeded.

Happily back on her feet, the woman told PREVENTION that comfrey truly "worked wonders."

Herbalist Juliette de Baïracli Levy calls comfrey ". . . another of the small company of 'wonder herbs', being good for almost every ill of mankind," and recommends eating several small leaves daily, cut up and eaten with other salad greens.

During the Middle Ages, comfrey was a popular remedy for mending broken bones and battle wounds. It earned the name "knitbone" because of the ability of its leaves, when applied directly as a poultice or salve, to reduce swelling around fractures and promote bone union. A decoction made by simmering an ounce of ground comfrey root in a quart of water for 30 minutes was taken internally to treat dysentery, diarrhea, and stomach ulcers. As a remedy for bleeding hemorrhoids or other internal bleeding, one-half ounce of witch hazel leaves was added to the preparation. Comfrey root tea has long been used to treat lung troubles and whooping cough. In parts of Ireland, comfrey was eaten as a cure for circulation troubles and to strengthen the blood.

Modern herbalists recommend a hot strong decoction of comfrey tea for bad bruises, swellings, sprains, and boils. Jethro Kloss recommends a poultice made of the fresh leaves for sore breasts, wounds, ulcers, burns, and gangrene. Where the skin is lacerated, of course, the poultice should never be uncomfortably hot.

Audrey Wynne Hatfield (*A Herb For Every Ill,* J. M. Dent & Sons, London, 1973) makes a comfrey poultice by chopping up the leaves and mixing them with boiling water. When they are cooled, she sandwiches them between gauze and applies to the skin. She notes, however, that "repeated applications may irritate, so apply lanolin first." She testifies that "with this treatment, my own fractured tibia [shin bone] was completely mended within eight days."

A comfrey ointment may be prepared by mixing a small portion of a concentrated comfrey decoction with a skin salve. Comfrey mixed with honey and vitamin E or wheat germ oil would make an admirable ointment to speed healing of minor burns and skin ulcers.

As Levy pointed out, comfrey also makes a beneficial addition to the daily diet. Science has discovered that comfrey is a rich source of calcium, potassium, phosphorus, and trace minerals. The leaves contain sizable amounts of vitamins A and C. Surprisingly, the plant also contains some vitamin $B_{12}$—usually found only in animal sources.

But the most important ingredient of comfrey is allantoin, believed to be a cell proliferant that can strengthen skin tissue and help heal ulcers. Charles J. Macalister, M.D., an English physician, wrote a fascinating treatise on comfrey and its allantoin back in 1936. Entitled *Narrative of an Investigation Concerning an Ancient Medicinal Remedy and Its Modern Utilities*, the slim book was republished in 1955 by the Lee Foundation for Nutritional Research, 2023 W. Wisconsin Ave., Milwaukee, Wisconsin 53201.

Dr. Macalister first became aware of comfrey through personal observation and medical reports of cases where comfrey was used to treat skin ulcers. One case, published in the *British Medical Journal* of June 8, 1912, related that an 83-year-old man with marked arteriosclerosis and other serious health problems developed an ulcer on his left foot, which rapidly spread and eventually exposed the very bones. The patient became delirious and was taken home to die. "He was then treated with four-hourly fomentations made with decoction of Comfrey root. The ulcer immediately began to fill up rapidly and was practically healed by the end of April [about four months after the beginning of treatment], and the patient's condition made corresponding improvement."

Chemical research showed that the active constituent of comfrey was a white crystalline substance readily soluble in hot water, but not cold, and identified as allantoin.

Allantoin is also present in the urine of pregnant women, and in plants is "generally found in parts which are related to growth, either active or potential." From this and other evidence, including the fact that allantoin is found in maternal milk, Dr. Macalister concluded that the substance is probably intimately related to the process of growth and the multiplication of cells.

Dr. Macalister was also struck by the "very interesting analogy" between the presence of allantoin in the fetal allantois, a tubelike sac which eventually becomes part of the placenta, and its presence in the root of the comfrey plant. "In the earliest months of pregnancy," he wrote, "dating from the third week onwards, the allantois becomes relatively large, and the amount of allantoin contained in it corresponds to some extent with the size of the sack [*sic*]. The vessels of the chorion conveying the maternal blood to the fetus pass through the allantois and probably derive the allantoin from it, to be utilized in the metabolism connected with growth and development. As pregnancy advances, the allantois diminishes in size and at length, shortly before the child is born, it becomes vestigial and the amount of allantoin infinitesimal."

And in the comfrey plant? In the earliest months of the year—January to March—Dr. Macalister explained, the rhizome, or small, relatively horizontal roots of the comfrey plant, contain a very high proportion of allantoin—from 0.6 to 0.8 percent. A few months later, it drops to 0.4 percent. By summer, when the plant is in full growth, practically no allantoin is in the rhizome "but it is discoverable in the terminal buds, leaves, and young shoots. This important fact may be regarded as evidence that the plant withdraws allantoin from its storehouse in the rhizome and utilizes it for purposes of cell-proliferation."

In numerous experiments with plants, Dr. Macalister writes, it was discovered that injecting a solution of allantoin into the bulbs of various plants caused them to grow much more rapidly than plants which were not injected.

He relates further experiences with using solutions of allantoin applied to serious skin lesions, which often produced truly remarkable results. As for gastric and duodenal ulcers, Dr. Macalister wrote that some results were good, and some uncertain, but it was his general impression "that allantoin and Comfrey are useful adjuncts to the general dietetic treatment."

Dr. Macalister in his own practice frequently used oral allantoin solution as supportive therapy for pneumonia patients and said that the patients in his wards, who were given allantoin, had a mortality rate 75 percent lower than that of patients in other wards who were not given allantoin. Blood counts, he said, showed that patients given allantoin had increased leukocytosis, or production of disease-fighting white blood cells, ranging as much as 83 percent higher than in the unsupplemented patients.

English folklore, to this very day, maintains that comfrey may be useful in fighting cancer. "A good many cases have been recorded where cancers, or sarcomatous growths are reported to have been benefited by treatment with Comfrey," Dr. Macalister says. However, he continues, scientific tests failed to show that either comfrey or allantoin has the ability to stop cancer or change a malignant cell into a normal cell. On the other hand, he admits, a survey of the results of using decoctions of comfrey and solutions of allantoin in cases of alleged malignancy "brings out the suggestive observation that nearly every case in which benefit seemed to ensue was treated either with the decoctions alone or sometimes with the addition of small amounts of allantoin." While this certainly proves nothing, he says, it does suggest that there may be something about either natural allantoin or the whole comfrey plant which is "superior" to synthetic allantoin. (Traditional herbalists would insist this distinction is true with every herb.)

In any event, when preparing a comfrey decoction, it is important to use distilled water, Dr. Macalister says, because allantoin is very sensitive to the action of alkalies. This might not be a great problem when you aren't isolating the allantoin, but only making a strong decoction. However, if you can get distilled water, or water which has only a minimal content of calcium and magnesium, you might be better off using it.

He offers two other guidelines. First, never boil water containing comfrey, because it may destroy the allantoin. Second, make solutions fresh each day, as older solutions are less useful.

**Growing Comfrey** • Ordering root cuttings through the mail is by far the cheapest and best method to begin raising comfrey. Plant cuttings about 2½ feet apart, three to six inches deep. Few growers have any success at all raising comfrey from seed. Once established, however, comfrey thrives in almost any soil or situation, although it does like added limestone or powdered dolomite. The plant is a hardy perennial, whose roots can withstand temperatures as low as 40° below zero. Keeping comfrey alive is no problem, but eradicating it is! A new plant will arise from the smallest portion of a severed root left in the soil.

In your garden, comfrey will be a fast grower that stands erect and tall, rough and hairy all over. Some varieties tower to five feet or more, but you can expect plants two to three feet high. Their roots are white and juicy and grow deep down into the soil where minerals are concentrated.

Keep in mind that the allantoin is concentrated in that part of the plant which is growing most rapidly. In winter and early spring, it's stored in the rhizome. As the plant grows, it moves up into the leaves, and eventually into the buds and young shoots. So, harvest some roots from your comfrey bed before spring growth. The leaves probably contain the most allantoin while they are still growing.

The tender first leaves can be used as salad greens. They are slightly fuzzy, though, so you'll want to chop them into tiny pieces if you're adding them to salad. Another possibility: run one or two fresh leaves through the juicer and mix with vegetable cocktail or tomato juice. Or you can make comfrey tea by adding one teaspoon of dried leaves to a cup of hot water. It seems best, though, to use the leaves fresh, rather than dried.

Larger, older leaves are coarse and unpleasant for eating, which should remind you that by this stage in the plant's growth, the allantoin is mainly in the buds. You don't have to worry about stunting the plant when you cut the younger leaves—if you leave a two-inch stub, you'll be amazed how quickly the plant grows back.

To get at the roots, clean them carefully and let them dry slowly in the sun, turning often. Once they're dried, they can be stored in a tight container. When you're ready to use them, powder or grind them and dissolve in hot but not boiling water, to form a mucilage that can be applied directly to the skin or taken internally as a tea.

## Garlic

The sun, the Cross, and garlic are the only three things reputed to scare away vampires. The famed pungent odor of garlic, however, is not necessarily the "active ingredient" in this particular usage of the herb; both the ancient Egyptians and Greeks regarded garlic as having supernatural powers.

That attitude towards garlic has lingered, like its aroma, down through the ages. Even today, there are people who maintain that garlic has so many beneficial properties that it should be regarded with suitable awe and used in generous amounts at the first sign of almost any illness.

It's generally accepted that garlic acts as a diuretic, stimulant, expectorant, and sweat promoter. For centuries, it has been a common European remedy for colds, coughs, and sore throats. During the 17th century, garlic was credited with protecting many European households from the ravages of the Great Plague. In New England during Colonial times, garlic cloves were bound to the feet of smallpox victims. Cloves were also placed in the shoes of whooping cough sufferers. For intestinal worms, raw garlic juice or milk which had been boiled with garlic was often drunk. A clove or two of garlic, pounded with honey and taken two or three nights successively, is good for rheumatism, herbalist lore tells us.

In World War I, garlic was used as an antiseptic in hospitals. Pads of sphagnum moss were sterilized, saturated with water-diluted garlic juice, wrapped in thin cotton, and applied as bandages to open wounds.

Garlic has long been recognized as one of the best natural worm remedies. Its rich content of allicin, found in the pungent volatile oil, is said to be responsible for this particular action. A number of people have told us of their success in ridding their dogs of worms by feeding them garlic. You can't depend upon it to always do the job, however. The same goes for treating worms in humans.

Arnold Krochmal tells us that "a fresh poultice made of the mashed plant, applied three times daily, has been used to treat snake bites, hornet stings, and scorpion stings." Other traditional uses which he mentions include browning garlic in honey and butter and eating it to treat kidney and bladder troubles, and placing the raw garlic clove against the gum to treat toothache.

Levy says that "the Gypsies worshipped this plant (*moly*) for its remarkable medicinal powers. It is one of the most powerfully antiseptic herbs known."

Hatfield says of garlic that "the herb's effects are to induce perspiring, stimulate energy, prompt urination, loosen congestion, cleanse the stomach, and aid digestion." It's also used for arthritis, rheumatism, sciatica, and sinus infections.

European and Russian physicians, but not, as far as I know, American physicians, have reported that garlic has two outstanding medical properties. One is that it tends to open up blood vessels and reduce blood pressure in hypertensive patients. The other property is antibiotic, and several researchers have found that garlic in large amounts can be effective against bacteria which may be resistant to other antibiotics. Because of this, garlic is sometimes called "Russian penicillin." According to reports, however, unlike penicillin, garlic only attacks pathogenic bacteria and does not destroy the body's normal flora.

You can use garlic in different ways. Many people take several garlic perles daily. Encapsulated in gelatin, the garlic is not released until the capsules are digested by the stomach, so the garlic odor on the breath is minimized, but not entirely eliminated. If you buy whole garlic cloves, or grow your own, which is remarkably easy, you will have other options. Crushed or bruised, the cloves can be added to almost any kind of food or hearty beverage. You can mash up the bulbs to apply to insect stings or express the juice and add small amounts to hot water or honey. The combination of honey and garlic is particularly popular, although if inflammation is present, the garlic may make it worse.

One of the nicest ways we know to eat garlic is to enjoy a piping hot bowl of garlic *soup* (believe it or not!). We tried this recipe from *Maurice Mességué's Way to Natural Health and Beauty* and found it surprisingly delicious.

> Cut up half-a-dozen cloves of garlic and sauté in oil, being careful not to let them burn. Add a quart of stock (I used beef stock) and let it come to a boil for just a few moments. Then lower the heat. Separate two eggs and add the whites to the hot liquid, stirring rapidly. Mix the yolks with two tablespoons of vinegar and then pour them in. Add salt and pepper if you want and some croutons if they're handy.

If the garlic aroma on your breath bothers you after eating garlic, try chewing up a few sprigs of parsley or some caraway seeds.

**Growing Garlic** • Garlic is easy to grow but requires a fairly long growing season. As early in the spring as possible you should buy some garlic bulbs, split them into cloves (there are usually eight to twelve cloves to a bulb) and plant each one separately. Put the cloves about two inches down into the soil, pointed end up, and six inches apart, leaving a foot between rows. Garlic will grow in almost any sunny spot, but it prefers moist, sandy soil. A dressing of well-rotted manure is helpful. Keep the weeds out, and you should be gathering the pungent bulbs by late August or September. After harvesting, braid the stalks together and hang up to dry.

## Camomile

It may take a few cups of camomile tea until you get used to the taste, but once you do, you will never want to be without a tightly sealed container of camomile flowers in your pantry. In our house, we use it as a beverage, often mixed with peppermint tea, and as a soothing and relaxing tea whenever minor illness appears.

The herbalist Kloss said that "everyone should gather a bag full of camomile blossoms as they are good for many ailments." He went on to enumerate its uses, which include helping indigestion, or poor appetite, a tonic for troublesome monthly periods, and an excellent wash for sore and weak eyes, as well as sores and wounds. Made into a poultice, it can be used for pains and swellings. Kloss also declares it "splendid for kidneys, spleen, colds, bronchitis, bladder troubles. . . ."

Dr. W. T. Ferni, in *Herbal Simples* (1897), declared that "no simple in the whole catalog of herbal medicines is possessed of a quality more friendly and beneficial to the intestines than Camomile Flowers."

Maude Grieve says that camomile tea is especially good for women during menstruation. "It has a wonderfully soothing, sedative, and absolutely harmless effect. It is considered a preventive and the sole certain remedy for nightmare."

Camomile may even be good for the other plants in your garden. Grieve relates that ". . . it has been stated that nothing contributes so much to the health of a garden as a number of camomile herbs dispersed about it, and that if another plant is drooping and sickly, in nine cases out of ten, it will recover if you place a herb of camomile near it."

Alma Hutchens tells us that in Russia they call camomile by the "tender-sounding name of Romashka." The demand is said to be great, and Russians use it from cradle on for colds, stomach troubles, a sedative, colitis, a gargle, and topically for eczema and inflammation. In India, Hutchens adds, camomile is called Babunah and is especially valued for women's complaints as well as indigestion and for soothing children.

The fact that the herb is used in Russia and India for almost exactly the same purposes as it is in England and the United States is a good indication that camomile deserves its reputation as one of the most beneficial and trustworthy herbs. From personal experience and reading, my impression is that the two best uses for camomile are for soothing an upset stomach—small amounts are good for colicky babies—and for inducing sleep.

There are two kinds of camomile, which causes some people a good deal of confusion. One variety is known as *Anthemis nobilis,* or Roman camomile. *A. nobilis* is a low-growing perennial, seldom topping more than nine inches in height. It is often nearly prostrate and is strongly scented.

The other variety is known as *Matricaria chamomilla,* or German camomile. One of the major importers of camomile told me that he gets the herb from Hungary for the most part, and it is *Matricaria,* not *Anthemis.* Which herb is the most useful? That depends on whom you ask. If you ask an herbalist in Germany, he or she will tell you that *M. chamomilla* is the real herb, while Roman camomile is only a weed. Ask an herbalist in England, and you'll probably get the exact opposite reply.

**Growing Camomile** • If you're going to grow camomile, it is much easier to use *Anthemis* because it's a perennial and can be easily managed by root division. If you want to grow German camomile, you will have to obtain seeds, which are very tiny and do not have an outstanding germination rate. The instructions we give, therefore, will be for *Anthemis,* which is the variety most easily available in the United States.

In the garden, camomile is perhaps best known for its applelike fragrance and flavor. It is a low-growing, creeping or trailing plant whose leaves give it a feathery appearance. The flowers resemble daisies; there are large yellow center discs surrounded by creamy white petals. Camomile is sometimes called the "herb of humility" because it seems to grow best when it's walked on. In England, it was planted as a fragrant lawn.

To cultivate camomile purchase some mature, *double-flowered* (more potent than single-flowered) plants, and in March, divide each into a dozen or more smaller plants by pulling apart the roots into smaller clumps. Plant each of them in rows 2½ feet apart, with a distance of 18 inches between the plants.

Camomile doesn't require especially fertile soil, but you might want to add some dried cow manure (available at many lawn and garden centers) to insure an adequate supply of nitrogen.

When the plants bloom, you're ready to pick and dry the flowers. You'll need an airy spot, away from direct sunshine. Spreading the flowers on an old window screen is an ideal solution—not just for camomile flowers, but for any other herb as well. That way, air circulates underneath and all around the leaves or flowers, speeding the drying process.

To brew camomile tea, bring a cup of water to a boil, remove from the heat and drop in about two teaspoons or more of the dried flowers—depending upon how strong you like your tea—and allow to steep for about 10 minutes. Be sure there's a tight lid on the container to prevent steam (and medicinal value) from escaping. Then strain off the flowers and enjoy a warm and soothing drink.

## Peppermint

Peppermint, the source of menthol, is one of the oldest household remedies and grows easily in almost any garden. Its brisk aroma and stimulating taste make it a fine beverage in itself, but its wonderful ability to make the stomach happy means it will be doing double duty after a large meal. If you have the chills-fever-upset stomach syndrome, there are few things that will do you more good than a hot cup of peppermint tea, perhaps mixed with camomile. An alternative during a cold or the flu would be an equal amount of peppermint and elder (perhaps spiked with a little yarrow or boneset).

Kloss recommends peppermint tea for headaches. Drink a few strong cups and lie down.

In many respects, peppermint is similar to spearmint, except that it is more powerful. Grieve recommends spearmint when a child has an upset stomach or is nauseous, because it is milder than peppermint.

**Growing Peppermint** • In the garden, peppermint likes moist, rich soil but isn't very fussy about it. Because it often cross-pollinates to produce small variations from plant to plant, peppermint is best started by cuttings or root division of a purchased plant. The cuttings should be spaced at least two feet apart because runners spread rapidly. In fact, peppermint is such a vigorous grower that you must watch your peppermint patch carefully if you don't want it to completely take over your garden or lawn. If you're growing peppermint along with other herbs, it's best to give the peppermint a separate bed.

Hand weeding among the runners is very important, especially to keep out grasses and clover. A thin mulch will help keep the weeds down, but don't make it too thick, or it will hamper the development of young shoots.

Peppermint is ready for harvesting when the lower leaves begin to yellow. The entire plant, including shoots of runners, should be clipped one inch from the ground. Don't leave any stems with leaves; disease might take hold. With luck, you can harvest the plants twice more in the season. After the last harvest in fall, cover the exposed roots with a two-inch thick blanket of compost to protect and fertilize them for next year.

If you want dried peppermint, strip the leaves from the stems and set them aside in a warm, shady spot. When dry, crumble the leaves and store them in tight jars. Good peppermint tea can also be prepared from fresh leaves. Cover a cupful of chopped, fresh herb with two cups of boiling water, let steep for just five minutes, strain, and serve with a squeeze of lemon.

In the Middle East, mint is considered primarily a salad material. You can use it in this way, too, by chopping up a half-cupful of fresh mint leaves very fine and thoroughly mixing them with other greens in a tossed salad. Or try adding chopped mint leaves to cream cheese.

## Cayenne

Most people don't think of the hot red pepper—which is what cayenne is—as a medicinal herb. But herbalists love cayenne, and they don't limit their enjoyment to putting it on hoagies and steak sandwiches.

Kloss calls cayenne "one of the most wonderful herb medicines that we have" and terms it a "specific" for fevers. Take some in capsules, he says, followed by a glass of water. Other authorities highly recommend cayenne, often called by its Latin name *Capsicum,* as a gargle for sore throat, a powerful stimulant, and a hangover remedy. West Indians soak the pods in hot water, add sugar and the juice of sour oranges, and drink freely when feverish. This seems to make a lot of sense, as the cayenne would induce cooling perspiration, the sugar supply energy, and the oranges add lots of vitamin C and bioflavonoids.

Levy calls cayenne "a supreme and harmless internal disinfectant."

R. C. Wren calls it "the purest and most certain stimulant in herbal *materia medica. . . .* A cold may generally be removed by one or two doses of the powder taken in warm water."

To make a powerful liniment for sprains and congestion, gently boil one tablespoon of cayenne pepper in one pint of cider vinegar. Bottle the unstrained liquid while it's hot. One authority says that to relieve the pain of a toothache, first clean out the cavity of the tooth, then make a small plug of absorbent cotton saturated with oil of capsicum. Press this into the cavity. It will probably burn like the devil at first, but it's said to be a good remedy, and the effect long lasting.

Cayenne from Sierra Leone in Africa is said to be the most pungent and medicinal. Common paprika is the most mild form of cayenne but is also the highest in vitamin C content.

Mature hot red peppers are bursting not only with heat, but nutrition. Ounce per ounce, they have more vitamin C than anything else you can probably grow in your garden: 369 mg. per 3.5 ounces. The same goes for vitamin A content: a whooping 21,600 units. In tropical areas, where people eat goodly amounts of hot peppers every day, they're also getting important amounts of iron, potassium, and niacin from these spicy pods. (Sweet green peppers, when they turn red, are also highly nutritious, but are inferior to the hot variety on every count.)

**Growing Cayenne** • Although cayenne is native to the tropics, you can grow it with good results in temperate latitudes. In fact, it should do as well as tomatoes or eggplant would in your garden, reaching a height of two feet or more by late summer and bearing long, podlike fruit. Cayenne grows best in soil that is quite rich. But even if you have average garden soil, you can get satisfactory results by fertilizing with compost, rock phosphate, greensand, and wood ashes.

The hot red peppers have a long growing season (14 to 18 weeks) so it's best to start them indoors from seed. Get the Long Red Cayenne variety. About two weeks or more after the last frost— when the soil has warmed up some—you should set the young plants out in the garden 12 to 18 inches apart, allowing three feet between rows. The plants will need plenty of water during the early stages of growth, but a thorough straw mulching will protect them against drought later in the season.

Cayenne peppers are ready to be harvested when the fruit has turned uniformly bright red. Don't pull the peppers off; cut the stems one-half inch from the pepper cap. Hot peppers keep best if they are dried immediately and then stored in a cool, dry place. So string them up on a line to dry. Or you can pull the entire plants and hang them upside down in a well-ventilated place until the peppers dry.

When perfectly dry, the peppers can be ground into a fine powder.

## Sage

"Sage is singular good for the head and braine; it quickneth the sences and memory . . . and put into the nostrils, it draweth thin flegme out of the head," the herbalist Gerard wrote several centuries ago. Today, sage is still highly valued, although primarily as a gargle and mouthwash for sore throat or inflamed gums. Made into a poultice, it is recommended for ulcers, sores, and other skin eruptions. Its astringent quality will also help staunch the flow of blood from small wounds. Whether or not it will do anything for your memory, no one really knows, but tradition says that it will. David Conway states that sage "is also powerfully nervine [relaxing to the nerves] and will stop any involuntary trembling of the limbs." Maybe. Levy reports that sage is "believed" to quell "vicious sexual desires," but at the same time "will also restore normal virility when the failure is not due to venereal disease." It seems you can't go wrong with sage!

More realistically, sage does seem to be helpful for sore throats and is widely recommended for colds and coughs. Red sage, if you can get it, is preferred by some herbalists.

But you don't have to be sick to enjoy the bracing effect of sage. Try adding half an ounce of fresh sage leaves to the juice of one lemon or lime. Sweeten with honey and infuse in a quart of boiling water removed from the heat. Strain and serve either hot or ice cold.

If you have an electric blender, try mixing a cup of fresh sage leaves into a half-quart bottle of Claret or Burgundy. Run it on high speed until the leaves are pulverized and thoroughly suspended in the wine. Then put the wine back in the original bottle. During winter months, sip small amounts, perhaps diluted with a small amount of water, as a tasty tonic.

**Growing Sage** • Sage is a hardy perennial but after three or four years it tends to become woody and tough. Sage is easy to start from seed because the seeds are large and can be spaced and observed well in their early growth. Place the seeds a foot apart in the early spring. Sage likes a sunny area without strong wind and plenty of water, especially when it's young. Companion-planting experts recommend putting sage next to rosemary in a garden for a beneficial effect on both. Harvest leaves from high up on the stem no later than September. The first year you won't get much, but by the second year, you'll be able to get at least two cuttings. Dry the leaves in the shade until they're crisp. If you're going to use them for tea, just crumble them. If you want to use them for seasoning, rub them through a fine screen.

Sage leaves can also be used fresh. Rubbed on the teeth, they are said to keep them remarkably clean. Chopped fine, they may be added to a salad or mixed with butter or cream cheese.

## Horseradish

Like garlic, hot peppers, and onions, horseradish is usually thought of as a food or a spice rather than a medicinal herb. But like its pungent companions, horseradish has a solid reputation as a healing herb.

Externally, fresh chopped or grated horseradish has been mixed with a little water and applied as a heat-producing and pain-relieving compress for neuralgia, stiffness, and pain in the back of the neck. Conway says that chopped horseradish is antiseptic, relieves local discomfort, and encourages healing.

The classic internal use of horseradish is to treat kidney conditions where excessive amounts of water are retained. Horseradish is believed to be one of the more potent herbal diuretics. A traditional preparation consists of one ounce of fresh, chopped horseradish root, one-half ounce of bruised mustard seed, and a pint of boiling water. Let the herbs soak in the water in a covered vessel for four hours, then strain, and take three tablespoons three times a day. Horseradish can also be eaten spread on some bland food like bread or fish, mixed with vinegar, or diluted in almost any way imaginable. One favorite way to take it when you want to flush fluids out of your system is to mix it with white wine.

A syrup made of grated horseradish, honey, and water is one of the standard remedies for hoarseness.

Lelord Kordel tells us that horseradish was high on the list of Gypsy remedies. Gypsies, he says, take horseradish for coughs, colds, and bronchitis, and eat the leaves of the plant to combat food poisoning. "They add horseradish to vegetable juices to stimulate digestion and to aid the passing of urine through faulty kidneys. For rheumatic pains, they either eat the horseradish or mix it with boiled milk as a compress."

**Growing Horseradish** ● Horseradish is a perennial and propagation is by root cuttings only. Cuttings should be made from straight roots and should be six to seven inches long and include a bud—although any piece of root will develop buds and shoots. For this reason, horseradish should be planted in the corner of the garden that will be kept strictly for horseradish.

Horseradish prefers wet, clay soil and must be planted early for a good fall crop. The ground should be deeply tilled in January and fertilized with rotted manure or compost. Plant your root cuttings in February, 12 to 15 inches deep and 12 to 18 inches apart each way. The horseradish bed should be weeded regularly.

Expect to harvest your crop in the fall. Wash the roots and store them in damp sand in a root cellar. They should last through the winter and can be grated fresh as needed. Or, if you wish, you can leave the roots in the ground where they grew and simply dig them up when you want them.

## Catnip

Catnip can be thought of as nature's Alka-Seltzer. Herbalists recommend it highly for upset stomach, nervous headache, and promoting perspiration to cool a fever. Krochmal relates that "In Appalachia, a tea made from the plant is used for treating colds, nervous conditions, stomach ailments, and hives. . . ." Its use may well have been learned from American Indians, who, Michael A. Weiner tells us, often used it for infant colic. Kloss describes catnip as one of the oldest household remedies, mentioning among other uses, a catnip infusion as an enema for babies with intestinal colic and for "hysterical headaches."

Grieve says that catnip produces free perspiration and is very useful in colds, fever, restlessness, and nervousness. Conway reports that catnip is an antispasmodic and "is used in Wales to stop persistent coughs and hiccups. . . . The dosage is one or two tablespoonfuls daily in the standard infusion, which is prepared from the whole plant above ground."

When preparing catnip tea, never boil it. Just let it steep in a covered vessel. And do not drink too much hot catnip tea, because in excessive doses, it can produce nausea. Catnip tea is probably best taken with camomile and peppermint, sweetened with honey. This should be an excellent combination for relieving the symptoms of colds, headaches, and indigestion.

**Growing Catnip** ● Catnip is a delicately perfumed herb with heart-shaped, downy-haired leaves that look as if they have been coated with blowing dust. Catnip prefers a rich soil but will do all right almost anywhere that the soil is light and there is ample sunshine. Adequate moisture is no problem, either.

A hardy perennial that requires no attention, catnip will last for several years if its bed is kept free of weeds. If you're interested in raising your own catnip, spring is the best time to get started, either planting seed or root dividing an older plant into three or four new ones. New divisions should be transplanted immediately, but watch out! If not protected, they can easily be destroyed by enthusiastic cats. Sown from seed, however, the herb won't attract cats unless the plant is bruised. Rows should be spaced 18 inches apart, and the seedlings thinned to 12-inch intervals. Catnip grows fast and appreciates a mulch of hay, straw, or cocoa hulls.

Harvesting can begin anytime after the plant matures and blooms, but before any yellowing begins. Strip the leaves off the plant and set out on screens or newspaper to dry. Don't leave the drying leaves in the sun, or catnip's volatile oils will be lost. When the leaves are thoroughly dry (after three days to a week), crumble them into pieces but *not* a powder. Discard all large stems, then pack in tight containers and store in a dry place.

## Rosemary

"Take the flowers and put them in a lynen clothe, and so boyle them in fayre cleane water to the halfe and cole [cool] it, and drynke it for it is much worth against all evyls in the body."

So says *A Lytel Herball,* written in 1550.

Prime among the "evyls in the body" which we moderns worry about is heart trouble. And herbal tradition, if not modern science, has it that rosemary is good for the heart. Levy, who says she uses it "more than any other plant," calls rosemary "a proved supreme heart tonic, one of the few powerful heart tonics which is not a drastic drug."

More modestly, Grieve says that the young tops, leaves, and flowers of rosemary made into an infusion make a good remedy for headache, colic, colds, and nervous diseases. Both tension and depression are said to respond to the charms of rosemary.

Levy tells us that the Arabs sprinkle dried powdered rosemary on the umbilical cord of newborn infants "as an astringent and antiseptic." She likes it internally for high blood pressure, headaches, and threatened abortion, and externally for wounds and stings.

Mességué believes rosemary is effective against rheumatism, paralysis, weakness of the limbs, and vertigo. He also thinks that rosemary sprinkled into bath water is very stimulating for sickly children and old people. But bath water isn't the only place you can sprinkle your rosemary if you want to be stimulated. Rosemary wine is very popular in Europe. Here are two simple ways to make it:

Chop up some leaves and green sprigs and cover with light wine. Let stand for four or five days, strain off the wine, and drink it. Or simply put about two ounces of rosemary into a bottle of Bordeaux and let it steep for a few days.

A third-of-a-teaspoon each of rosemary, anise, and peppermint, steeped in a cup of hot water, produces a pleasant mouthwash. One ounce each of rosemary and sage infused in a pint of water for 24 hours makes a hair tonic for treating dandruff. Water in which rosemary has been boiled is said to benefit the skin when used as a wash. And oil of rosemary, made by soaking the plant's tops and leaves in a good vegetable oil for a week, can be rubbed directly on sore or sprained areas.

Rosemary is tangy enough to flavor beef, veal, and other meat dishes. If you grow your own, you can put fresh cuttings directly on roasts and poultry.

**Growing Rosemary** ● Rosemary is a perennial evergreen shrub that grows as high as four feet. Its woody stems with boughs of dark green needles and blue flowers make it a very pleasing ornamental bush. The herb requires a well-drained, alkaline soil. If the growing bed isn't naturally chalky, added lime, eggshells, or wood ash will help. Rosemary needs to be looked after and watered occasionally; it is vulnerable to dehydration. Plants should have a sheltered, southern exposure where they will get maximum sunlight. In winter they should be protected against the cold by burlap or a small, plastic greenhouse arrangement. Because seeds often fail to germinate (and those that do take three years to produce a mature bush), rosemary is best started by cuttings or root division of established bushes. Cuttings may be taken in February or March and again in May or June after the plant has flowered. Just take a six-inch tip of a new growth and bury its lower four inches in vermiculite. The sprouted cutting will be ready to transplant in two to three months.

## Coltsfoot

Coltsfoot is the herb to take when you're trying to get over a chest congestion, with or without a cough.

It has been used in many ways. People once snuffed the powdered leaves into their nostrils to relieve nasal obstruction and headache. A strong decoction of the green leaves, sometimes with the roots, is probably the most popular way to take coltsfoot. It may be sweetened with honey or licorice.

Grieve calls coltsfoot "one of the most popular of cough remedies," which is generally taken with horehound, marshmallow, and other herbs. In fact, she points out, the Latin name for coltsfoot, *Tussilago,* means "cough dispeller." In England, the dried leaves of coltsfoot are often smoked by asthmatics or others with congestion.

Rather than smoking coltsfoot, I would suggest standing over a simmering pan of coltsfoot and breathing deeply of the vapors. Hot coltsfoot tea should also be taken, mixed with slippery elm and perhaps some sage.

To make your own cough syrup, cover one ounce of *fresh* coltsfoot leaves with a pint of water and boil down until just a cup remains. Then strain and add honey, bringing the syrup to a boil. Bottle it, and you've got a centuries-old, homegrown cough remedy to be taken in tablespoon doses as needed.

**Growing Coltsfoot** • Named for its horsehoof-shaped leaves, coltsfoot grows so abundantly in wild places and pastures that many people consider it a troublesome weed. But its very tenacity, combined with its reputation as an outstanding healer, makes it a good selection for the medicinal herb garden. Coltsfoot is indifferent to poor soil. It grows well in both wet and dry conditions. All it really needs is full sun.

You can raise coltsfoot quite easily, either from seed or from root cuttings. Once established, the plants spread out and make an excellent ground cover. Orange-colored blossoms appear as early as February, even before there are any leaves. Both the flower stalks and leaves are used by herbalists, the former being collected in February, the latter in June or July. The material can be dried by spreading out on newspapers or screens in a dry, well-ventilated area.

# Dangerous Herbs

Never take any herb internally (or externally, for that matter) unless you know exactly what it is and what it may do. Unfortunately, there are some books which recommend herbs known to be toxic with little or no warning. One paperback book, which presents a mishmash of herbal remedies from Dr. W. J. Simmonite and Culpeper, even recommends squill, an herb which you may well find in your local hardware store in the rat poison department.

The following list is not meant to be comprehensive, but it does present some of the more common and a few of the uncommon herbs with toxic potentials.

In general, it is safe to say that you should never use the following herbs for a home remedy: jimsonweed, daffodils, spurge, arnica, wormwood, mandrake, hellebore, squill, poison hemlock (looks like parsley), tobacco (internally), tonka beans, aconite, white bryony, nux vomica, calabar bean, camphor (internally), ergot, ignatius beans, bittersweet, gelsemium, henbane, celandine (externally), belladonna (deadly nightshade), foxglove (source of digitalis), and mayflower.

Some herbs may be used with safety in small amounts but one should be very cautious with them. These include tansy, rue, valerian, lobelia, goldenseal, and bloodroot. Tansy is narcotic and may cause abortion. Valerian in excessive doses may cause headaches and even delusions (never boil valerian). Goldenseal should present no problems if taken in weak doses, something on the order of one-quarter teaspoon in a cup of hot water.

Levy warns that pennyroyal should not be taken by pregnant women.

# 'Quack' Salad and Cancer
## by Jim Duke *

Retiring at age 65, my father looked forward to a full life of golf, something his insurance career would not fully permit. Cancer cut him down less than a year later, just as it did at least two of his

*Jim Duke is a professional botanist who runs a small vineyard called the Herbal Vineyard in Fulton, Maryland. There he cultivates over 100 different kinds of herbs and 60 varieties of grapes. "It's a kind of Noah's Ark of the vegetation world," he says.*

brothers, both shortly after age 65. He didn't smoke or drink, and he advised against such habits. Childishly I told him they'd have a cure for cancer before my time came. That was when I was around 20. He died when I was nearly 30. Still no cure or prophylaxis for all cancers was in sight.

By the time I was 40 I feared my prediction had soured. There was no cure for most cancers. So I kicked the three-pack-a-day smoking habit. But the tars of 25 years of intensive smoking coat my lungs.

My father and his brothers died of cancer of the lower bowel. They had graduated from the fibrous farm diet they lived on as kids in the Deep South to the refined bread, meat, and potato diet of modern America. It seems generally accepted now that lack of fiber in the American diet correlates with cancer of the lower bowel. That's why you'll often find me eating unhusked cereals and seeds. I need the fiber that the food processing industry goes to such pains to remove (with considerable energy expenditure).

Repeating now that science has not yet come up with a cure for all cancer, I have resorted to folk medicinal lore which has given science such esteemed and powerful drugs as atropine, cocaine, henbane, ipecac, morphine, and reserpine. Now I have listed for myself and others who might like to live dangerously 30 salad plants that have been reported by Dr. Jonathan Hartwell of the National Cancer Institute (in the journal *Lloydia*) as folk cures for cancer.

| | | | |
|---|---|---|---|
| absinthe | chicory | flax | salvia |
| arnica | chive | garlic | stinging nettle |
| atriplex | chufa | hot pepper | tamarind |
| beet | colocynth | licorice | tansy |
| black walnut | crimson clover | onion | tea |
| borage | crown vetch | peanut | tomato |
| calendula | cucumber | poke salad | |
| celery | cumin | safflower | |

Of the 30 species cited in my "quack" salad recipe, over half possess some compound that has been useful in some treatment of some type of cancer.

Now I'll be the last one to say that tossing all these ingredients will cure or even alleviate cancer. I'll be the first to say, however, that you can make a decent salad combining these ingredients, using large portions of the standard salad ingredients and smaller portions of the strangers. I have sampled at least one leaf each of these plants and survived. I imagine I am helped more than hurt by having eaten these items. All plants manufacture important vitamins, and probably all manufacture some ingredients that are toxic if consumed in large quantities. Several thousand have been used in folk "treatment" of cancer, and many of these have scientific merit in the treatment of one cancer type or another.

I can't guarantee that the "quack" salad will cure or even prevent cancer. I imagine most people would be healthier if they ate such a salad once a day. I will surely nibble on these on my daily visit to my "quack" salad greenhouse. When time permits, I'll mix up the salad, using lemon juice, hot pepper, and garlic as a salad dressing. This is a dressing used by several Indian tribes of Latin America, among them the Cuna Indians of Panama. All three of the dressing ingredients show up in folk "cures" for cancer.

If even 10 percent of these folk treatments for cancer in "quack" salad have, in fact, some effect on some type of cancer, I figure I'm improving my odds by indulging my flight into folk fantasy. Genetically, the cancer odds are stacked against me. I quit smoking to change my odds. I eat sunflower seeds to improve my odds. And I'll eat "quack" salad, hoping to further improve my odds.

## Pharmacognosy, The Scientific Approach to Medicinal Herbs

Herbal medicine does not, as many of us suppose, begin and end with folk traditions. Although its beginnings have tentatively been traced back thousands of years, and for most of its history, herbalism has been closely linked with religion, astrology, and superstition, there is also a purely scientific approach to the world of herbs, known as pharmacognosy.

A pharmacognosist has expert knowledge of the chemical constituents of plants, how to go about identifying new chemicals and even molecules which occur in plants, and how various cultures use plants to their benefit, with particular interest in their medical applications. A pharmacognosist may, for instance, travel through a rural area such as Appalachia, or a remote jungle area, learning how the residents use plants for healing, and observing their actual use. He would then collect these herbs, take them back to a laboratory, and subject them to various sophisticated analyses.

Most typically, a pharmacognosist is interested in isolating and describing the active ingredients or "bioactive molecules" of plants. And his or her investigations might lead to attempts to synthesize these bioactive molecules, or to experiment with changing them slightly to achieve certain desired effects, such as increased activity, less toxicity, greater stability, and so forth.

Surprisingly, a recent survey revealed that close to 50 percent of all prescriptions written today contain drugs which are either directly derived from natural sources or synthesized from natural models, as the sole ingredient or as one of the several ingredients. To a pharmacognosist, there is no meaningful difference between a drug which has been synthesized and the natural substance on which its design is based. And the decision—made by drug companies—as to whether a given medicinal substance ought to be used in its natural state or synthesized is almost entirely an economic one. One herbal "drug," for instance, might be so easy to grow and harvest that it would not be worth the investment to synthesize it. Another natural "drug" might be very difficult to obtain in the wild but very easy to synthesize in the laboratory. Still another herbal "drug" might be expensive to collect in the wild, but its "bioactive molecules" may either be unidentified or simply too complicated to synthesize, so the wild sources must be used.

Traditional herbalists are strongly opposed to the use of "bioactive molecules" instead of preparations made from whole herbs. They argue that even if the "active" ingredients are chemically identical, the other constituents naturally found in the plant are there for a purpose, either to help the "active" ingredients or to help protect against possible overdoses or side effects.

I asked one pharmacognosist what he thought of popular or traditional herbalism, and he explained that while it certainly had some validity, doctors cannot use herbs unless they are absolutely certain of their purity, potency, amount, and availability to the body. Therefore, it is impossible for them to use preparations made from whole herbal materials, because these properties simply cannot be measured in an herb when it is still in its "crude" form. To do otherwise with a potent herbal substance such as atropine or digitalis, for example, would be to risk a possibly fatal overdose—or a possibly fatal *under*dose.

As for commonly used herbs such as garlic, peppermint, sage, and so forth, this pharmacognosist said that in general, his profession believes that they *do* have certain medicinal properties, but they are relatively weak and not sufficiently dependable to use in a medical setting.

I thought it would be a good idea to include in this volume an actual example of the kind of work that pharmacognosists do. I am therefore presenting here a report on saffron (true saffron, not American saffron or safflower), which was written by Dr. Ara Der Marderosian. My interest in this herb was triggered by some very sketchy reports about its possible value to the circulatory system, but ultimately, because the research so far is very preliminary and because the herb is fantastically expensive (and liable to be diluted with safflower), I decided not to pursue the matter further for the time being. But Dr. Der Marderosian's report constitutes an excellent example of the kind of knowledge and research involved in pharmacognosy.

Actually, I had to delete certain portions of Dr. Der Marderosian's report because of space considerations and the extremely technical nature of some of the material. You should understand that what follows is not a complete report, and that the original contained a good deal more technical information, including charts showing the molecular structure of some of the substances discussed.

## A Pharmacognosist Looks at Saffron: New Medical Findings on Crocin and Crocetin from Crocus sativus L. (Iridaceae)

**by Ara Der Marderosian, Ph.D.**

*Professor of Pharmacognosy*
*Philadelphia College of Pharmacy and Science*

". . . I must have saffron, to colour the warden pies . . ."

*The Winter's Tale,* act iv, scene iii, Shakespeare

Plants have been long known from almost all historical writings to possess "curative" or healing qualities. In the Bible, for example, over 100 plants are mentioned which have uses beyond their usual edible properties. One of these is saffron, also known by its botanical name, *Crocus sativus* L. (Family Iridaceae). The stigmas of this plant have been valued for their vivid orange red color as a food dye and for the characteristic aroma they possess. The crocus is first mentioned in the Song of Solomon of the Bible (4:13-14) and throughout history has been widely suggested and used in medicine as a diaphoretic (to induce perspiration), carminative (to expel gas), and as an emmenagogue (to induce abortion). While the first two of these properties may be attributed to certain principles of the plant, there is little or no evidence for any bona fide abortifacient effects.

The thin, dried stigmas of the flowers make up the true saffron of commerce, long recognized as the world's most expensive spice. The wholesale price in recent years has ranged from $80 to $120 a pound in large quantities in major ports of entry like London and New York. At gourmet shops and other retail food outlets, it brings anywhere from 80 cents to over one dollar a gram (approximately ⅟₃₀ of an ounce). Bought in bulk at the retail level, true saffron currently costs well over $200 a pound.

It is interesting to note that the word "saffron" has its origins in the Arabic word "zafaran" which means yellow. The Arabs introduced the cultivation of saffron into Spain about 921 A.D. At one time, before the advent of the synthetic coal-tar dyes, it was widely used as a natural dyestuff for cloth. One still can note its use as a dye among the people of the underdeveloped countries and, curiously, also among latter day "do-it-yourself" craftsmen, e.g., those who do rug hooking and knitting using home-dyed material or yarn in the more affluent countries. The pigments of saffron are so persistent that one part of crocin, its major pigment, has the ability to color up to 150,000 parts of water with definite yellow color.

Botanically speaking, the plant is thought to be native to Asia Minor and southern Europe. While rather small, it is distinctively showy with its vivid orange red, funnel-shaped stigmas centered in the midst of bluish to violet colored lily-shaped flowers. There are also several horticultural forms. It is a bulbous (technically a corm) perennial, growing usually six to ten inches in height. The leaves are long and slender, somewhat cylindrical and tapering at the ends.

In order to insure rapid and uniform growth of standard plants, saffron is propagated vegetatively. The young cormlets that form annually at the base of the bulblike "mother corm" are planted at six by six-inch intervals in previously well-plowed, harrowed, and cultivated soil. Under ideal conditions, well-established plantings yield eight to twelve pounds of dried saffron on an annual per-acre basis.

At the time of blooming, harvesting must begin immediately because the flowering period is relatively short—about 15 days. Because no mechanical picking device has yet been developed which can selectively collect the brilliantly colored tripartite stigmas, they must be picked by hand just as the flowers open. *It takes over 200,000 dried stigmas, gleaned from some 70,000 flowers, to make up one pound of the true saffron.* One can readily see why the cost of producing this material is so high.

In order to preserve the saffron, it must be thoroughly dried in the sun or at low heat to drive off moisture. The stigmas lose about 80 percent of their weight in this step, but it's needed to prevent molding when they're preserved in tightly sealed containers. Since light can bleach saffron, it should be kept in dark containers. At this point, it is ready for market and appears as matted masses of compressed, threadlike, dark reddish brown strands possessing a pleasantly aromatic odor and a spicy, pungent, bitter taste.

Saffron has historically been used for numerous purported medical effects. Some of these are very interesting and include such uses as saffron tea "to revive the spirits and make one optimistic." In fact, in England, during the 16th century, a happy, jovial person was said to have been "sleeping in a bagge of saffron." Irish women colored their bed sheets with it to "strengthen their limbs," and it was even added to the canary's drinking water so it might sing more cheerfully. For several hundred years saffron was used as a stimulant, emmenagogue, or antispasmodic (dose: 0.3 to 1.5 grams or 5 to 20 grains) and as a valuable aid in the treatment of many diseases including measles, dysentery, and jaundice.

Perhaps its high point in medical use was the 1620s, for in that time there appeared a weighty tome entitled, *Crocologia,* by J. F. Hertodt (Gena, Germany), which expounded on the efficiency of saffron as a panacea for all ills ranging from dental pain to the plague. Its use today has declined to the point where only occasionally it is encountered in use in India and other parts of Asia as a stomachic (stimulating secretory activity of the stomach) and stimulant tonic.

Some of the other medical qualities attributed to saffron include use as a sedative, expectorant, aphrodisiac, and a diaphoretic in exanthematous diseases (e.g., measles) to promote eruptions. With respect to its use as an abortifacient or emmenagogue, there have been recorded instances of several fatalities due to improper use. In particular, the saponin-containing corm, or underground parts, are very toxic to young animals. It is also recorded that stigmas in overdoses possess narcotic or severe sedative effects.

It has been known for some time that the stigmas of saffron are a rich source of the yellow pigment and vitamin, riboflavin. Physiologically speaking, riboflavin phosphate or riboflavin adenine nucleotide acts as a coenzyme in several enzyme systems for the purpose of hydrogen transport in the essential and ubiquitous Krebs cycle in body cells. In addition, the coenzyme functions in the degradation of fatty acids and the oxidation of pyruvic acid in the nervous system.

It is known that deficiency of riboflavin can lead to cheilosis (fissures at the angles of the lips), glossitis (inflammation of the tongue), and keratitis (inflammation of the cornea). Hence, saffron could conceivably be useful in riboflavin deficiency diseases where other sources of this vitamin were unavailable.

Saffron contains several other substances, with crocin being recognized as the major yellowish red pigment or carotenoid. Crocin is actually a mixture of glycosides. More specifically, the two major principles are known as crocetin, a carotenoid-dicarboxylic acid and α-crocin, a di-gentiobiose ester of crocetin. These are also known as flavonol glycosides. While primarily found in abundance in the stigmas and top of the styles of the crocus, these substances also have been described in other species of crocus in the Iridaceae family and in gardenias. In certain species of gardenias, a substance known as gardenidin has been shown to be identical with crocetin.

What is interesting from the chemical and pharmacological point of view is the fact that the chemical structures of crocetin, α-crocin, and cis- and trans-crocetin dimethyl esters bear resemblance to the prostaglandin type structures. The prostaglandins are derivatives of prostanoic acid with some 16 different derivatives known. While there are few presently accepted medical uses, certain of these prostaglandins have been proposed for the treatment of abortion, peptic ulcer, sterility, contraception, induction of labor, thrombosis, hypertension, asthma, and nasal congestion. It would be interesting to study the saffron for some of these prostaglandin effects to see if they can be produced at all, in higher dose levels.

Perhaps the most interesting recent development regarding the medical use of saffron is the fact that crocetin has been found to increase oxygen diffusivity. A patent has even been granted on the use of crocetin to increase the diffusivity of oxygen into solutions such as blood plasma, hence reducing local hypoxia when injected into animals.

Further, the specific intramuscular injection of crocetin (0.01 mg/kg) decreased the incidence of atherosclerosis in rabbits fed a one percent cholesterol diet for four months. Serum cholesterol levels were reduced by as much as 50 percent, due apparently to crocetin's ability to increase oxygen diffusion through blood plasma. The results of these experiments indicate that hypoxia, due to reduced diffusion of oxygen at the blood-tissue interface, may play an important and perhaps initiating part in the pathogenesis of atherosclerosis.

These experimental observations lead to speculation as to whether there is any relation, so far as cardiovascular diseases are concerned, between the crocetin-induced oxygenation effects, and the low incidence of heart disease in parts of Spain where saffron is a staple in the diets.

Epidemiological evidence has shown that heart disease has a low order of incidence in places like Valencia in Spain, where rice dishes containing liberal quantities of saffron are consumed daily. It certainly would be rewarding to study the diets of other cultures where saffron is consumed daily to see if this is not simply a chance occurrence.

Obviously, there are many questions raised here, particularly in attempting to relate an observation based on *injecting* a principle from a plant and its effect on one species of animals, to some possible beneficial action of *ingesting* the plant part in man.

Only further research can show whether this latest finding is useful. However, as with many previous leads to medical uses of plants (e.g., reserpine from Indian snakeroot and the digitalis glycosides from foxglove) we may one day find saffron (or its derivatives) recommended for control of atherosclerosis in humans.

## Bibliography

Claus, Edward P. et al. *Pharmacognosy.* 6th edition. Philadelphia: Lea & Febiger, 1970.

Gainer, John L. "Increasing Oxygen Diffusivity." U.S. 3,788,468, 5 pages long, 1-29-74. As cited in *Chemical Abstracts* 81: 45530m, 1974.

Gainer, John L., and Chisolm, G. M., III. "Oxygen Diffusion and Atherosclerosis." *Atherosclerosis* 19 (1974): 135-138.

Grisolia, Santiago. "Hypoxia, Saffron, and Cardiovascular Disease." *Lancet,* 6 July 1974, pp. 41-42.

Hegnauer, R. *Chemotaxonomic Der Pflanzen* III and IV. Basel and Stuttgart: Birkhauser Verlag, 1973.

Madan, C. L.; Kapur, B. M.; and Gupta, U. S. "Saffron." *Economic Botany* 20: 377-385.

Osol, Arthur et al. *United States Dispensatory.* 25th edition. Vols. 1-2. New York: J. B. Lippincott Co., 1960.

Rosengarten, Frederic, Jr. *The Book of Spices.* Philadelphia: Livingston Publishing Co., 1969.

Stecher, Paul G., ed. *Merck Index.* 8th edition. Rahway, N. J.: Merck & Co., 1968.

Uphof, J. C. T. *Dictionary of Economic Plants.* 2nd edition. New York: Stechert-Hafner Service Agency, 1968.

# Herbal Formulations for Mind and Body

**Author's Note:** True herbalism is more sophisticated than folk medicine. While folk tradition ordinarily relies on wild-growing local herbs, and uses them one at a time, herbalism draws on a much greater variety of plant materials and employs them in concert, in carefully measured amounts, to achieve its more ambitious aims.

For the most part, the herbal information in this book is in the tradition of folk medicine, rather than the art of herbalism. To suggest some of the methods and materials of true herbalism, I asked Leslie J. Kaslof to prepare the following brief report. Kaslof has been studying and experimenting with herbal formulations for many years. He has accumulated a vast library of herbal works and has done first-hand studies of herbs used by Mexicans and Mexican Indians. Kaslof's "Herb and Ailment Cross Reference Chart," published under the auspices of United Communications, is a unique contribution to the literature of medicinal herbs. Recently, he founded the International Institute for Biological and Botanical Research (G.P.O., Box 912, Brooklyn, New York 11202), an educational foundation which hopes to bridge the gap between scientists engaged in plant research and practitioners of medicinal and other healing arts.

**by Leslie J. Kaslof**

The joining together of herbs in a formula may be analogous to bringing together a group of people in hopes of accomplishing a multifaceted project. If each member of the group were of a forceful, volatile nature, each attempting to express the same idea with equal drive, and each having nearly identical talents, little would be accomplished. So it is with formulating herbs: to bring together only equally active substances would be to defeat the purpose. A "systems" approach is more conducive to equalization and revitalization of body and/or mind than trying to "overpower" a single bodily part.

In general, a simple way for the serious herb student to formulate is to use three parts of herbs actively concerned with the specific disorder, one part passive or soothing to injury (demulcent); one part nourishing, strengthening, and aromatic; and finally, one part eliminative (causing perspiration, urination, or defecation).

A more basic approach would be to blend four or five herbs, with two or three being specifically active, and the remainder being chosen for their quality of soothing or, if necessary, inducing perspiration or some other form of elimination.

For example, in alleviating upper respiratory congestion, you might be using such specifically active herbs as horehound, comfrey, and elecampane. To add a soothing dimension to the tea, you might add some marshmallow root and Irish moss.

In preparing herbs for use, unless otherwise indicated, a teaspoon of the herb is added to a cup of boiling water, covered, and allowed to steep for five to seven minutes. Reheat if necessary. Then strain and drink. Honey may be used, but sugar is not suggested.

In the formulations that follow, I have attempted to combine some of my research into traditional herbalism with the results of personal experiences. If you decide to try any of them, as part of your own personal herbal research work, it is probably best to make no more than one or two cups at a time. Remember, for every teaspoon of herbal material you use, use one cup of water. That means that in some cases you may be adding ingredients in very small amounts, perhaps only a fraction of a teaspoon. For instance, if a formula has 12 "parts," and you want to brew one cup, each part would measure one-twelfth of a teaspoon. To brew two cups, let each "part" equal one-sixth of a teaspoon. Depending on the strength of the brew, and your inclination, you might want to drink from one to three cupfuls of the tea a day, probably a half-cupful at a time.

In doing this kind of personal herb research, it is best to continue the program for a substantial number of days, carefully observing the effects both while you are taking it, and just as important, during the days and weeks that follow. Keep in mind that each plant and/or formulation will tend to produce an effect somewhat different in each individual.

**Cerebral Tonics** • These preparations do not include the mind-altering substances, and no great dramatic change will be noticed. They are specifically designed to revitalize and strengthen the powers of thought and concentration. These tonics may profitably be taken as an adjunct to deep breathing, yoga exercises, massage, meditation, etc.

1.  The Cerebral Tonic Stimulant consists of five herbs formulated to stimulate mental activity and concentration ability over a period of time.

> Sage (*Salvia officinalis*). Leaves, 3 parts.
> Rosemary (*Rosmarinus officinalis*). Leaves, 8 parts.
> Yerba Mate (*Ilex paraguayensis*). Leaves, 6 parts.
> Goldenseal (*Hydrastis canadensis*). Root, 2 parts.
> Cayenne (*Capsicum annum* or *frutescens*). Powdered fruit, 1 part.

2.  The Second Cerebral Tonic Stimulant is similar to the first except that it excludes the sage and adds three new herbs. This combination adds a dimension of mental exhilaration and endurance to the formula.

> Rosemary (*Rosmarinus officinalis*). Leaves, 4 parts.
> Yerba Mate (*Ilex paraguayensis*). Leaves, 3 parts.
> Goldenseal (*Hydrastis canadensis*). Powdered root, 1 part.
> Cayenne (*Capsicum annum* or *frutescens*). Powdered fruit, 1 part.
> Valerian (*Valeriana officinalis*). Powdered root, 1 part.
> Virginia Snakeroot (*Aristolochia serpentaria*). Powdered root, 1 part.
> Calamus (*Acorus calamus*). Crushed root, 2 parts.

3.  Cerebral Tonic Nervine is formulated to relax the mind and help bring about a state of mental harmony.

> Rosemary (*Rosmarinus officinalis*). Leaves, 4 parts.
> Sage (*Salvia officinalis*). Leaves, 2 parts.
> Goldenseal (*Hydrastis canadensis*). Powdered root, 1 part.
> Skullcap (*Scutellaria laterifolia*). Powdered herb, 3 parts.
> Valerian (*Valeriana officinalis*). Powdered root, 2 parts.

**Glandular Tonifier and Strengthener** • Following herbalist principles, this formula is specifically designed to increase cellular and glandular activity, and assist in the removal of congested material from the system. The active ingredients are considered to be among the most efficacious systemic purifiers. Research with this formula is indicated as an aid in helping the body overcome infections and toxins.

Burdock (*Arctium lappa*). Root or seeds, 4 parts.
Echinacea (*Echinacea angustifolia*). Root, 3 parts.
Pipsissewa (*Chimaphila umbellata*). Leaves, 6 parts.
Plantain (*Plantago major*). Leaves, 4 parts.
Prickly Ash (*Xanthoxylum americanum*). Bark or berries, 3 parts.
Yellow Dock (*Rumex crispus*). Root, 4 parts.
Yarrow (*Achillea millefolium*). Flowers, 3 parts.

**Cardiac Tonic and Strengthener** • Based on herbal traditions, this preparation is worthy of research as an aid in improving the tone and endurance of all circulatory tissue.

Hawthorn (*Crataegus oxyacantha*). Berries, 4 parts.
Marigold (*Calendula officinalis*). Flowers, 2 parts.
Motherwort (*Leonurus cardiaca*). Powdered herb, 2 parts.
Lily of the Valley (*Convallaria majalis*). Leaves, 2 parts.
Goldenseal (*Hydrastis canadensis*). Powdered root, 1 part.
Cayenne (*Capsicum annum* or *frutescens*). Powdered fruit, 1 part.

**Reproductive Organ and Tissue Tonic** • Herbal tradition values several plants for restoring or assisting potency. This formula goes beyond stimulation and includes plants which should help strengthen and normalize tissues involved in the reproductive system.

Damiana (*Turnera aphrodisiaca*). Leaves, 8 parts.
False Unicorn Root (*Chamaelireum lutum*). Crushed root, 6 parts.
Ginseng (*Panax quinquefolius*). Root, 3 parts.
Saw Palmetto (*Serenoa serrulata*). Berries, 2 parts.
Irish Moss (*Chondrus crispus*). Whole or flakes, 2 parts.
Motherwort (*Leonurus cardiaca*). Leaves, 3 parts.
Prickly Ash (*Xanthoxylum americanum*). Berries or bark, 3 parts.

# A Critical Review of Correspondence Courses in Herbalism

**Author's Note:** The idea for this section of the book came from many inquiries I have received over the years asking about schools of herbal medicine. I was never able to give helpful responses to these questions, so I decided it would be a good idea to write to every such institution whose name I could find, and ask them to send me information on their programs, including the actual courses.

Here are the major lessons I learned from this project:

There is no school in the United States or Canada that we could locate which offers an in-residence course of study in herbalism. Although one school—Dominion—does have seminars during the summer, all the schools are essentially geared only to provide correspondence courses.

There are numerous herbalism schools in Britain, including several which have in-residence programs, and at least one that demands long years of apprenticeship. But none of these schools offers correspondence courses.

Herbal schools or "colleges" are almost always very small operations, usually consisting of a faculty of one or two people. The courses are more often than not simply books, sometimes divided into "courses" instead of chapters.

Because of their small size, these institutions cannot be depended upon for much of anything. If you deal with them, it is always necessary to use caution, writing first and receiving full details before signing any agreements or checks.

All the material I received from these schools was sent for evaluation to Leslie Kaslof, who has long been a student and researcher in herbalism. After finishing his evaluation, which appears below, Kaslof had this to say: "It would be a mistake if anyone were to take any of these courses with the idea that they were going to qualify her or him to practice herbal medicine. These courses just don't do that. And although some of them will give the student a certificate or diploma upon completing the course, and sometimes upon passing a test, it should be emphasized that such certificates are legally absolutely meaningless.

"One of the things that bothered me about some of these courses is that by providing information on physiology and biology, some of these courses tend to give the idea that they are preparing the student to treat people. Usually, the physiology material is on a high school level and often contains errors at that.

"These courses should be considered not much different from a good book or books on the subject. They do not provide professional training."

For what they are worth, then, here are Kaslof's remarks on the schools whose materials I was able to obtain.

**by Leslie J. Kaslof**

**Dominion Herbal College (1962) Ltd.**—*7527 Kingsway, Burnaby— British Columbia V3N 3C1 Canada* ● The Dominion Herbal College was established in 1926 by the British-trained naturopathic doctor and master herbalist, Herbert Nowell, who researched and wrote the original course. Dr. Nowell, at various times, taught botanical medicine at universities in Boston, Toronto, and England.

Charles Nelson, B.A., M.A., the dean of Dominion, told us that "Among the graduates of the Dominion Herbal College are Jethro Kloss, author of *Back to Eden;* Dr. Edward Fewer, M.D., lecturer and teacher; and Dr. Bernard Jensen, naturopathic author and teacher now based in Escondido, California."

The school was reorganized in 1962, but since that time, very little seems to have been added to the original work.

The first part of the course is concerned with anatomy and physiology and we found it to be quite outdated. The herbal section of the course has been a source of inspiration to herbalists and students for many years and it still has much to recommend it. Divided into sections dealing with different medicinal properties of herbs, such as diuretic, from five to ten herbs are discussed in each section, with a description of their action and a formula with directions for preparation. At the end of each section there are about half a dozen questions which are to be answered and submitted to the college for marking.

There are some excellent formulas throughout this course, and it is evident that the late Dr. Nowell was indeed a talented and sensitive herbalist. It seems to me that Kloss, in his classic *Back to Eden,* derived a good deal of his information from this course.

We are told that the college has seminars during the summer, with lectures and field trips for students. After a final examination, a diploma is awarded naming the recipient a "Chartered Herbalist." This school has asked us not to mention the price of the course, but comparatively speaking, it is in the middle range of the various courses I have seen.

**School of Natural Healing**—*Box 352—Provo, Utah 84601* ● This is a voluminous work, consisting of about 1100 multicolored mimeographed pages of lectures, personal experiences of the author, Ray Christopher, along with information derived from assorted herbal texts.

Instructions are given concerning the various means of preparing herbs, their dosages, administration, and other practical details. The predominant therapeutic properties of each plant are discussed, along with how they are best combined with other herbs. One section deals with gathering plants, including the best parts, and when to pick them.

The bulk of the course consists of chapters with headings such as "The Healing Astringent Herbs," "The Healing Diuretic Herbs," etc. Within each of these categories are listed from seven to twelve herbs with their identifying characteristics, parts used, properties, symptomatic use, dosage, preparation, specific formulation, and administration.

The text is not designed with questions to be answered, nor, to my knowledge, is there any kind of certificate issued.

I have had and used this work by Ray Christopher for many years, and it has sometimes proven extremely useful in obtaining obscure information I was not able to find elsewhere, as well as supplying some very basic, reliable knowledge. The text was $30 when I first bought it, but I am sure it has probably increased in price somewhat since then. I have been told that the course is now in the process of revision.

Taking all this into account, whether the current course or the revised edition is obtained, it would be a substantial addition to any natural therapeutics library.

**The Institute of Herbal Philosophy**—*Box 968, 115 East Foothill #10—Glendora, California 91740* ● The Institute of Herbal Philosophy is operated by Gene Matlock, an herbalist and professional schoolteacher. His course consists of 128 pages and is quite easy to read. I found many things in Matlock's course that were exciting, and others that were objectionable.

In the introductory pages of the book is the statement: "Why don't you cash in on herbalism? . . . Herbalism is the greatest unknown home fortune maker in this or any other country" etc. It goes on to describe how many people have allegedly built businesses working with a few herbs in their home, garage, or barn.

This approach I found repugnant. Besides, it is very doubtful that the average person is going to make a "fortune" by growing or selling herbs. On the other hand, if you do want to try to make a small business out of your interest in herbs, the first lesson in this course does give some practical and sometimes ingenious ideas for selling herbs.

That portion of the course which deals with herbalism rather than opportunism has much to recommend it, however. For instance, one section compares various cultural herbal systems, from the ancient Aztecs to present-day Chinese medicine. Each culture's individualistic approach to healing is then related to the whole, so that each system's individual contribution may be appreciated.

The chapter ends by giving various medical terms in Aztec and Mayan, and explaining their meanings. The school's basic philosophy is said to be taken from and based on these ancient Indian doctrines.

Each chapter dealing with herbs and their uses concludes with some positive suggestions under the repeated title of "Learning How to Think Like an Herbalist." This in turn is followed by a short synopsis of the chapter and from five to ten questions, most requiring lengthy dissertations, which when submitted to the school become their property.

One lesson is said to present the "great secret of herbalism," which basically deals with various degrees and types of stress, how to recognize these degrees in people, how they are to be treated, and the importance of a well-tuned and balanced nervous system to the human economy.

The price of the course at present is a little over $50, which, considering there is some information here which is not generally available elsewhere, seems to be reasonable. For those who are into it, there is a certificate of achievement issued upon completion of the course.

**The Qui-tsi-tsa-las Spiritual Sanctuary**—*Box 46506, Vancouver— British Columbia V6R 4G7 Canada* ● This school is in a state of transition, and their revised course was not available to us. We were informed, though, that it will incorporate Ray Christopher's original herbal correspondence course which at this time is still available from the school in Provo, Utah.

The director of the school, Norma Meyers, told us she was president of an organization called the Green Leaf Herbal Guild of British Columbia, composed of herbalists and laypeople dedicated to the continuation of herbal healing. Along with the Canadian Herbalist Association of British Columbia, that group is attempting to protect the right of herbalists to practice under the common law tradition of Great Britain as set forth by King Henry VIII.

At this time, we can't say anything very informative about the course of this school, except that we are told they have seminars and field trips during the spring and summer. Recent advertisements we have seen indicate the price of instruction is relatively high.

**Bernadean University**—*Las Vegas, Nevada* ● After looking over the entire Bernadean course, which includes chapters on physiology, chemistry, biology, bacteriology, toxicology, pathology, Swedish massage, hypnosis, and information about the various body systems (these sections consisting of three to four pages each), I decided to consult with some professional associates. They determined this information to be of a first to second year high school level—and presented in a very general way, at that.

The herbal section, which takes up the second half of the roughly 120-page course, presents an uninspiring compilation of general information which may be generally obtained through one or two good books on herbalism.

Do not be deceived by the word "University" in the title of this course. The institution is in fact more of a personal business or shop than a university. Neither is the material up to the level of anything remotely approaching a college. One chapter, for instance, describes an herb as "being good for the bites of poisonous beasts and mad dogs," and this was not quoted in historical context, but rather as a contemporary fact.

One more point should be noted here, and that is that the cost of the course works out to be somewhere in the vicinity of $880. This entitles one, upon completion of the course, to a diploma as a Doctor of Naturopathy. That is as dangerous as it is ludicrous, because some people might complete this course and feel justified in advising or even treating people, who under more enlightened circumstances would do a lot better taking care of themselves.

We wrote to more than a dozen other herbal schools, mostly in England, but we received little or no useful information from them. We were informed by the Academy of the Science of Man in England that they had a correspondence course, but upon sending an application, we received no response.

We did receive some very warm correspondence from the National Institute of Medical Herbalists at 149 Hunts Street, Small Heath, Birmingham, 20, England, and subsequently I had an opportunity to visit their office. It is unfortunate that they no longer have a correspondence course, but they are still quite active in England and operate an apprentice-type program and clinic as well. The Institute was founded in 1864 and trains Practitioners of Herbal Medicine with a four-year course which, after examination, qualifies them to become members of the Institute.

This seems to be the only school of herbal medicine in the United States, Canada, or England which truly trains people in the art and science of herbal healing. They are presently trying to raise the required funds to build a new college, a research facility, and a new clinic.

> **Author's Note:** By reading the annotated bibliography of herbal medicine and folk remedy books, which follows, the reader will be able to select a number of books for serious study which, together, should serve at least as well as most of the courses described here. A good selection might include Clymer's *Nature's Healing Agents;* Grieve's *A Modern Herbal;* Hutchens's *Indian Herbalogy of North America;* Kloss's *Back to Eden;* and Levy's *Herbal Handbook for Everyone.* To round out your studies somewhat, you could add the *Rodale Herb Book* and Kordel's *Natural Folk Remedies.*

# An Annotated Bibliography of Herbal Medicine and Folk Remedy Books

This bibliography is not meant to be a complete listing of books which deal in whole or part with herbal healing. Such a bibliography would make a book in itself (and probably a good one at that). Rather, this listing is meant as a practical guide for those who wish to pursue the subject further. The emphasis here is very heavily on the *practical* aspects of herbal healing. Many of the great classics of herbal medicine, some written hundreds or even thousands of years ago, have been omitted because they are not what I would consider "practical" books. In general, the herbal remedies discussed by these earlier authors which have the most to recommend them have been picked up and preserved by the later writers, whose works appear in this bibliography. The person who wishes to approach herbalism from an historical point of view is urged to visit a large public or university library. Likewise, those whose main interest in herbs is their identification or cultivation, rather than their medicinal qualities, are urged to seek out the appropriate books or visit a big bookstore or library. In recent years, many new books have been published on all aspects of herbs.

Brown, Alice Cook. *Early American Recipes.* New York: Bonanza Books, 1966.

Offers a very convenient way of becoming acquainted with how early Americans—through the 19th century—used herbs, without having to go back to the original sources. Included are some 85 recipes for herbal remedies, the source noted in each case. There is also a list of herbs used for various diseases taken from Joseph Taylor's *Nature the Best Physician; A Complete Domestic Herbal,* published in 1818. In addition, the book covers herb gardens, herbal perfumes, and culinary uses of herbs, presenting the information in the words used by the original authors.

Clymer, R. Swinburne. *Nature's Healing Agents.* Philadelphia: Dorrance and Co., 1963. (First published in 1905.)

The advanced student of herbalism will want a copy of this classic book by Dr. Clymer. For others, it may be confusing, because his approach to herbs was that of the homeopath, and the formulas are given in terms of tinctures (alcoholic solutions) to be administered in carefully measured doses ranging from one-half drop to one teaspoon. On the other hand, many of Dr. Clymer's formulas can be translated into the more usual infusions and decoctions with a little imagination. Although he held the M.D. degree, he considered himself a "Natura Physician" and a follower of the "Thomsonian" system. Dr. Samuel Thomson was an early 19th century physician whose theories and practices have been much adopted by our present-day naturopaths and homeopaths. Emphasized in this system is the desirability of cleansing the body of toxins by means of induced regurgitation and enemas. Dr. Clymer even regards the enema as a useful way of nourishing the patient, by injecting him with small amounts of liquefied and filtered vegetables, malted milk, beef broth, and virtually anything else he feels like eating, if that is the right word for it. Except to the student of herbal medicine history, the most valuable part of this book will be Dr. Clymer's formulas for common ailments, many of which seem to be excellent even if you translate them from tinctures into common teas.

Conway, David. *The Magic of Herbs.* New York: D. P. Dutton, 1973.

A good overall introduction to herbs, including chapters on herbalism and astrology, how herbs are prepared, and a lot of information on the religious and magical background of various herbs. The author is identified as a practicing herbalist, but this fact is not immediately evident from his discussion of medicinal herbs, which does not seem much different from that in books written by nonherbalists.

Coon, Nelson. *Using Plants for Healing.* Great Neck, N.Y.: Hearthside Press, 1963.

A straightforward listing of herbs along with relatively brief information on their healing uses. If you have other books on herbs, you may find this one useful simply because the herbs are listed in alphabetical order based on their Latin names. A 10-page chapter on "Medicines in House and Garden" gives a number of useful tips. Another plus factor is that the author points out which herbs and remedies he has personally used with success.

Eichenlaub, John E. *A Minnesota Doctor's Home Remedies for Common and Uncommon Ailments.* Englewood Cliffs, N.J.: Prentice-Hall, 1960.

This book, by an M.D., is loaded with advice, much of it bad. A few examples: The author suggests that a person with chronic joint pains who weighs more than 170 pounds should take 15 aspirin a day regularly, "even if you need them over a period of years." Then he says that some people worry about whether or not aspirin might subtly harm their health when taken for a long time. Dr. Eichenlaub declares: "The answer is, *absolutely no!*" He says further that unless there are very clear-cut symptoms, the dosage he is recommending "is entirely harmless." Perhaps Dr. Eichenlaub didn't know this back in 1960, but 15 aspirin a day taken month after month and year after year can cause significant blood loss in many people and give others bleeding ulcers. In addition, this dosage of aspirin, taken throughout the day as Dr. Eichenlaub recommends, destroys much of the vitamin C in the body and therefore invites trouble which could be more serious than the original problem.

Dr. Eichenlaub also advises people with constipation to avoid "like the plague" raw vegetables, cabbage, and bran cereals, on the grounds that they are "dry-bulk" foods. Again, perhaps he did not know this in 1960, but it is just these foods which are today recommended as the very best preventive and cure for chronic constipation, when taken with sufficient water or juice.

Another bit of bad advice is telling people to cut their own corns and calluses with a razor blade unless they have "diabetes or disease of the arteries." Even if you don't have these diseases, self-surgery is always dangerous. Furthermore, many people have diabetes or disease of the arteries and do not realize it—until they give themselves a nasty gash in the foot and find that for some strange reason it won't heal!

Grieve, Maude. *A Modern Herbal.* New York: Dover Publications, 1971. This is a soft-cover republication of a work originally published in 1931.

Grieve's two-volume herbal is the supreme practical guide for those seriously interested in medicinal herbs. Her book has obviously been exhaustively and meticulously researched, and the material is presented in a very clear and systematic fashion. Included is information on the chemical constituents of herbs, where they are grown, how to cultivate them, how to prepare them, and what conditions they are recommended for. Aside from being the most comprehensive modern treatise on herbs I have seen, it also makes fascinating reading. Its only shortcoming is that it does not discuss the best ways to combine herbs, which is a rather important topic since herbs are best taken in combinations. However, this information can be gathered from other books, such as Kloss's *Back to Eden* and Clymer's *Nature's Healing Agents.*

Huson, Paul. *Mastering Herbalism.* New York: Stein and Day, 1974.

One of the more ambitious—and successful—herb books of recent vintage. It will be especially interesting to those who want to learn every last wrinkle about traditional herb lore. Here you will find information on how to make herbal incense, herbal aphrodisiacs, herbal witchcraft potions, so-called elixirs of life, and how to plant and harvest your herbs by the phases of the moon. Covered also are the more usual topics of healing herbs, cooking herbs, and herbs for beauty and perfume. For those who are looking for a relatively complete and systematic approach to healing with herbs, this book is not as good as some others. But if you want to know how to make Pears Bordelaise, tansy pudding, and Persian incense; which herbs can be smoked to achieve a dopelike effect; and the 10 herbs the author feels are the most likely to produce a true aphrodisiac effect, then this book may be well worth buying.

Hutchens, Alma R. *Indian Herbalogy of North America.* Canada: Merco (620 Wyandotte, East, Windsor 14, Ontario), 1973.

"A study of Anglo-American, Russian, and Oriental literature on Indian medical botanics of North America with illustrations, glossary, index, and annotated bibliography." Written in consultation with herbalist N. G. Tretchikoff, and Natalie K. Tretchikoff, who contributed the Russian material and bibliography, this is one of the best books on herbal medicine available, with entries on over 200 herbs. The type is large and easy to read, and the illustrations well defined. There are clear instructions on how each herb is used, and even a notation for each herb on its solubility in water, boiling water, or alcohol. The information on how herbs which grow in North America are also used in parts of Asia adds color and interest to the book. Those who wish to pursue the study of herbal medicine will find the annotated bibliography very helpful.

Hylton, William H., ed. *The Rodale Herb Book.* Emmaus, Pa.: Rodale Press, 1974.

Here is the most comprehensive "how-to" book on all aspects of herbs I have seen. While it does not contain the enormous number of details about individual herbs contained in Grieve's book, the information here is much easier to get at and more concisely presented. Chapters written by experts in specific areas of herbalism offer step-by-step instructions on how to buy, plant, cultivate, harvest, store, and even freeze herbs; how to use herbs for cooking and making vinegars, butters, teas, and liqueurs; how to use aromatic herbs for sachets, baths, powders, oils, perfumes, and insect repellents; how to use colorful herbs for dyeing; how to plant formal and informal herb gardens; and even how herbs can be used in the garden to keep insects away. The best section for our purposes is the 200-page-long "Herbal Encyclopedia," which gives instructions on the cultivation and medicinal uses of herbs. Large type, glossary, index.

Jarvis, D. C. *Folk Medicine,* 1958, and *Arthritis and Folk Medicine,* 1960. Both books originally published by Holt, Rinehart and Winston, New York, and subsequently published in softback by Fawcett Publications, Greenwich, Conn.

Dr. Jarvis's two books may be the best-selling volumes on folk medicine published in recent years. They may also be the most nonsensical published in the 20th century. His basic premises:

Apple cider vinegar will prevent or cure almost any disease known to man—or beast. What's a little bit of arthritis compared to the fury of a mad bull? But bulls will not only be calmed by cider vinegar, says Dr. Jarvis, but will greedily slurp it up if it's put in their water or on their feed.

Second, it is vitally necessary to keep the system on the acid side, says Dr. Jarvis. Get just a little bit over on the alkaline side, and calcium will collect on your joints like bird droppings on a public statue.

Third, the way to keep your system on the acid side is to drink plenty of apple cider vinegar—several teaspoons in a glass of water with every meal.

Fourth, the most vital mineral to health is potassium. And the best place to get your potassium is—you guessed it—from good old apple cider vinegar.

In reading Dr. Jarvis's books, I was especially struck with his stories about how all animals instinctively love apple cider vinegar and thrive on it. I immediately went out and put some cider vinegar in a fresh bowl of water for my huge Newfoundland dog. She took one sniff of the stuff and turned away. When I gave her a bowl of fresh water, she lapped it up eagerly. That's when I began to get suspicious about good old Dr. Jarvis and his miraculous apple cider vinegar.

Then, I noticed in chapter 9 of *Arthritis and Folk Medicine* he points out that "the blood is always alkaline because of the presence in it of sodium bicarbonate. . . . The normal reaction is faintly alkaline." Yet, throughout both of his books, he rails endlessly about the disaster that is going to befall you if your body becomes alkaline. He seems to forget that it already is. And if it wasn't *supposed* to be that way, it wouldn't be. In fact, it is very difficult to play games with the pH of your body. The mechanisms that control it are very powerful and exquisitely sensitive. Variations, except in the presence of serious disease, are normally very small.

Dr. Jarvis also talks about the importance of keeping the urine acid (with cider vinegar) in order to avoid kidney stones. We asked Charles E. Nuttall, M.D., a nephrologist at the University of Kentucky College of Medicine, about that. According to this kidney specialist, "Vinegar (acetic acid) is not an effective means of acidifying the urine, because it is converted by oxidative metabolism to water and volatile carbon dioxide. Nor is an acid urine always desirable, since it can precipitate uric acid stones. On the other hand, many infections of the urinary tract may be more easily eradicated if the urine is acid, and here the time-honored folk remedy of cranberries (hippuric acid) is effective."

As for apple cider vinegar being a great source of potassium, that is simply ridiculous. If Dr. Jarvis had looked on page 65 of the *Composition of Foods* (Agriculture Handbook No. 8, United States Department of Agriculture), he would have seen that 100 grams, or 3½ ounces, of cider vinegar contains 100 mg. of potassium. Skimming through the rest of this authoritative book, he would discover that the same amount of orange juice contains 200 mg.; raw elderberries, 300 mg.; raw mushrooms, 400 mg.; roasted peanuts, 700 mg.; and blackstrap molasses, 3,000 mg. To get the same amount of potassium that you would from half a cup of roasted peanuts, you would have to drink—if you could—at least three whole cups of apple cider vinegar! The fact is that there are very few unprocessed foods which have *less* potassium than cider vinegar!

Kaslof, Leslie J. "Herb and Ailment Cross Reference Chart." United Communications, Box 320, Woodmere, N.Y. 11598.

A one-of-a-kind chart, cross-indexing 87 symptoms or ailments and over 150 herbs, with annotations and plant illustrations as line drawings. Some 30 inches wide and 40 inches deep, the chart is most useful in suggesting topics for further reading on the uses of herbs for ailments, but it also makes a unique wall hanging and an intriguing conversation piece.

Kloss, Jethro. *Back to Eden*. Beverly Hills, Calif.: Woodbridge Press, 1939. A softback revised edition was published in 1973 by Lifeline Books, P.O. Box 1552, Riverside, Calif. 92502.

Jethro Kloss was the Walt Whitman of herbalists. The new softback edition of his classic, which runs on to some 700 pages, is packed with every imaginable kind of information about maintaining health and curing illness. Kloss wrote with a passionate conviction; not surprisingly, you will find in Kloss's dietary and general health advice many passages that seem arbitrary, outdated, excessively emphatic, or simply incorrect.

On the other hand, the hundreds of herbal remedies, and especially the combination herbal therapies which Kloss presents, are a goldmine of potential usefulness. Kloss is one of the few herbal writers who actually practiced this art extensively. At various times in his life, he seems to have been not only an herbalist, but a medical assistant as well. There is virtually no disease he did not tackle with utter confidence that he would cure it. And if you believe him, he rarely failed.

To make the best use of the wisdom of Kloss, I would suggest consulting him along with several more modern authors. That would help to keep you from getting carried away with Kloss's sometimes excessive exuberance.

Kordel, Lelord. *Natural Folk Remedies*. New York: G. P. Putnam's Sons, 1974.

I recommend this book highly as a companion to the more systematic herbal remedy books. Kordel has managed to squeeze in more remedies and recipes to the square inch of text than any other author I can think of. And surprisingly, the majority of them are good ones. They reflect not only the most "promising" remedies Kordel has collected in his extensive travels and reading but also much of the latest information in nutrition. His herbal burn remedy from Germany, for example, is a mixture of wheat germ oil, honey, and comfrey leaves. If this doesn't work, I doubt that anything else will. His Icelandic remedy for breaking up a cold consists of chopped onions, barley water, and some cod-liver oil. I can't even imagine what this would taste like, but my guess is that your cold wouldn't like it. If you want something that tastes better, try his Polish cold remedy, which consists of one cup of milk heated until it's scalding hot, to which you add one tablespoon of honey, a teaspoon of butter, and one-half teaspoon of grated fresh garlic. The book is filled with such practical but slightly exotic remedies for the colds, headaches, aches, pains, and pimples that bother us. In short, a most valuable companion book to some of the more classic works in the herb field.

Krochmal, Arnold and Connie. *A Guide to the Medicinal Plants of the United States.* New York: Quadrangle, 1973.

This handsomely produced book, featuring excellent photographs and careful line drawings, will be more appreciated by the botanist or hunter of herbs in the field than the person looking for practical information about herbal medicine. No information is given about preparing the herbs or the dosages to be used. The editorial assumption is that the information in this book will only be used for identification purposes.

Law, Donald. *The Concise Herbal Encyclopedia.* Edinburgh, Scotland: John Bartholomew and Son, 1973.

Not nearly as authoritative as the title suggests, this book nevertheless has enough remedies listed to make it worth reading. However, it is flawed by numerous emphatic statements about health and disease which are either fallacious or completely arbitrary. For example, Law states that constipation "is one of the most dangerous conditions"—which it isn't—and in his discussion of anemia, he fails to mention that food, such as liver, is what is really indicated, not nettle tea or "honey and lemon juice."

Levy, Juliette de Baïracli. *Herbal Handbook For Everyone.* London: Faber and Faber, 1966.

Here is one of the very best of the nonencyclopedic type books on herbs currently available. The author has used herbs herself for decades—in veterinary and human ailments—and has added some interesting items to herbal literature based on her own experiences and the remedies she learned from Gypsies. This may be the very best of the smaller books on herbs.


Lucas, Richard. *Nature's Medicines.* West Nyack, N.Y.: Parker Publishing Co., 1966.

One of the more heavily promoted herb and remedy books, but not one of the best. It is largely a hodgepodge of information taken from a variety of sources, such as newspapers and magazines. It emphasizes unproven remedies with a sensational aura to them but ignores many others which are more reliable. Looking in the index, for example, there is no mention of such stalwarts as camomile, dandelion, plantain, pennyroyal, tansy, etc. And it doesn't seem to make much sense to talk about the tiny traces of antibiotic activity found in wheat seeds, without even mentioning the health-building and curative potencies of wheat germ and wheat germ oil.


Mességué, Maurice. *Of Men and Plants,* 1973, translated and adapted from the original 1970 French edition, and *Maurice Mességué's Way to Natural Health and Beauty,* 1974. Both books published by Macmillan, New York.

Subtitled "The Autobiography of the World's Most Famous Plant Healer," *Of Men and Plants* is the only herb book I know of which has a "plot." And the story of Mességué's experiences in healing paupers, drunks, generals, and famous actresses with herbs is at least as compelling as the information about the herbs themselves. One difficulty is that Mességué uses herbal foot and hand baths almost to the exclusion of all other approaches. This is largely at variance with the way other herbalists work, but if we are to believe the author, these herbal baths of his can do near-miracles. If you want to try some of these baths, an appendix offers the "basic preparations" that he uses. Regardless of how you feel about soaking your feet in herbs instead of drinking or applying them, you will find this book fascinating to read.

His follow-up book, packed with simple remedies based on familiar herbs, fruits, and vegetables, is in many ways more practical than his first book. This volume is highly readable, contains some excellent recipes (I tried a few), and in general, combines the lore of folk medicine with much common sense and a knowledge of current medical practice.

Meyer, Joseph E. *The Herbalist.* First published in 1918, the book was subsequently revised and enlarged by Clarence Meyer and was in its tenth printing by 1973. Available from Indiana Botanic Gardens, Box 5, Hammond, Ind. 46325.

The first half of the book, dealing with individual herbs, is notably lacking in really useful medicinal information. However, the second half of the book is loaded with practical tips on how to combine herbs into botanical formulas, how to make infusions and decoctions, salves, poultices, tinctures, etc. There are also many color drawings of herbs, but their clarity leaves something to be desired.

Simmonite, W. J., and Culpeper, Nicholas. *The Simmonite-Culpeper Herbal Remedies.* England: W. Foulsham and Co., 1957. Published in the United States in a softback edition by Award Books, New York.

This book is a mess. First, the cover of the softback edition proclaims that the herbal remedies presented have been "proven effective by modern medical findings!" That's not true. Second, it is impossible to tell which portions of the book were written by Dr. Simmonite, a 20th century herbalist, and which sections by Culpeper, the famed astrologer-physician of the early 17th century. That destroys whatever value the book may have as an historical document. Worst of all, there are no cautions given after recommending such potentially dangerous herbs as celandine, valerian, tansy, rue, or even squill, an herb so powerful that it's still used today to kill rats.

Talaiseul, Jean. *Grandmother's Secrets—Her Green Guide to Health From Plants.* London: Barrie & Jenkins, 1973. Translated from a 1972 French edition by Pamela Swinglehurst.

The title is clever but don't be misled. This is the usual sort of herb book, average in every respect. In 286 pages, the author deals with herbs one at a time, devoting a page or two to each. If you have read several other herb books, you will find little that is new here. But if you are in England or France, and can get this book easily, it will give you your money's worth.

Weiner, Michael A. *Earth Medicine—Earth Foods.* New York: Macmillan, 1972.

"Plant remedies, drugs, and natural foods of the North American Indians." This is a fine book detailing herbal remedies used by a number of Indian tribes for some 65 ailments. However, by its very nature, it is bound to be of more use to the advanced student or one who is interested in the history of herbs, than to someone seeking directly practical information. A handsomely produced book, and one which makes a good addition to any library of herbal books.

Wren, R. C. *Potter's New Cyclopaedia of Botanical Drugs and Preparations.* Rustington, Sussex, England: Health Science Press, 1907. Revised and enlarged by R. W. Wren in 1956.

This venerable book has a place in the library of any serious student of herbal medicine. The presentation is systematic, easy to understand, and easy to read. The lack of illustrations is not a serious drawback, since many other books have them. The value of the book would probably be improved, however, if the entries on the major herbs were expanded somewhat and if fewer of the directions for preparing herbs were not given in homeopathic jargon. If you have Grieve's *A Modern Herbal,* you can probably get along without this book.

# Hernia

Believe it or not, there is an herb called rupturewort (*Herniari glabra*). According to the old-time herbalist Gerard, "It is reported that being drunke it is singular good for Ruptures and that very many that have been bursten were restored to health by the use of this herbe. . . ."

Like I said, believe it or not.

Many people find that a truss takes care of their problem nicely, particularly when surgery for some reason seems undesirable. Which reminds me of a small store which used to be located on Philadelphia's Ninth Street, a few blocks north of Market, which sold nothing but trusses and had a large sign in the window proclaiming "Your Rupture Is Our Rapture."

# Hiccups

First, try this remedy suggested by the eminent anthropologist Ashley Montagu. I don't know if his remedy is any better than others, but Montagu's advice about everything else is so excellent that it wouldn't surprise me if his hiccup cure is equally outstanding. Besides, he says it has never failed.

Fill a glass with water and place in it a metal object such as a spoon, fork, or knife. Then slowly sip the water while holding the upper part of the handle against the temple. The bottom part remains in the water. The hiccups should cease within the minute.

Should the first cure fail to work, try this. Fill a cup with water and get a teaspoon. Hold the handle of the spoon between your teeth, lengthwise, then drink some water.

Still got them? Then it's time for the heavy artillery!

Take the teaspoon that you used in the second cure, dry it off, fill it with ordinary white granulated sugar, and eat the sugar.

Edgar E. Engleman, M.D., of the University of California School of Medicine in San Francisco, and two colleagues, said that eating one teaspoon of dry sugar "resulted in immediate cessation of hiccups in 19 of 20 patients." Some of these patients had hiccups for several days, and one for six weeks. Five had received other forms of therapy (including breathing into a paper bag, an old standby) without success. Sometimes, hiccups cured in this way will return in a few hours but repeated treatment proves universally successful.

If you're worrying about that one patient whose hiccups weren't cured by sugar, he recovered spontaneously eight hours later.

# Hives

An eruption of hives may be caused by almost anything, including emotional stress. Most often, though, it seems to be an allergic reaction to foods. Simply by observing what was eaten before an outbreak, you should be able to pinpoint the offending agent without too much difficulty.

What can complicate the matter, though, is that you may be reacting not to a food *per se*, but to a food additive. This is especially true of people who have hives nearly all the time. In a study at the University of Uppsala, Sweden, persons who had frequent cases of hives were tested with various substances. Half of them had adverse reactions to food dyes and preservatives in amounts that could easily be present in a daily diet. Most of those who were hypersensitive to dyes and preservatives also reacted to aspirin. In a follow-up study, 75 patients were warned to stay away from artificially colored and preserved foods. As a result, 24 percent became completely symptom-free, 57 percent had no hives as long as they avoided additives (but broke out when they went off the diet), while 19 percent were only slightly improved or unchanged.

As a result of this work, which was conducted by Dr. Lennart Juhlin, Swedish law now requires that all additives be listed along with official code numbers and quantities used (*Skin and Allergy News*, November 1975).

A reader from North Dakota told us that he had been suffering with hives for a year and had gone to several local doctors without gaining any relief. He did know that he was allergic to aspirin and that his hives would become worse after taking the medication. He then discovered in reading about the work of Dr. Ben Feingold (see HYPERACTIVITY, later in this book) that margarine may contain the additive Yellow 5, which can also cause allergic reactions. He then eliminated colored margarine completely from his diet and also watched other foods which contained artificial colors or preservatives.

"I was soon rid of the hives and I am not taking any medication," he told us.

# Homeopathy

Homeopathy is a medical specialty based on the principle that "like cures like," or the Law of Similars enunciated by Dr. Samuel Hahnemann, the German physician who fathered the art of homeopathy in the early 19th century.

"If a medicine administered to a healthy person causes a certain syndrome of symptoms, that medicine will cure a sick person who presents similar symptoms," Hahnemann declared, and proceeded to prove this hypothesis to his own satisfaction by administering homeopathic medications to many patients.

If this theory strikes you as a bit slippery, look at it this way. If you had a fever and you went to your family physician, the first thing he would try to do would be to find the reason why you have a fever. Then he would probably advise taking aspirin to reduce the fever. Aspirin is what is known as an "antipyretic," which means that it acts against fevers. That is the logic of its use.

The homeopath, on the other hand, operating on the principle that "like cures like," would probably prescribe some substance, of either herbal or chemical origin, which in a *healthy* person would actually *cause* a fever. He would give you this substance in a very tiny amount, most likely in the form of a pill which is not only tiny but contains the medication in a highly diluted form. And what this medication is going to do, he would say, is stimulate the natural resistance of your body to rise from its lethargy and defeat not only the fever induced by the medication but the fever that brought you to his office.

Everything clear?

We must admit that the principles underlying homeopathy, like those of acupuncture, are essentially incomprehensible to the student of modern physiology and medicine. The big difference is that while the *results* of acupuncture therapy—positive and negative—have been presented in hundreds of articles in journals and at medical conferences, precious little of a scientific nature has been presented which would encourage belief in homeopathy. Or for that matter, disbelief.

Anecdotes of the successful use of homeopathy are not lacking, from both clients and practitioners, but anecdotes—*by themselves*—are hardly enough evidence to conclude that homeopathy succeeds more often than it fails.

Looking again at the principles of homeopathy in action, imagine that you have been stung by a hornet and your whole arm is swollen and you're beginning to feel very weak. A typical M.D. would probably administer an antihistamine and perhaps epinephrine (adrenaline) to short-circuit the inflammatory reaction. The homeopath might well give you some tiny pills containing a diluted extract of hornet or bee venom. At least that is what one practitioner of the art told me he would do. And as I said to him, I simply can't understand why the body would react in a special way to the ingestion of a very tiny amount of poison when it is already loaded with larger amounts of the same poison.

Likewise, if a person had lead poisoning, the administration of tiny amounts of lead would seem to be useless, inasmuch as lead poisoning typically develops slowly over a period of months or years as the person ingests tiny amounts of lead on a daily basis until it accumulates to the point where symptoms of nerve damage appear. If the body does not react therapeutically to these small daily ingestions, why would it respond otherwise in the office of a homeopath?

Having said that, let me point out that nearly all homeopaths are also M.D.'s—they are supposed to be, although I know one who isn't—and hopefully, an M.D. is going to know how to deal with an acute illness in a reasonable way and is not going to use homeopathy in situations where the results would be doubtful. And in fact, the impression I have after checking up on some doctors who practice homeopathy is that they do not use the homeopathic approach in all cases. Some are just as likely to take the same approach to a given illness as any other M.D.

What I am getting at is that there may well be a considerable gap between the theory and practice of homeopathy. In practice, the pure homeopathic remedies seem more likely to be used on minor or chronic conditions where drug therapy is probably of little value, or as a last resort after all else has failed.

Another plus for the *practice* of homeopathy is that homeopathic doctors are not only trained in traditional medicine, but in herbal medicine and nutrition as well. They also devote considerably more time to each patient than most other practitioners, not because they are more considerate, but because there is such an enormous number of homeopathic remedies—kept in bottles which line shelf after shelf of any practitioner's office—that diagnosis and the choosing of the appropriate medications may be quite a lengthy process.

The number of homeopathic physicians in the United States is very small. Recently, though, more of them have been coming to my attention for some reason or other, and I notice that most of them seem to have excellent medical credentials. They appear to be enthusiastic, open minded, and eager to learn as much as possible about such therapies as acupuncture and biofeedback.

One homeopath on the West Coast admits that there is no scientific validation for homeopathic theories. But he insists that after completing medical school and serving an apprenticeship with a leading homeopath in Europe, he was completely convinced that homeopathy is basically correct and can sometimes perform "miracles." A friend of mine would agree with that assessment: a homeopath apparently cured his son of a very serious illness after a great many specialists at a very large hospital had failed to do the child much good. In this case, the homeopathic treatment consisted largely of herbs.

It would be wonderful if homeopathy could be tested as extensively and fairly as acupuncture. I see no signs that this will happen, however, and it seems that homeopathy will remain essentially a mystery for years to come.

# Hyperactivity

A child who is forever getting into things and straining at the bit to dash across the room or run outside is not necessarily hyperactive. The child who is truly hyperactive in a pathological sense has an attention span obviously shorter than other children and his behavior is more bizarre than simply energetic. In school, he is likely to disrupt the entire class by repeatedly jumping out of his seat, throwing things around the room, and generally acting as if he were "possessed."

That still leaves a considerable gray area between a child who is ill behaved and a child who is actually *ill*. Thousands of children who drive their teachers to distraction are given a drug to help control their behavior, but how many of them really need medication is the subject of considerable debate.

The most promising natural approach to true hyperactivity was developed in the late 1960s by Ben F. Feingold, M.D., who at the time was chief of the allergy department at the Kaiser-Permanente Medical Center in San Francisco. Dr. Feingold had already been achieving good success with children whose allergies did not seem to be caused by the usual allergens by putting them on a diet which excluded all artificially flavored and colored foods. Soon, he began to notice that a surprisingly large number of these children (and some adults as well) were observed to suddenly "outgrow" behavior problems of a hyperactive nature along with their skin allergies.

Years of further testing and research resulted in the publication of a book, *Why Your Child Is Hyperactive* (Random House, New York, 1975) in which Dr. Feingold presents a dietary plan to help control hyperactivity.

It is not a simple diet. It excludes many processed foods and virtually all "junk foods" because they contain synthetic coloring and flavoring agents. It also excludes aspirin preparations, a number of over-the-counter remedies, including artificially flavored vitamin pills. In addition, it eliminates a rather large number of fruits because they contain substances which are similar to aspirin, which is one of the prime offenders. Excluded are almonds, apples, apricots, berries, cherries, grapes and raisins, nectarines, oranges, peaches, plums, and prunes. Tomatoes and all tomato products, as well as cucumbers and pickles, are also prohibited.

Adherence to this diet must be strict if results are to be achieved; a single piece of additive-laden cake, for instance, eaten at a birthday party, can trigger symptoms which may last for three days! If you wish to try this diet, please read Dr. Feingold's book, where the diet is given in its complete form along with other vital information.

We cannot say at this point that Dr. Feingold's diet has been proven to work on most children. However, in 1975, a double-blind study carried out by C. Keith Conners, Ph.D., indicated that the diet was of definite value. Dr. Conners divided 15 hyperactive children into two groups for a period of 12 weeks. One group received a normal or control diet containing the usual processed and additive-laden foods. The other group received the special elimination diet described by Dr. Feingold.

Because the study was double-blind, neither the investigators nor the children (nor their parents and teachers) knew which diet was being followed. At the end of the study, observations by all concerned revealed that there was a significant reduction in hyperactive symptoms only in those children who were eating the Feingold diet.

Dr. Feingold's ideas about hyperactivity and diet have been sharply attacked by a number of government figures and nutritionists. This is hardly surprising, since for years they have maintained that there is nothing, absolutely nothing, deleterious about "approved" food additives. They have demanded further extensive tests of Dr. Feingold's diet, but it is worth keeping in mind that the driving force behind these "scientific" tests now being carried out is the Nutrition Foundation, a group established and funded by the Coca-Cola company, the Life Saver company, and most of the other giant manufacturers of either processed foods or food additives. Need we say more?

# Hypnosis

**by B. Joan Arner**

It's a real shame that hypnosis as a therapeutic tool is still largely a stranger to us. To some, the very word probably conjures up images of Boris Karloff drilling his gaze into the eyes of a young girl. At least, there is the basic idea that hypnosis means one person *imposing his will* on that of another person—even if only to make a night club audience laugh at the subject's hilarious antics.

In the healing context, hypnosis is precisely the *opposite* of one person imposing his will on another. Rather, hypnosis means trying to impose your *own* conscious desire to be well upon your *own* body and mind. Certainly, there is a hypnotherapist involved, but in perspective, all the therapist is doing is helping the client achieve some goal which the *client* desires.

Doctors today who are interested in treating the whole patient like to talk about "taking control of your own health." And despite the need for a facilitating therapist, there is probably no therapy which more dramatically permits a person to "take control" of his or her own health than hypnosis.

Consider an actual case, involving a teenage girl. "I have never seen so many warts on one individual in my life," Thomas A. Clawson, Jr., M.D., wrote later in a scientific journal. "Her face and body were literally covered with pinhead size warts. There were hundreds of them, including five large ones on her arms."

A dermatologist had referred this particular case to Dr. Clawson, of Rancho Mirage, California. The dermatologist had failed for several years to get results in treating the girl; if one wart disappeared several appeared in its place.

And now Dr. Clawson proposed to treat this stubborn problem through hypnosis. Although the girl's mother was skeptical, she agreed to the attempt.

When the doctor had induced hypnosis, he told his patient, "Catherine, your subconscious mind has the ability to control the blood supply to any part of the body. Now I want you to stop the blood supply to each wart on your body."

After repeating this suggestion three times, Dr. Clawson awakened the girl and advised her to come once a week for hypnosis.

As if magically, the number of warts decreased from week to week. All were gone within two months. Three and a half years later not one wart had recurred, Dr. Clawson wrote with a colleague, Richard H. Swade, Ph.D., in *The American Journal of Clinical Hypnosis,* January 1975.

This dramatic episode points up a fact with important implications: No longer a trick for charlatans or performers, hypnosis is finding a valued place among the tools of the health professions. And this is true although no one knows for certain how it works or what its limits are.

One plausible theory is that hypnosis bypasses the conscious, "logical" mind. At the subconscious level, the subject is open to all sorts of suggestions from the hypnotist. The subconscious mind accepts all these suggestions as "true," since it has no way of judging objective truth or falsity.

The suggestions the subconscious accepts and acts upon would almost defy belief if they were not attested to by reputable scientific researchers. For instance, in the example given above, Dr. Clawson suggested to his patient that she could control the flow of blood to her warts. Normally, of course, blood circulation is not under the control of our individual will. Can hypnotism give us that control?

## Control Over Blood Clotting

Emphatically yes—and for that we have the testimony of doctors and dentists who work with hemophiliacs or "bleeders." For hemophiliacs, any minor cut is a crisis, because their blood does not clot normally. In such patients control of blood flow is nothing less than a matter of life and death—and in many cases such control has been achieved through hypnosis.

Dr. Oscar N. Lucas, a dental surgeon, is one practitioner who uses hypnosis in his work with hemophiliacs. He reports being able to extract up to six teeth at one sitting from severe hemophiliacs, without blood transfusions, using hypnosis as an aid.

Dr. Lucas has observed that emotionally tranquil hemophiliacs tend to bleed less severely than those who are under emotional stress. He uses hypnotic suggestion to induce calm in his patients, since for many victims of hemophilia the prospect of a tooth extraction is as traumatic as the anticipation of major surgery would be for the average person.

He goes so far as to say, "During the pre-extraction period the hemophiliac is very afraid, emotionally distressed, and fearful of the hemorrhage that follows the dental extraction. *This pre-operative period of anxiety in a hemophiliac may frequently be the cause of failure to produce hemostasis* [clotting] *in a dental extraction even after the best performed surgical technique and the correction of the clotting defect by blood, plasma, or A.H.G.* [antihemophilic globulin] *has been done"* (emphasis mine; *American Journal of Clinical Hypnosis,* April 1965).

In other words, scientists now recognize that the mind or emotions can have a great influence on "involuntary" body functions such as blood circulation and clotting. They are also, as in Dr. Lucas's work, beginning to see that to some extent at least—and no one is sure yet to *what* extent—they can "control the emotional controls" through hypnosis.

## 'Plastic Surgery' by Hypnosis

If incidents involving the control of blood circulation by hypnosis seem unbelievable, they pale before the work of James E. Williams, director of the Greg Harrison Mental Health and Retardation Center in Longview, Texas, and vice-chairman of the Texas Board of Hypnosis Examiners. For Williams's results seem to indicate that hypnosis can be used as an aid in causing body organs to grow even after they have attained what would normally be full size. Specifically, he conducted a series of experiments in which hypnosis was used to increase breast size in women (*Journal of Sex Research,* November 1974).

Dr. Williams, a psychologist, told us he was approached in 1964 by a woman whose son's grand mal epilepsy seizures had been alleviated by hypnosis, and who wanted to know whether the technique could be used to increase bust size. In response he conducted a study using volunteer female students of North Texas State University, Denton, Texas. His technique involved hypnotizing members of his experimental group and giving them suggestions regarding breast growth.

The women, undergraduate and graduate students, ranged in age from 18 to 40 years, with an average age of 24. Each was hypnotized for about one hour, once a week, for 12 weeks. The treatment procedure, Dr. Williams explained, "consisted of a series of suggestions for regression to a period when the breasts were developing, and the sensations of breast growth were suggested during this period. Suggestions were then given for time projection to an unspecified future date, and the subject was directed to visualize her body image with increased breast size."

Following each treatment, a series of measurements were taken with calipers and a tape measure to note changes both in the total bust measurement and the size of the breasts themselves. Measurements were confirmed by other subjects involved in the experiment. The measurements taken following the last three treatments were averaged and considered to be the "result."

At the beginning of the experiment, the average bust size, measured after exhalation, and taken on the horizontal plane of the nipples, was 33.64 inches. At the end of the experiment, it was determined that every individual had experienced enlargement of the breasts, with increases ranging from one to 3½ inches. The average increase was 2⅛ inches.

The possibility that this increase represented enlargement in chest size, rather than breast size, was ruled out by differential measurements. It was determined that, on the average, the chest size of the women had actually decreased during the experiment, while their breasts had increased in size. Further, the increase was symmetrical.

In further work on the same subjects, Dr. Williams told us that the women had maintained these gains.

Breast size among women is, of course, a matter with complex psychological overtones, and the "natural plastic surgery" effect reported by Dr. Williams may provide an alternative to various bust enlargement methods now in use. And if hypnosis can produce growth in other organs "on demand," the medical applications of Dr. Williams's work may prove to be far broader than anything that can be imagined at present.

## Control Over 'Habits' Such as Bed-wetting

The use of hypnosis in simpler cases—those such as habits involving purely psychological factors—has long been well known. Even so, it is worthwhile taking a look at some of the more spectacular research work in this field, if only to remind ourselves of the possibilities. Many of the habits hypnosis has helped to overcome shorten life or make it miserable, and the victims of such patterns of behavior need all the help—and hope—they can get.

To a child, for instance, few things can be more humiliating and uncomfortable than bed-wetting (nocturnal enuresis). To combat the problem parents have tried everything from bribery to ridicule, and in between many have purchased gadgets such as alarm systems which disturb the child's sleep cycle. Doctors have been driven to trying such drugs as imipramine, which has only temporary effects and which has caused deaths among children when taken accidentally. (Imipramine has not been approved by the FDA for children under the age of 12.) Caught in a web of stresses, it is not uncommon for the child who is a bed wetter to develop an emotional disturbance.

Among these not-very-attractive alternatives, can hypnosis provide a better way to deal with bed-wetting? Indications are that in many ways it can.

Karen Olness, M.D., Assistant Professor of Medicine and of

Child Health and Development at George Washington University, Washington, D.C., decided to try teaching self-hypnosis to a group of 40 children as a means to overcome this particular problem (*Clinical Pediatrics,* March 1975). The children, 20 girls and 20 boys, ranged in age from 4½ to 16 years. Only two of the group were teenagers. These two were taught a standard self-hypnosis technique. The rest of the children were shown a special method adapted to their age.

With a marking pencil, a clown face was drawn on the right or left thumbnail, depending on the child's preference. A quarter was then placed between the thumb and forefinger, and the child was asked to hold the quarter up in front of his face in such a way that he was looking at the face on the thumbnail. "He was then told that he was to focus only on the face and that, as he did so, the quarter would slowly become heavy and would slip down and fall," Dr. Olness explains. "When this happened he would feel very relaxed and his eyes would close." If the quarter fell on the floor, the child was told not to worry about it but was instructed to put his hands on his legs and answer questions by raising his "yes" hand or his "no" hand. Usually, the quarter would fall within five minutes, and a number of questions were asked, such as, "Do you like the color yellow?", "Do you like to eat ice cream?" and, finally, "Would you like to have dry beds every night?"

If the child answered in the affirmative, he was told that he could use the trick that was now in progress to teach himself to wake up every time he needs to urinate, and to go to the bathroom. In doing the "trick," the child would tell himself, after the quarter fell out of his hand: "When I need to urinate I will wake up all by myself, go to the bathroom all by myself, urinate in the toilet, and return to my nice dry bed." This was repeated several times and the child was praised for being such a quick learner. He was also told that by learning to do this trick and not urinating in bed, he would be very happy when he woke up in his dry bed.

The 40 children had been followed for periods ranging from 6 to 28 months at the time Dr. Olness reported on her study. Thirty-one appeared to have been cured completely of bed-wetting, 28 in the first month of treatment. Six others improved, while of the remaining three, one learned self-hypnosis with great difficulty and did not practice it very often, and a second had had a urinary tract operation at age four and showed only marginal improvement. The third learned self-hypnosis easily but gave a "no" answer twice when asked the question, "Would you like dry beds?" He was referred for psychiatric evaluation.

Some of the parents reported that as their children gained bladder control they also improved in their schoolwork and in general behavior—an instance in which overcoming one undesirable habit leads to benefits all around.

But if hypnosis holds out hope for many sufferers, it is not a plaything or an entertainment. We know very little about the mechanism of the mind or how hypnosis affects it. Unfortunately, some hypnotists are trained only in hypnosis and have no idea at all of the workings of the mind and body. *It is always advisable to choose a hypnotist who is a trained doctor, clinical psychologist, or dentist.* Usually a call to your city or county medical, psychological, or dental association will provide you with several names, or you may send a self-addressed stamped envelope to the American Society of Clinical Hypnosis, 2400 E. Devon, Suite 218, Des Plaines, Illinois 60018.

# Hypoglycemia

Hypoglycemia, also known as functional hypoglycemia and low blood sugar, has been the subject of many heated debates. Some doctors claim that the condition is quite common, occurring in about one out of every ten people, while others call it rare and still others deny its very existence.

Doctors who do find hypoglycemia in their patients associate it with such symptoms as nervousness, irritability, chronic fatigue, dizziness, headaches, and to a lesser extent, a host of physical complaints, such as aching joints and racing pulse. The skeptics look at such cases and say they are either classic examples of neurosis or hypochondria, or just the "ordinary" aches, pains, and worries of everyday life.

Doctors who "believe" in hypoglycemia counter that when the normal sugar level of the blood drops, the first organ to be affected is the brain, and when the brain is starved of its only fuel—glucose—it's not surprising that the symptoms mimic those of neurosis and many other conditions which involve the nervous system.

But why should hypoglycemics have low blood sugar? Very

basically, the leading theory is that in most cases the insulin-secreting portion of the pancreas is overactive, so that when sugar enters the bloodstream, it is not only controlled (shifted into tissues) by insulin, but *over*controlled; i.e., too much of it is removed from the bloodstream. In some cases of mild low blood sugar, doctors may prescribe eating a piece of candy to boost the sugar level. And while this may be bad advice in the long run, it's said that the heavyweight boxer, Muhammad Ali, for instance, eats candy when his blood sugar drops and is apparently—so far—none the worse for it. In other cases, however, eating candy is—ironically—the very worst thing to do.

In these cases, the infusion of sugar into the bloodstream reverses the symptoms temporarily, but before long, perhaps in a few hours, the activity of insulin called forth in reaction to the high sugar levels becomes so intense that all the new sugar is swept out of the bloodstream, and with it, some of the scant amount of sugar that was there to begin with. This is sometimes called reactive hypoglycemia.

At least, that is how the theory goes at present; like every other medical theory, it is subject to change. In any event, we still haven't answered the question of whether hypoglycemia is a "real" condition which afflicts a substantial number of people, or rather a phantom disease that is nothing more than a convenient explanation for symptoms which cannot be explained by physical damage to the pancreas, the nervous system, or other organs.

## The Doctor Who Has Never Seen Functional Low Blood Sugar

Let's suppose that you had heard someone mention hypoglycemia and were wondering what it was, and if it could possibly be responsible for some chronic and troublesome symptoms which your doctor has not been able to help. Then, you look in the newspaper, and read the words of a rather well-known physician who declares: "I have never seen a case of functional low blood sugar in 30 years of practice." That sounds pretty convincing, doesn't it?

Well, it so happens that a man by the name of Stephen Gyland who had been troubled for several years with unprovoked anxieties, dizziness, weakness, and difficulty in concentrating, went to the clinic where that well-known doctor was on the staff, and was told that his problems were a result of a brain tumor.

But Stephen Gyland is an M.D. himself, and when he persisted in an attempt to find the true cause of his problems, he learned that he did not have a brain tumor at all. What he had was functional low blood sugar, the condition which that well-known doctor said he had never seen in 30 years of practice.

The incident is related in *Low Blood Sugar and You* by Carlton Fredericks, Ph.D., and Herman Goodman, M.D. (Constellation International, New York, 1969), the classic book in the field of hypoglycemia (which may shortly be republished in a revised edition). It seems that Dr. Gyland, who practiced in Tampa, Florida, became ill with a variety of symptoms and sought medical help. As Dr. Gyland himself said in a letter he wrote to the *Journal of the American Medical Association* (July 18, 1953): "During three years of severe illness, I was examined by 14 specialists and 3 nationally known clinics before a diagnosis was made by means of a six-hour glucose (sugar) tolerance test, previous diagnoses having been brain tumor, diabetes, and cerebral arteriosclerosis."

After adapting a hypoglycemia diet, Dr. Gyland's symptoms simply faded away.

The glucose tolerance test which Dr. Gyland mentioned is generally done in the following manner. For three days, a high-carbohydrate diet is eaten. On the fourth day, the level of blood sugar is tested in a fasting state, and a drink containing a great amount of sugar is given. Then, on an hourly basis, blood samples are drawn and checked for sugar content. It's advisable for the test to continue for five to six hours. Typically, in a hypoglycemic, the blood sugar level does not increase at the normal rate. And in many cases, the initial rise is followed by a steep fall to below-fasting levels. This may not happen, however, for four or five hours and that is why the test should be that long.

Because the glucose tolerance test is somewhat of a nuisance to take, and because the results are not always clear, many doctors who are extremely skeptical about low blood sugar to begin with will not order one for a patient. While I do not have the definitive answer to this problem, let me relate an anecdote which I think is pertinent. It was told to me by a good friend and former colleague, and retold several times, so I could get as many details from him as he could recall.

## A Case of Migraine from Low Blood Sugar

Jerry was a young art director in his twenties. He was extremely athletic and seemed to be in vigorous health, except that for several years he had been plagued with migraine headaches. Sometimes they would hit him at work, but more often they would strike at night, waking him up from his sleep with excruciating pain. Aspirin "wouldn't touch the pain," and drugs helped but little. It appeared to be a classic migraine, seizing hold of half his head (I forget which side he mentioned) and causing tears to flow from one eye.

Naturally, he frequently visited his family physician, but eventually, he was simply told that nothing more could be done for him. Finally, when the headaches began hitting him several times a week, and his family physician was out of town, he decided to visit a clinic which specialized in difficult diagnoses. After his initial examination, he was hospitalized for three days and given innumerable tests. After two days, there was still no evidence of a tumor or any other physical cause of his migraines. On the very last day, though, he was given a glucose tolerance test. Several hours later one of his doctors came waltzing into his room and announced that his blood sugar had plunged to an extremely low level, and it was obvious that he was hypoglycemic.

In questioning him about this incident, I asked him if the test itself produced a migraine, and he replied that he did not recall that it did. This is significant, because some doctors assume that if the symptoms are not provoked by the glucose tolerance test, then they are not a result of low blood sugar.

In Jerry's case, his doctors put him on a strict hypoglycemia diet. Basically, this means eating from four to six small meals a day, each of them containing a generous amount of protein. Sugar in any form is completely forbidden. Besides no ice cream and cake, this means no processed foods of any kind to which sugar has been added. And in a strict diet, it even means no oranges or grapes because of the large amount of natural sugars these foods contain. Coffee, tea, and alcoholic beverages are also forbidden.

He immediately went on his diet, and for the first time in years his headaches ceased completely. Gradually, he was able to "loosen" the diet a bit, until he discovered the point at which trouble started again. In time, he found that he was able to drink a bottle of beer without any problems, but occasionally he would be caught by surprise. He also found that drinking a glass of milk first thing in the morning and last thing at night was excellent, apparently because milk is rich in protein and also contains a small amount of natural sugar (in the form of lactose) which very gently raises blood sugar levels.

In the years since he made that discovery, Jerry has remained free of headaches, but often wonders about other people who might be plagued with similar problems and who were told by their physicians—as he was by his—that there is no hope except drugs.

He added a final ironic note to his story. "You know, when I was having all those headaches, my mother used to tell me that I might not get them if I ate a good breakfast before leaving the house in the morning. That used to make me angry, and I would snap at her that migraine headaches had nothing to do with diet. But now, looking back, I have to admit that my mother's old-fashioned obsession about eating a good breakfast before leaving the house was right on the button. In fact, if I had listened to her, most of my problems would have been solved."

Dr. Fredericks and others who have investigated blood sugar problems recommend a daily supplement of brewer's yeast, perhaps a tablespoon a day, because of its B-complex vitamins and its relatively high content of chromium, a trace element which helps to normalize blood sugar metabolism. If you are overweight, try by all means to slim down, because that can also be a great help.

A clinical psychologist who is knowledgeable about hypoglycemia points out that if you or your doctor do not wish to bother with a glucose tolerance test, there is a simple alternative. Simply put yourself on a strict hypoglycemia diet for a week. If you notice a tremendous difference in how you feel, you can be fairly certain that you are hypoglycemic, and in that case, you can continue the diet. After a while, you can try eating oranges and grapes again if you wish; chances are, you will be able to handle them. Basically, though, eat all you wish of milk, cheese, cottage cheese, vegetables, fruits (except sweetened or dried), and lean meats. Be sure to eat immediately upon awakening and shortly before going to bed.

For more detailed information on a hypoglycemia diet, you can consult the book by Drs. Fredericks and Goodman.

# Infertility

Textbooks say that laboratory rodents made deficient in vitamin E will become sterile, but that this finding has no relevance for human beings. Whether that assertion is true or not, however, I am not so sure.

I personally know of one case in which a young married couple was unable to have children. Tests revealed that the man had an extremely low sperm count, which all but precluded the possibility of impregnating his wife. On the advice of a friend, he began taking several hundred units of vitamin E daily. A month later, his wife was pregnant. And while that incident certainly proves nothing, it's worth keeping in mind that their total investment was about $2.

A woman wrote to us with an even more dramatic story. At the age of 19, she said, she ceased having monthly periods. Because she wanted a family, she sought out medical help and "for the next four years I underwent various tests, took medications, but still no change took place."

Jumping ahead six years, the woman said that she read about a new drug. Even though it was experimental, and there were risks involved, she decided to try it. "After two years of extensive, expensive, painful, and discomforting tests, I became pregnant."

When their son was two years old, the couple decided they wanted another baby, and the woman once again began getting injections of the drug. This time, however, it did not lead to conception.

One year later, she became keenly interested in nutrition. She stocked up on raw wheat germ and began using it liberally in everything, and then also began taking some wheat germ oil concentrate.

"About one week later, I started experiencing severe cramps and my husband suggested I stop taking it for a while. Then two weeks later I had my first menstrual period since the age of 19—16 years ago!"

Her periods continued for several months and then stopped. The woman believed she was no longer ovulating and became quite depressed. Then she also became nauseous, which she attributed to the flu. "I decided to call my new doctor. He became quite excited, having studied my past records, and was quite interested in my case. He insisted I come in for a checkup and pregnancy test. A pregnancy test! I hadn't even thought of that—well, not too much, for fear of another disappointment.

"I dreaded that Friday morning appointment. I knew I would be extremely frustrated if the tests were not positive. I was tempted to break my appointment. But I kept it, and the tests proved positive!"

Then, the woman asked, "Why, oh why, with all their medical knowledge, did not one of the doctors suggest this possible deficiency?"

The answer, of course, is that the textbooks say it's impossible: wheat germ and its vitamin E can't help. And that's why it took this woman 11 years and about $1,500 to conceive her first child, and a few months and a few dollars to conceive her second.

I certainly don't want to hold forth the expectation that vitamin E or wheat germ is going to do the trick for every infertile woman, or even a substantial fraction, but clearly, from a purely practical point of view, it should at least be given an honest try.

In fact, inasmuch as fertility and successful pregnancy require the participation of all nutrients, anyone—male or female—with reproductive problems would be well advised to insure that vitamin and mineral intake is *more* than adequate. Some European research also suggests that the bioflavonoids, not considered vitamins in the United States, can also help in cases where women have previously had spontaneous abortions or miscarriages. Apparently, the bioflavonoids work in concert with vitamin C to increase the strength of small blood vessels.

## High Temperatures Can Wilt Sperm

An article in the *Journal of the American Medical Association* on March 4, 1974, suggests that there is something that can be done for some men with low sperm counts. Research conducted by Howard W. Gabriel, III, Ph.D., associate director of the Health Planning Council of Southcentral Kansas at Wichita, found that an unusual number of men with low sperm counts were for various reasons causing excessive heat to build up in their scrotums, where sperm are produced. Sperm can only be manufactured at temperatures somewhat lower than the normal body temperature (that's why there is a scrotum), and in the presence of excess heat, sperm production is slowed down or halted.

Dr. Gabriel found that this excessive heat could result from taking hot showers or baths, sauna or steam baths; the use of tight-fitting underwear or athletic supporters, tight or dark-colored pants; the use of electric blankets at night; or occupational exposure to very high temperatures.

Dr. Gabriel suggests that taking a cold bath for half an hour can not only cause a rise in the sperm count but also make the sperm livelier. One man who had tried unsuccessfully to impregnate his wife for two years was able to do so three weeks after he began taking baths in 65° F. water. During the time that he was infertile, his job had exposed him to extreme heat for several hours each day, and he was also in the habit of taking long, warm baths on a daily basis.

Although it may seem bizarre, one doctor obtained impressive results by giving tranquilizers to women patients in which no particular reason could be found for their infertility. In cases where conception did not result, he also gave tranquilizers to the husbands and succeeded in producing still more conceptions.

What was apparently happening in these cases was that the anxieties and guilt reactions aroused in some people who are not able to conceive children as rapidly as they wish makes it all the more difficult for them to conceive a child.

A number of people have told me that they have attempted to conceive a child by various methods but were unable to do so for several months. But, when they discarded the "plan" and all the expectations and anxieties that went with it, and resumed sexual relations on a random, impulsive basis, conception quickly followed.

# Insect Bites And Stings

When my daughter was very young, she was running in the grass and a bee stung her on the sole of her foot. It was very painful as well as frightening to her. A quick call to a doctor's office got us these words of advice from his nurse: pour some cold water into a pot, dump in some baking soda, stir, and add a tray of ice cubes. Soak the foot.

The swelling and pain were stopped almost instantly after we plunged her foot into this icy bath.

(If the stinger of the honeybee remains in the skin, it should be scraped out, not pulled out.)

If you don't have baking soda or cold water handy, try applying a fresh-cut slice of raw onion to a sting. Hold it or tape in place and you may find swift relief.

No onion? Try smearing the sting with honey and then putting an ice bag on top, or else plunge the honey-smeared part in ice cold water. Wheat germ oil may work just as well as honey.

Some people swear by plantain, the common broad-leaved weed, for treating all kinds of insect bites. It may help as much for a bee-sting as for the itching of a mosquito bite. Plantain fanciers use this tried-and-true technique: Tear off a few leaves, bruise or break them, and then heat (but don't burn) them with a match until the leaves are wilted. Squeeze the juice from the weed and apply it to the sting or bite.

If you are bitten by a venomous insect, such as the brown recluse spider, you are well advised to seek immediate medical attention. Dr. Frederick Klenner has used massive doses of vitamin C to treat venomous bites. By massive doses, I mean thousands of milligrams.

The itching of mosquito bites may be relieved by applying a poultice of cornstarch, fresh lemon juice, or witch hazel. One reader told us that she was quite sensitive to mosquito bites and would get swollen lumps "that remain and itch for weeks." Nothing helped her, she said, until she applied a mixture of alcohol and PABA, the B vitamin. This solution provided almost instant relief from itching, she said, and the swollen bites disappeared in less than a day. Such solutions are now widely available either in drugstores or from health food sources in the form of a suntan lotion. The ingredients should state that the lotion contains both PABA and ethyl alcohol.

Let's digress for just a paragraph or two from our format as a "healing" book and suggest that a good way of *preventing* bites from most insects is to take large amounts of thiamine, or vitamin $B_1$. If you are going on a picnic, for instance, take one 100 mg. tablet or the equivalent before leaving the house. If you're going camping, take a bottle and swallow one tablet two or three times a day. When you take this much thiamine—far more than a normal supplemental amount—the body excretes part of the overload through the pores of the skin. It seems that the thiamine has an odor that most insects can't stand. I would consider this to be a highly reliable preventive measure, especially for mosquitoes and flies. It also keeps fleas off pets. If your pet is small, you may find that simply adding some brewer's yeast to the diet will be enough to rid him of fleas.

Rubbing crushed pennyroyal leaves on the skin is also said to keep away mosquitoes and gnats. Mességué, the herbalist, adivses hanging a bouquet of dried tomato leaves in all rooms of your house to keep out bothersome bugs. One woman told me that she unexpectedly drove all the ants out of her pantry when she placed a box of goldenseal tea bags in it.

# Insomnia

Over-the-counter sleeping pills are one of the biggest rip-offs in the drugstore. A study of the most popular brand revealed that besides being ineffective, it produced worse side effects than Librium, a prescription tranquilizer.

But if you do suffer from insomnia, take heart, because there are a number of excellent and purely natural relaxation inducers that can help you.

One is plain warm milk. Dr. Julius Segal of the National Institute of Mental Health has pointed out that milk contains generous amounts of the amino acid tryptophan. When this amino acid was given to volunteers in sleep research experiments, Dr. Segal said that they fell asleep with unusual speed, awoke less during the night, and spent more time than usual in the deep phases of sleep. Dr. Segal recognizes that a warm glass of milk also has an emotionally soothing effect, but he thinks its sedative quality goes further than this. Even animals can be sedated with large doses of tryptophan, and it seems unlikely that any psychological effect would be involved.

If warm milk is not your cup of tea, why not *try* tea? Not ordinary tea, which contains caffeine, but an herb tea.

One of the best is camomile. Long recognized by traditional herbalism as a harmless sedative, camomile was tested by Lawrence Gould, M.D., and colleagues, who reported their findings in the *Journal of Clinical Pharmacology* (January 10, 1974). Actually, the purpose of their test was to see if camomile tea had any ill effects on cardiac patients who had undergone ventricular catheterization as part of their treatment. The tests showed that drinking camomile tea had no significant cardiac effects. But there *was* a positive reaction of a different kind: "A striking hypnotic [sleep-inducing] action of the tea was noted in 10 of 12 patients," the medical team reported. "It is most unusual for patients undergoing cardiac catheterizations to fall asleep. The anxiety produced by this procedure as well as the pain associated with cardiac catheterizations all but preclude sleep. Thus," their report continues, "the fact that 10 out of 12 patients fell into a deep slumber shortly after drinking camomile tea is all the more striking."

It seems that if someone can fall asleep right after undergoing a painful medical procedure, the more garden-variety traumas of everyday life ought to be easy work for a nice warm cup of camomile tea.

Other herbs valued for overcoming insomnia are hops, passionflower, catnip, basil, violets (the leaves), and lemon verbena. Catnip seems to be especially valuable if you're being kept awake by pain. Kloss says that catnip should be steeped, but not boiled, and flavored with some honey.

Personally, I have found that a bowl of garlic soup prepared with chicken broth makes me very warm and sleepy.

Kordel, in his excellent book *Natural Folk Remedies,* relates that he found this recipe for a nightcap in Spain: Dissolve two tablespoons of honey in a glass of buttermilk and stir in the juice of one lemon, mixing well. This might be good for people who have lactose intolerance and cannot ordinarily drink milk without making their bowels rumble, as fermented milk is more easily digested.

## Try Exercise and Napping

Drinking herbal tea or milk should not be the only part of your program if you have insomnia. Exercise—the right kind—may be just what you need to relax you. This doesn't mean exercising before going to bed. On the contrary, the best time to exercise is in the morning or afternoon. A good long walk of several miles fills the bill perfectly.

One mistake a lot of people make is to assume that all sleep must be gotten at night. Actually, many have found that the answer to getting more rest is an afternoon nap. One advocate of the daily siesta is Dr. Uros Jovanovic, whose work has been discussed in the *German Tribune.* "People need to take a nap some time between 1 P.M. and 3 P.M. to maintain full efficiency," Dr. Jovanovic says. An afternoon nap should be not less than 20 minutes long or more than 90 minutes."

An unsuspected benefit of the afternoon nap is that many people find it helps them sleep better at night. Dr. Philip M. Tiller, Jr., of Louisiana State University School of Medicine, conducted experiments during the late 1960s, in which several hundred women complaining of being tired, nervous, and generally run down were all induced to take a one- or two-hour afternoon nap. They were also told to try to sleep at least nine or ten hours at night. He determined that the afternoon nap, far from interfering with nocturnal slumber, actually helped the women get a better night's rest. On this regimen, about two-thirds of the women reported significant improvement in their symptoms.

At first, you will probably find it very difficult to nap during the afternoon if you aren't used to it, but you will soon learn to enjoy it. And if you can't actually fall asleep, just lie still. It will help you to relax and ease your tensions.

You may also want to use the techniques of meditation to help you fall asleep. Although these techniques were not designed to put you to sleep, they can have that effect if you practice them while lying in bed. Dr. Herbert Benson, author of *The Relaxation Response* (William Morrow and Co., New York, 1975), says he personally finds that meditating "works beautifully" if you wake up in the middle of the night (see MEDITATION).

# Itching

Itching in the rectal area, politely called pruritus ani, can be absolutely maddening. If you have this condition, you have probably been to several doctors already and tried every over-the-counter medication available. But natural remedies can often do what no drug can.

Not long ago, a reader told us that he had been afflicted with sores and irritation in the anal area for over two years. He went to all kinds of doctors and each one gave him a different ointment. He went so far as to name five of them by their brand names and said that was only the beginning of the list. Nevertheless, the condition did not clear up. In fact, it grew steadily worse. "I was on my way to becoming a partial invalid because of the pain and deterioration of the entire area. Finally I was given X-ray treatments but this did not clear it up. A few of the drugs gave me temporary and partial relief for a day or so, but back again came the sores with ferocious intensity.

"In desperation, I decided to use natural vitamins and home treatment. For the first time in two years I have cleared it up *completely* and it has not returned for six weeks. The real miracle is *wheat germ oil*."

He went on to explain that he scrupulously washed himself several times a day with warm water, dried himself, and then applied the wheat germ oil.

After his letter was published in PREVENTION, another reader wrote in to say that this technique put an end to the torment he had suffered for over 15 years. Doctors had told him that his condition was caused by antibiotics killing off the beneficial bacteria in his bowels. He tried buttermilk, yogurt, and various salves but in no case was the benefit lasting. Then he took the advice of the other reader and washed himself with soap, rinsed it off, dried with tissue, and applied the wheat germ oil to the affected parts. The sores and itching vanished.

Some foods, such as citrus fruit and sugar, are said to sometimes cause pruritus ani. Another cause—oddly enough—may be cigarette smoking. At least, one reader told us that he suffered with pruritus ani for many years until he stopped smoking and was amazed to realize that his bottom no longer itched. This makes sense, because heavy smoking reduces blood circulation in the peripheral and genital areas and poor circulation can in turn cause intense itching.

Application of vitamin E oil has also helped many itches.

For more or less temporary itches, try making a paste of baking soda and water. Or use oatmeal or cornstarch instead of the baking soda. Fresh lemon juice or witch hazel lotion are also good for an occasional itch. Personally, when I have a mosquito bite that itches, I put some water (or saliva) on it, sprinkle on some salt and then rub it in. If it's really a bad itch, I then pour on some witch hazel or wintergreen alcohol. Some people, though, will find the salt treatment too irritating to their skin.

See also DERMATITIS and ECZEMA.

# Kidney Stones

Calcium oxalate stones, the most common kind, can often be prevented. It appears that they occur, in the vast majority of cases, because of a double nutritional deficiency. Adequate daily supplements of the two deficient nutrients—magnesium and vitamin $B_6$—may be all that's needed for a person to rid himself of this often agonizing ailment.

Harvard investigators Drs. Edwin L. Prien, Sr., and Stanley F. Gershoff, first announced their successful use of the double supplement in the *American Journal of Clinical Nutrition,* May 1967. Of 36 patients who previously had formed at least two urinary stones a year, the investigators reported, 30 either had no further stone recurrence or markedly decreased recurrence during the five years or more they were protected by a daily supplement of magnesium oxide and pyridoxine ($B_6$).

Judging from the latest word from Drs. Prien and Gershoff, the chances of success are high indeed. In their article published in the *Journal of Urology* (October 1974), the authors report on an expanded study, involving the cooperation of 64 urologists and (initially) 265 carefully selected patients, all with a long history of chronic stone formation. In the course of the investigation (approximately five years), 98 patients were lost to the study for a variety of reasons.

Of those who stayed with the program and continued to take the protective nutrients, only 17 were considered failures and continued to form stones as in the past. Eighteen others continued to have pain symptoms (though milder than before) and probably—say the investigators—passed small fragments of stone or "gravel" in their urine. The remaining 132 were symptom-free and stone-free.

All of 89 percent benefited, and 79 percent found complete protection—simply by regular ingestion of two harmless nutrients!

"A number of patients, having become free of stones," Drs. Prien and Gershoff write, "stopped treatment and began having stones again within a few weeks, only to become free of stones again when they resumed treatment."

## What's In a Stone?

The content of stones varies geographically and even with the stage of "civilization" a country has reached. But in North America, the Harvard researchers say, the major substance making up urinary stones is calcium oxalate. "About a third of the urinary calculi are composed of this substance and another third contain major amounts, usually associated with calcium phosphate," they note. Oxalic acid and calcium—both normal constituents of urine—combine to form this relatively insoluble crystal.

But oxalic acid from the diet forms only a minute portion of the oxalic acid present in urine. Drs. Louis Hagler and Robert H. Herman, Army research scientists writing a three-part series on oxalate metabolism in the *American Journal of Clinical Nutrition* (July, August, September 1973), explain that only about two percent of dietary oxalate is absorbed and eventually excreted in the urine. Most of the urine's oxalate is synthesized by the body itself.

"The urine is normally supersaturated with respect to calcium oxalate," Drs. Hagler and Herman state. Then why do most people *not* get urinary stones, the authors question, and "in what ways do stone formers differ from the normal?"

It seems very clear that nature must normally provide some protective device so that, despite the supersaturation of urine with calcium oxalate, most of us never have kidney stone trouble. And if this natural protection is largely provided by dietary magnesium and vitamin $B_6$, we might guess that stone formers "differ from the normal" in terms of their greater requirement for these two nutrients.

## Magnesium and $B_6$

Not that they need extravagant amounts. In working with stone-forming patients, the Harvard team successfully used 300 mg. of magnesium oxide—actually less than the Recommended Dietary Allowance (RDA) of 350 mg. As for vitamin $B_6$, patients received 10 mg., which is five times greater than the RDA. But much recent research on this B vitamin suggests that 10 mg. is probably much closer to the human physiological need for the nutrient than the meager 2 mg. declared adequate by the National Research Council and the Food and Drug Administration.

Magnesium, Drs. Prien and Gershoff have shown, makes the urine more solvent in respect to oxalates. With greater solvency, the fluid can hold the crystals in solution with less risk of precipitation or aggregation—that is, the clumping together of particles.

Vitamin $B_6$, on the other hand, has no effect on the solubility of oxalate in the urine, but appears to help control the body's production of oxalic acid and therefore to limit the amount reaching the kidneys

# Lactose Intolerance

By the time you know you are intolerant to lactose, or milk sugar, you already know what to do about it:  don't drink milk or any other dairy product.

The problem is, a great number of people, possibly numbering into the millions, are intolerant to lactose and don't know it. All they know is that they get terrible cramps and diarrhea. Many have gone to a succession of doctors and found little or no relief. It is likely, in fact, that a good number of people who are intolerant to lactose have been misdiagnosed as having colitis or simply "nervous bowels."

Curiously, it seems that the majority of people who dwell on this globe are intolerant to lactose, and that the ability to digest large quantities of milk and other dairy products is found mostly among Europeans. Blacks and Orientals have a very high incidence of lactose intolerance, ranging from 70 to 97 percent. Jews of Eastern European extraction also have a high incidence of lactose intolerance.

All these people have very little of an enzyme known as lactase, which is necessary to digest lactose.

The standard test for lactose intolerance consists of ingesting, on an empty stomach, the amount of pure milk sugar found in a quart of milk, with a blood sample taken before the drink and then three later samples at hourly intervals. The test not only indicates your tolerance to lactose, but if your intolerance is mild or severe. If it is mild, then you may well be able to drink milk in moderate quantities. Most people, at least in the United States, are in this category. Fermented dairy products such as buttermilk and yogurt are also more easily handled.

We found out more about lactose intolerance in an interview with Dr. S. Philip Bralow, a gastrointestinal specialist at Jefferson

Medical College and Hospital in Philadelphia. He told us that "It's true that lactose intolerance is often misdiagnosed as regional enteritis or colitis," even though there are differences between lactose intolerance and those diseases. However, enteritis and colitis may also be misdiagnosed as lactose intolerance. Further, "a great number of patients have both lactose intolerance *and* a GI disorder, so the two may be related," he pointed out.

"The symptoms of lactose intolerance—diarrhea, cramps, and so forth—also tend to make the regional enteritis or colitis worse. Likewise, people who have inflammation of the small intestine may have a deficiency of lactase, but when the inflammation quiets down, they may have enough lactase to be normal."

In general, people past the age of 50 are not plagued by severe bouts of lactose intolerance, either because they've learned not to drink much milk or because they've adapted to the ingestion of reasonable amounts. "Apparently there's an adaptive mechanism in some cases," Dr. Bralow says. "If a person drinks small amounts of milk over a long period of time, the body can eventually start producing enough lactase to break it down."

Anyone who suspects that his GI troubles may be related to lactose intolerance can find out easily enough. Eliminate milk, cheese, ice cream, and any processed food which contains dairy products or milk sugar. If your problem rapidly begins to disappear, you know you are on the right track. In any case, the results of such a trial should be discussed with your doctor or a gastrointestinal specialist.

Those who can't eat any kind of dairy product regularly should pay special attention to their calcium needs. Salmon and sardines with their bones are good sources of calcium as are mature beans, nuts, and dried fruit. Bone meal or calcium gluconate are supplemental forms of this mineral. There is some indication that lactose-intolerant people may be at special risk of developing osteoporosis, or severe thinning of the bones, in later life because they have not consumed enough calcium. This possibility can be minimized by insuring a calcium intake from all sources which totals about 1,200 mg. a day. If you aren't drinking any milk at all, that probably means getting about 1,000 mg. of calcium a day from supplements.

# Leg Pains

Under this heading, we will discuss a number of conditions which can cause agonizing pain in the calf, including Buerger's disease and intermittent claudication.

Women or men who wear high-heeled shoes may get a terrific cramp in the calf without warning. This may well be a result of a contraction of tissue caused by walking with the heel in an abnormal position. The very least you could do is to quit wearing high-heeled shoes except on special occasions. A more vigorous approach to the problem involves gradually stretching the calf muscle.

Stand several feet in front of a wall with your palms flat against it. Lean forward while keeping your legs rigid, until you feel a stretching sensation in your calves. Slowly and gently, rock back and forth. Don't do too much at once or you may find that your calves will be very painful the following day. Do this simple exercise several times a day, and you will gradually notice that you can stretch them more and more.

Another way of stretching the calf muscles is to sit on the floor with your legs out in front of you and extend your heel out as far as it will go, while withdrawing the top of your foot. You can do this simple movement in any position, at any time. Just do it regularly, gently, and with gradually progressive stretching.

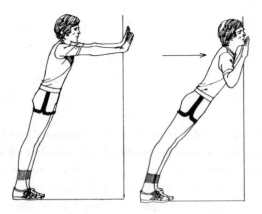

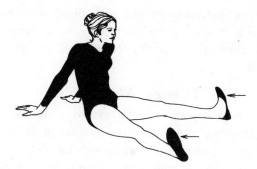

For those of you who have taken up jogging and find that you get pains in the tendon or calf region, I suggest this same approach, which I can say from experience works well. I can also say that if you overdo these stretching exercises, your jogging will become more painful than ever, at least until your tissues get used to this stress.

## Nocturnal Leg Cramps

Another kind of leg pain hits you in the middle of the night and may make you leap up from your sound sleep into a state of excruciating pain. I suffered from this condition for a few years as a teenager, and I found that when my calf muscle was all knotted up, the only thing that would bring relief was to hop out of bed and bounce up and down on the toes of the affected leg. However, the trick is to prevent the cramps from occurring in the first place.

Dr. Samuel Ayres and Dr. Richard Mihan, both of Los Angeles, say the answer is vitamin E—300 to 400 units daily. In 1974, they published the results of seven years of study involving 125 patients who suffered from nocturnal leg cramps. On vitamin E therapy, the cramps were completely or almost completely controlled in 103 cases, while 13 other patients reported some degree of improvement.

"The response of nocturnal leg and foot cramps to adequate doses of vitamin E is prompt, usually becoming manifest within a week, and occurring in such an overwhelming number of cases that it appears almost specific for this ailment," the authors concluded (*Southern Medical Journal,* November 1974).

Calcium also seems to be indicated as a preventive measure for leg cramps—and other types of cramps as well. Letters we've received indicate that many people, particularly women (who seem more prone to these leg cramps than men), have learned to control the pains by chewing up several bone meal or dolomite tablets before bedtime.

## Leg Cramps While Walking

Intermittent claudication is not exactly a disease, but a kind of syndrome resulting from obstructed circulation in the legs and is characterized by increasing pain while walking. The pain builds in intensity until it becomes impossible to continue walking, and then disappears when the muscles are rested.

Knut Haeger, M.D., a vascular surgeon, discovered in a lengthy series of experiments involving a great many patients that 300 to 400 units of vitamin E daily combined with daily walking, does two things: first, it greatly increases the distance the person is able to walk before feeling pain, and second, it significantly increases the flow of blood to the lower leg.

Patients who exercised as much as they could but did not take vitamin E were not helped nearly as much. Dr. Haeger, who summed up his experiments and previous publications in an article written for PREVENTION in March 1975, said he believes vitamin E itself was not responsible for the increased flow of blood in patients. Rather, he theorizes, the vitamin E permits the muscles to do more work before they become painful, and as more exercise becomes possible, the blood flow is permanently increased.

Do not expect to overcome intermittent claudication in a week or two. Dr. Haeger found that results take several months.

People with poor circulation in their legs may achieve much more than relief of walking pain by taking vitamin E. Dr. Haeger wrote in PREVENTION that "During the years in which we conducted the study, it was necessary to amputate 12 legs because of intractable pain and/or gangrene. This was, of course, done as a last resort, only after more conservative treatment and operative techniques had failed. In the group of patients who were taking vitamin E, there was only one amputation case out of 95 surviving patients. But of 104 patients who did not receive vitamin E, there were 11 amputations. This difference is very significant."

## Buerger's Disease

In Buerger's disease the blood vessels of a limb, usually the legs, are inflamed with clot formations. Deprived of adequate circulation and nourishment, the lower legs may become cold and painful and if injured, heal poorly. The condition may occur simultaneously with the intermittent claudication discussed earlier.

Although Buerger's disease is a serious condition, and may be complicated by other diseases involving the circulatory system, there is reason to believe that purely natural remedies can—at least in some cases—be of enormous help.

Basically, such a therapy (to be done in addition to whatever your doctor prescribes) is very similar to Dr. Haeger's therapy for intermittent claudication: vitamin E and plenty of exercise. Only with Buerger's disease, it seems that more vitamin E may be needed.

One reader told us that he apparently had Buerger's disease in his left leg, which was bluish purple in color. He had ulcers on his foot which refused to heal. The doctor prescribed several medications but they did not bring about any improvement. He was at the point where he was visiting a podiatrist every few days "to watch for any development of gangrene" when he began to take 600 I.U. of vitamin E daily.

He soon noticed a very slight improvement in the ulcers, and he began to increase the vitamin E until he reached 2,000 units daily. At that point, the ulcers began to respond dramatically and the color of his leg began to normalize. He then improved his total diet and a year later he felt "reasonably sure" that he had arrested the Buerger's disease—as well as his angina. As a further bonus, he found that he was able to reduce the amount of medication he was taking for the diabetes he had had for 40 years and was eventually able to eliminate it entirely.

A woman told us that a doctor decided to amputate the first three toes on her left foot after they became blue, abscessed and so painful that she was barely able to walk and scarcely able to sleep from the pain.

She had been taking vitamin E, 800 I.U. per day, but she increased it to 1,600 and gradually to 2,400 units a day along with lecithin granules and 500 mg. of vitamin C. In addition, she massaged her foot and leg and got regular exercise. "Within three days the pain was almost gone and I was able to sleep and walk better," she reported. Gradually, her toes returned to their normal color.

There are some specific movements—called Buerger's Exercises —which help relieve some of the symptoms, especially when real exercise is too painful. They are performed as follows:

1. Lie on your back with your legs elevated about 45 degrees, with the help of some cushions or the back of a chair which has been turned upside down. Hold this position until your feet blanch—about two minutes.

2. Sit with your legs hanging down over the edge of the bed until they become flushed with blood—about a minute or two.

3. Lie flat on the bed, relaxing, and keep legs and feet warm with the covers or an electric blanket.

Repeat the cycle about four times per session, for three sessions daily, and add active exercises such as walking or cycling.

# Legg-Calvé-Perthes Disease

Also known as osteochondritis deformans juvenilis, this disease usually hits children and seems to involve an inflammatory process that prevents normal calcification of the top of the thigh bone. Apparently, the medical view is that mineral supplementation will not help much, if at all. Fortunately, the degeneration ordinarily halts in time and the bone is recalcified.

For what it may be worth, we relate this anecdote from an Ohio woman who said that her otherwise perfectly normal 10-year-old son developed Legg-Calvé-Perthes Disease. "His right leg was put in a brace, and the left foot was built up with a special shoe. We were told by the specialist he would be like this for at least two or three years, and this was the only cure." Shortly after this diagnosis, the entire family, including the son, began to take supplements of dolomite and bone meal. Six months later, they took their son back for a checkup "and the specialist took his braces off and said our son was cured, and it was the quickest cured case of Legg-Perthes he had ever seen." Typically, when the parents mentioned the dietary change, the doctor refused to admit that these minerals could have been involved in the rapid cure, but, the reader stated, he did, in a fit of open-mindedness, exclaim, "It was something!"

# Leprosy

Dr. Olaf K. Skinsnes, Professor of Pathology and Director of Research at the University of Hawaii American Leprosy Mission, has discovered that vitamin C prevents the leprosy bacilli from utilizing one of the nutrients they need to grow. The effect of the vitamin was revealed during routine processing of leprosy biopsy specimens. Four of the patients from whom the specimens were obtained had been treated with 1,500 mg. of vitamin C in addition to their regular leprosy drug, dapsone. One patient had received only vitamin C. But in all five patients, the leprosy bacilli had been almost totally destroyed. As we write this, an extended series of trials with vitamin C is being conducted among leprosy patients.

# Lupus Erythematosus

Lupus is a disease of unknown origin which may appear either in the cutaneous form, in which a variety of skin lesions appear, or in the systemic form which can cause damage to many organs. The attention of a physician knowledgeable about this condition is imperative. In the case of cutaneous LE, for instance, it is important to avoid exposure to sunlight. Once the skin has been damaged by ultraviolet radiation, therapy is much less successful.

I do not know of any medical studies reporting improvement from a nutritional program, but a number of people who have had this condition report that a nutritional program *seemed* to help. People who have lupus, like those who have MS, may have spontaneous remissions, and so it is impossible to say for certain that improvement following a certain course of therapy was caused by that therapy. Nevertheless, the nutritional approach was so helpful to one woman, Betty Hull of Corpus Christi, Texas, that she founded a nonprofit organization, LEANON (LE Anonymous) which publishes the

"Lupus Lifeline." In the October 1974 issue, Ms. Hull outlined her personal nutrition program which she credits for getting her to the point where her condition went into remission and she was able to eventually get off drugs except for a few crises.

Basically, her nutrition program consists of drinking several glasses of carrot juice a day, to ensure a high but safe intake of vitamin A; B-complex tablets; individual B vitamins as follows: 100 mg. of PABA, 250 mg. of pantothenic acid, 100 mg. of niacin, 50 mg. of $B_6$ twice daily, and 250 mg. of choline; 3,000 mg. of vitamin C; 2,500 I.U. of vitamin D; 1,000 I.U. of vitamin E ("I had to begin slowly and increase very slowly, due to a history of high blood pressure"); six tablets of bone meal and six tablets of dolomite; two tablets of kelp; and one multimineral capsule.

Judging by some letters which Hull has published in her "Lupus Lifeline" and a letter we have received, this across-the-board approach to bolstering nutrition sometimes pays off in dramatic improvement. At least that's what the people say who have tried it.

Those who have lupus should keep in mind that remissions which may last for years are common. Have a hopeful outlook, because many who were terribly ill have recovered to enjoy many years of near-normal health.

# Meditation

On November 23, 1975, I had one of the most unusual experiences of my life. It happened in the ballroom of a hotel in New York City, but I wasn't dancing and there was no orchestra playing. There were a thousand people packed into the room with me, yet it was a deeply personal experience. And oddly enough, everyone else in that room probably had an almost identical experience.

What we were doing, all one thousand of us, was meditating.

Now, the average person has never practiced meditation, let alone in the crowded ballroom of a New York City hotel. But more than likely, you've had a similar experience. Perhaps it was during a period of silent devotion in a place of worship. Or at some kind of function where the master of ceremonies asked for a moment of silence to honor the memory of a departed friend.

There's a big difference, though, between that sort of thing and real meditation. The most striking, obvious difference is that after about 60 seconds, that jam-packed ballroom became completely— and I mean utterly—silent. No one was shuffling his feet. No one was clearing his throat. There were no nervous coughs and no whispering.

It was downright eerie. In my journalistic career, I've been to many places where silence had been called for, for one reason or another, but if you think about it, there is never *complete* silence. There is always at least one person in the group who manages to cough or clear his throat, which in turn sets off other people coughing, sighing, or shifting around in their seats. That would lead you to believe that perfect silence in a large group of people is physically impossible. There are just too many nervous impulses, twitches, itches, and spasms to achieve perfect calm and quiet.

But it isn't impossible. I saw that and experienced it. And that means that much of the restlessness and nervous habits that all of us develop as outlets for tension are *also* unnecessary.

More important, the tension itself is unnecessary.

We meditated for about five minutes, and when it was over, everyone seemed to be smiling with a kind of euphoria. We'd all been refreshed in a very profound, almost peculiar way.

But relaxation and refreshment in the normal sense of the word is just the beginning of what meditation can do for you. Herbert Benson, M.D., of Harvard Medical School and director of the Hypertension Section of Boston's Beth Israel Hospital, has shown in clinical studies that meditating for 10 to 20 minutes twice a day can be remarkably effective in improving total health and well-being, and more specifically, in reducing high blood pressure.

Dr. Benson was our instructor in that mass meditation exercise I described, and the best part about it all is that his instructions took approximately one minute to explain.

Before I pass along Dr. Benson's technique for eliciting what he calls the Relaxation Response, let me hasten to point out that "meditation" in this context does not mean what most of us think it does. It does not mean thinking profound thoughts about the nature of the universe or anything else. In fact, it means thinking about nothing, nothing at all.

Impossible, you say? You're right. Random thoughts are bound to pop into our heads no matter what we do, but total freedom from extraneous thoughts is not required in meditation. The idea is simply to prevent the *continuity* of thought; i.e., dwelling on one idea and considering its implications.

## How to Really Relax

Want to give it a try?

Good. It's remarkably simple. First, select a quiet room and sit in a comfortable chair. Adjust yourself so that you are as relaxed as possible. This will probably mean slouching forward a bit, resting your hands on your thighs, and keeping your feet flat on the ground, somewhat in front of the position of your knees. (Some of these tips are mine, not Dr. Benson's.)

Close your eyes. Now, consciously relax all your muscles, beginning with your feet. Move up through your legs, your stomach, your chest, your arms, your neck, and even your face, jaws, and mouth. When your jaw muscles are really relaxed, your lower teeth will probably not be touching your uppers.

Breathe through your nose, and draw the breath into your belly, which should be rising and falling. Become aware of your breathing, but don't make a big deal out of taking deep breaths. They aren't necessary. Breathe normally and naturally.

Now, as you breathe out, say the word "one" to yourself. Inhale. Exhale and again repeat the word "one."

Keep the muscles of your body relaxed and continue breathing rhythmically and easily in and out, repeating the word "one" with every exhalation.

Continue for 10 to 20 minutes. When you finish, sit quietly for a while and then gradually open your eyes.

As I said, it's only natural that stray thoughts are going to pop into your head. Don't worry about them; they aren't going to ruin your Relaxation Response. Just say to yourself, "Oh, well," and let the thought drift out of your mind. If it returns, don't worry about it and don't try to fight it. Just keep repeating the word "one," breathing easily and rhythmically and keeping your muscles relaxed.

After meditating, you'll feel like your "idle" has just been turned down to where it belongs. Just as with a car, you may not realize that your motor is racing until it's lowered. Then you can feel that the *energy* is still there, waiting to be called on, but there's less noise and shaking and smoke. You suddenly realize that what you had become habituated to accept as normal really wasn't, that the tension was abusing your body's most vital organs just as a racing auto motor damages the cylinders.

Actually, I had meditated before attending the symposium where Dr. Benson spoke. I had read his book, *The Relaxation Response* (William Morrow and Co., New York, 1975), and my first full-length meditation took place on the bus that was taking me to New York to the symposium. The time was dusk, which is usually one of the most trying times of the day from the point of view of exhaustion, hunger, and irritability, and I was amazed at how mellow, relaxed, and content I felt during and after that first meditation.

## How Your Blood Pressure Benefits

As a specialist in hypertension, Dr. Benson is naturally most interested in what that Relaxation Response can do for people with high blood pressure. He warns that hypertensives must not suddenly give up their medication in hopes that the Relaxation Response is going to take care of everything. In fact, all the patients Dr. Benson worked with were on their regular blood pressure medicine throughout the study. What the meditation did was to improve upon the benefit conferred by the medication, and it proved to be a very significant improvement indeed.

In one series of experiments, Dr. Benson selected 36 volunteers, all of whom remained with their original medication throughout the study. Prior to practicing the Relaxation Response, they had an average systolic blood pressure (the higher figure) of 146. The average diastolic blood pressure was 93.5. On the average, then, the 36 subjects had a blood pressure which could be expressed as 146 over 93.5.

After several weeks of regularly practicing the Relaxation Response, as we've described here, the average blood pressure fell to 137 over 88.9.

What that means is that the average blood pressure went from borderline high down to the normal range. The measurements were taken *before* each meditation, so the residual effect was being checked, not just momentary improvement.

In no sense, however, were these people "cured" of their high blood pressure. Their readings remained low only as long as they practiced their Relaxation Response regularly. When several subjects stopped meditating, their blood pressures returned to their initial hypertensive levels within a month.

Here's how Dr. Benson, in his book, puts the Relaxation Response in perspective. "Standard medical therapy means taking antihypertensive drugs, which often act by interrupting the activity of the sympathetic nervous system, thus lowering blood pressure. The pharmacologic method of lowering blood pressure is very effective and extremely important since . . . lowered blood pressure leads to lower risk of developing atherosclerosis and its related diseases such as heart attacks and strokes. The regular practice of the Relaxation Response is yet another way to lower blood pressure. Indications are that this response affects the same mechanisms and lowers blood pressure by the same means as some antihypertensive drugs. Both counteract the activity in the sympathetic nervous system. It is unlikely that the regular elicitation of the Relaxation Response by itself will prove to be adequate therapy for severe or moderate high blood pressure. Probably it would act to enhance the lowering of the blood pressure along with antihypertensive drugs, and thus lead to the use of fewer drugs or a lesser dosage."

Another thing meditation does, at least while it's actually in progress, is reduce the body's need for oxygen, the basic metabolic fuel. Yet, the amount of oxygen in the blood is not reduced, showing that your body isn't grinding to some kind of halt. It's just becoming more efficient. A better engine.

Perhaps you are more interested in simply falling asleep than cooling down the circuitry of your sympathetic nervous system. Although the Relaxation Response and similar meditative techniques were not designed to put you to sleep, they may do just that *if* you do them lying down in bed. Dr. Benson told us in New York that he uses the technique himself to go to sleep, although he says it can't really be called the Relaxation Response. He added that it also "works beautifully" if you have trouble getting back to sleep after you wake up in the middle of the night.

## Two Kinds of Meditation

Transcendental Meditation, which you have probably heard about, is virtually identical to Dr. Benson's technique except for a few details. In fact, those blood pressure patients we talked about were actually practicing TM under Dr. Benson's direction, rather than the Relaxation Response, which Dr. Benson subsequently developed as a simpler approach.

The question naturally arises: which technique is best?

Some people get pretty testy about it. One or two doctors at the New York meeting called TM a rip-off because people are charged $125 to receive some very simple instructions. The rest of TM, they claim, is just a lot of religion, philosophy, and yoga traditions that have nothing to do, necessarily, with effective and successful relaxation. On the other hand, the followers of TM are sometimes critical of variations on their technique, claiming that their method has been proved through the ages and should not be tampered with.

Dr. Benson refuses to be drawn into this fight. As he told one questioner, if you feel that TM is better for you, that the meetings you go to will increase your compliance, fine. But if you want to do meditation after simply reading the instructions on a piece of paper, that is fine, too. And if you'd rather say "Hail, Mary" instead of "one," that's fine, too. A mellow man, Dr. Benson.

To try to see for ourselves what differences there might be between TM and the Relaxation Response, we spoke with a colleague who enrolled in the TM program a few months ago and who has since been meditating twice a day without fail.

One obvious difference is that in TM, each person is given a special word or phrase to say, rather than just "one." This phrase is called a *mantra* and it is to be kept secret. And its repetition is not linked directly to the rhythm of breathing. Other than that, there does not seem to be any difference at all between the two techniques.

The person who enrolled in TM felt that he was too tense and wanted to learn how to relax. Did it work?

## A Calmer, Happier Person

"At first, for about a week, I had these wonderful subjective feelings after meditating," he said. "After that the euphoria seemed to wear off, but there are definite changes. For one thing, things don't bother me as much any more. Emotional storms blow over much faster or don't come at all. I sleep better, too. And although it may sound funny, I'm actually happier in my work. I didn't expect that to happen, even though they tell you that it will. Supposedly, practicing TM enhances your job satisfaction unless your job is really miserable. In that case, it can give you the confidence to seek another position."

When do you meditate, we asked. "I don't like to do it first thing in the morning, because I'm still too groggy. I wait until I shave and shower, then I meditate for 20 minutes. After work, but before dinner, I meditate again. You aren't supposed to meditate after a meal."

In one instance, he said, he meditated successfully while waiting in an airline terminal. And on a recent vacation that had him hopping around at a hectic pace, he found that those few minutes of meditation restored his energy remarkably well.

Personally, I find that meditating is a wonderful investment. I admit I don't do it regularly, but on the other hand, I find that even a minute or two at an especially overwrought moment can be a blessing. Once you get the hang of it, you can swing into a very relaxed state anytime you want to with just a few good breaths, almost like pushing a button.

The Relaxation Response isn't something you want to turn on when you're faced with a troublesome challenge. Don't try to use it as a crutch. Use it to train yourself to relax, and you'll find that those moments which do present great emotional challenges are much easier to handle.

# Menopausal Problems

The scientific literature on natural or nutritional approaches to easing the distress of menopause is almost nonexistent. The standard medical approach is to prescribe various forms of estrogen.

Estrogen, however, is apparently much less helpful than many people suppose. In a recent double-blind study conducted in England, doctors could find precious little difference between a group of women receiving estrogen and another group receiving a placebo, except that the estrogen was clearly more effective in eliminating hot flashes. As we write this, preliminary reports are appearing in the medical literature which suggest that the long-term use of estrogens is associated with an increased risk of uterine cancer, and the feeling in enlightened medical circles is that these hormones should only be given when there is a very clear need for them, and should be stopped as soon as possible.

Although there is little scientific support for the idea that vitamin E can be of help, several women have written to us that their hot flashes were extinguished shortly after beginning a vitamin E regimen. One woman began by taking 400 I.U. with each meal and found that the hot flashes disappeared completely after one week. She then tapered off to 400 units a day. A second woman reports that 800 units a day proved helpful. Since hot flashes apparently do not respond well to the placebo approach, it is possible that vitamin E is worth trying.

# Menstrual Problems

Vitamin B complex will often help reduce premenstrual tension and related problems. Carlton Fredericks, Ph.D., points out that the B vitamins, plus protein, are needed by the liver to convert the hormones released prior to menstruation into less powerful substances.

Dr. Fredericks some years ago conducted a study at Fairleigh Dickinson University (Rutherford, New Jersey), where about 200 women students with menstrual problems were given nutritional counseling. Advised on such facts of life as the value of milk and eggs for protein, and brewer's yeast and liver concentrates for B vitamins, the students found their "female troubles" diminishing within a few months.

The monthly premenstrual development of breast cysts, which occurs in some women, also responded to the nutritional approach, Dr. Fredericks says. And menstruation itself became less severe in both pain and duration in many students who followed the nutritional guidelines.

The same approach has worked for many other women, judging by some of the letters we've received. A typical letter states that the writer "tried the brewer's yeast, vitamin B plus iron pills, and what a change! My husband sure noticed the change and I felt so much better towards life. To test this I went for a month without them and believe me, never again!" Prior to this, she said, her periods would send her up the wall and she would "get so depressed that she thought of suicide."

Vitamin $B_6$, an important part of the B complex, has special value for premenstrual women suffering from edema, or fluid retention in the tissues. A pioneer in clinical studies of vitamin $B_6$, John M. Ellis, M.D., of Mt. Pleasant, Texas, tells of his consistent success with large doses of this nutrient in the treatment of severe premenstrual edema. In his book, *Vitamin $B_6$: The Doctor's Report* (Harper & Row, New York, 1973), he writes: "Over the years as I saw more and more patients, edema of the hands during the premenstrual period could be linked with evidence of abdominal distention, involuntary muscle spasms of the legs and feet, and swelling of the eyelids and face. In one group of women I treated for these disorders, four out of eleven of them had previously taken diuretics for control of edema, with little success. But when they took 50 to 100 milligrams [of $B_6$] daily, all their signs and symptoms were relieved. . . ."

The value of this approach was echoed by John J. Worthington, M.D., of Willow Grove, Pennsylvania, in a letter published in a medical newspaper in 1975: "I would urge physicians," he said, "to offer some of their female patients a 50 milligram pyridoxine [$B_6$] tablet twice a day as treatment for premenstrual tension. The marked improvement in the vast majority of cases is remarkable."

Further evidence that menstruation somehow creates a functional deficiency of vitamin $B_6$ was offered by Dr. B. Leonard Snider of Erie, Pennsylvania, at a conference of dermatologists in 1974. Dr. Snider reported that when 106 teenages troubled by premenstrual acne flare were given $B_6$ supplements, 76 reported that the flare was reduced by at least 50 to 75 percent.

Excess menstrual discharge, called menorrhagia, was treated with the bioflavonoids, or vitamin P, by a group of doctors at a French hospital who reported that these nutrients gave the women "good to excellent results" (*Family Practice News,* March 15, 1974).

Bioflavonoids, usually extracted for supplements from the inner peel and white pulpy portion of citrus fruits, are widely recognized in Europe for their ability to strengthen blood vessels, particularly the walls of the capillaries. In treating menorrhagia patients with bioflavonoids, the French doctors observed "progressive improvement, with the most marked improvement achieved by the third menstrual cycle."

When heavy menstrual flow is associated with fatigue which occurs throughout the month, that may be an indication of iron deficiency anemia. Liver and other meats, green leafy vegetables, peaches, and dried fruits are all good sources of iron. Dairy products are very poor sources. Iron supplements may be indicated, in daily amounts ranging from 50 to 100 mg., or even more on your doctor's advice. A good iron supplement also contains folic acid and vitamin $B_{12}$.

Some women have found that chewing several dolomite tablets, which contain calcium and magnesium, is remarkably effective in reducing menstrual pain and breast tenderness.

## Childbirth and Exercise—Natural Remedies

Sherwin A. Kaufman, M.D., in his book, *From a Gynecologist's Notebook* (Stein and Day, New York, 1974), points out that premenstrual tension and pain may become spontaneously cured once the woman has a baby. Menstrual cramps and other abdominal pain, he says, are usually caused by uterine contractions combined with a relatively narrow cervical canal. There is no better cervical "stretcher" than childbirth, he points out. "In addition, a uterus that has contained a pregnancy is generally less prone to undergo contractions during each period, hence less pain." From the strictly biological viewpoint, childbirth might be called a kind of "natural remedy" for menstrual problems, but Dr. Kaufman suggests that exercises can prove very helpful in minimizing the pain.

One exercise he suggests is alternate-leg toe touching. Stand with your feet at least 24 inches apart, with hands over your head, and swing your right arm down to touch your left foot. Try to reach around the foot and actually touch the heel. Repeat for the opposite side.

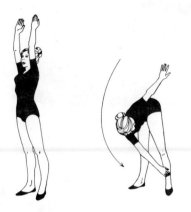

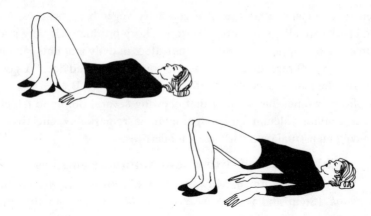

A second exercise is to lie on the floor on your back, with your knees bent and your feet flat on the floor near your buttocks. Lift the lower end of your spine off the floor as far as you can comfortably do so and repeat.

Finally, lie on the floor on your back, with your arms at your sides and palms up. Draw your knees up over your chest then slowly straighten your legs. Then bend your legs and return your feet flat to the floor as close to the buttocks as possible. Repeat a number of times.

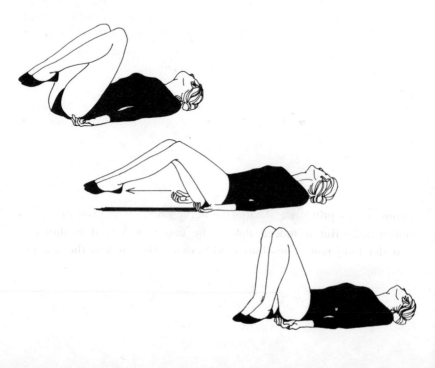

## Herbs May Help

Herbal tradition values several plants in assisting with problematic menstruation. Black cohosh and blue cohosh are both considered useful in expediting obstructed menstruation. They should be used moderately. A commercial product which has long been on the market contains black cohosh and a number of other herbs in an alcoholic base. The purpose of the alcohol is not simply to give the brew a zing, either. Black cohosh, like a number of other herbs, is much more soluble in alcohol than water. Little of the essence would be available from merely boiling this herb in water.

A hot cup of ginger tea is another old standby. So are motherwort and pennyroyal. Female regulator, also known as life root and squaw weed, is considered valuable in all kinds of minor gynecological upsets. Like black cohosh, it is most soluble in alcohol. If you're preparing this or a similar herb at home, first boil it in water, let it cool, add some brandy, and let it stand for a few days. In days of yore, many herbs were prepared in this fashion and it's hard to say how much of the resulting "relief" was from the herbs and how much from the brandy.

# Multiple Sclerosis

Multiple sclerosis, a disease of the central nervous system, is as puzzling as it is tragic. In some, it has a relatively benign course; in others, symptoms become progressively worse, producing loss of coordination, blindness, and even paralysis. However, the disease is characterized by spontaneous remissions which may last for months and even years. Why these remissions occur is not understood. They are especially peculiar in light of the prevailing belief that MS is caused by changes or lesions occurring to the myelin sheath, the protective covering of the brain and spinal cord. Because of the lesions in this protective sheath, the nerve impulses are not properly transmitted. But if indeed this is the cause of MS, it is difficult to understand how remissions could come about unless the lesions come and go, which does not seem to be the case.

These remissions are in some instances very dramatic, and a person who is barely able to take a step one year may be going for long walks the next. For this reason, it is devilishly difficult to evaluate therapies for MS, particularly when they are tried by individuals on themselves, rather than in large groups.

So far, there is no good scientific evidence that there is any natural—or medical—therapy for MS which can be considered reliable. In fact, some organizations go to great lengths to drive this point home to MS victims and attack anyone who suggests that there *is* a therapy as a prophet of false hope. If there is improvement, it's argued, it is simply a spontaneous remission and not the result of any particular therapy.

That is all well and good from the scientific point of view. However, I have learned that what MS victims want is not policy statements but any suggestion or clue of something that *might* help them. They aren't looking for cures, but for something that may improve their mobility by 50 percent or even 10 percent, and they don't care if the improvement does not last forever.

### Sunflower Seed Oil Tested

From this point of view, there are several reports that offer at least a ray of hope to MS victims. In Britain, a team of doctors has reported that two tablespoons of sunflower seed oil taken twice a day considerably reduced the severity of the disease and increased the periods of remission (*British Medical Journal,* March 31, 1973). The research was carried out by Dr. Harold Millar and his associates at the Royal Victoria Hospital in Belfast, Northern Ireland.

One of Dr. Millar's associates had been giving sunflower seed oil by mouth to 90 patients and had noted that the clinical course of the disease seemed to be improved. To determine if what they were observing were only spontaneous remissions, they divided 75 patients with MS at random into "treated" and "control" groups. Only patients who could walk, with or without aid, were included. All were at a clinically inactive phase of the disease at the start. Any patient who had already taken sunflower seed oil was excluded.

Two doses of an oil mixture were taken each day, morning and evening, for a period of two years. For the treated group, each dose consisted of two tablespoons of a sunflower seed oil emulsion providing 8.6 grams of linoleic acid. The control group received two daily doses of an emulsion similar in appearance and flavor but containing olive oil instead of sunflower seed oil. Each dose of this emulsion provided 3.8 grams of oleic acid (a nonessential fatty acid which can be synthesized by the body from saturated fatty acids) and just 0.2 grams of linoleic acid.

Patients were seen at intervals of two to three months and the severity of the disease at each visit was determined by reference to a specially devised scoring chart. Their progress was assessed according to sensory function, bladder and bowel functions, visual and mental function, and the patients' ability to cope with ordinary day-to-day tasks.

Dr. Millar's group determined the effect of the sunflower seed oil emulsion by counting the number of relapses suffered over a two-year period by the patients in both groups. There were 62 relapses among the 39 patients who did not receive the sunflower seed oil, but only 41 relapses among the 36 who received it. Not only were relapses less frequent in the treated group, they were much less severe. In fact, relapses—such as temporary loss of vision or weakness in the legs—were judged twice as severe in the untreated group and much longer in duration.

In all objectivity, it must be pointed out that the reason sunflower seed oil—rich in linoleic acid—was chosen as a supplement was that Dr. Millar had determined that MS victims have lower than normal quantities of linoleic acid in their blood. Subsequently, several other studies have indicated that this may not be the case, and that MS victims have the usual amounts of linoleic acid. This does *not,* however, throw out the clinical results, although it does cast doubt on the biochemical basis of the therapy.

## The MacDougall Treatment

A more comprehensive approach to MS has been popularized by Roger MacDougall, who was once in a wheelchair and almost blind, and at the time of this writing, is apparently completely free of symptoms. This did not happen overnight, but over a period of many years, during which he adhered strictly to a diet largely of his own design.

Basically, the MacDougall diet forbids absolutely all gluten-containing cereals: wheat, oats, rye, and barley—as well as any processed food containing even the smallest amount of these common cereals. Second, refined sugar is all but entirely eliminated. Saturated fats are also severely limited. This means no butter, cream, or rich cheeses. Skimmed milk, unsaturated margarines, and very lean meats are permitted, except that bacon, pork, duck, or goose is forbidden. So are alcoholic beverages and soft drinks.

Vitamin and mineral supplements are an important part of MacDougall's program, and he recommends taking generous amounts of every factor in the B complex family, vitamin C, vitamin E, lecithin, calcium, and magnesium.

I am in no position to say how many people who try this program are helped by it; probably, neither is anyone else. However, Norman A. Matheson, Ph.D., a British biochemist, had a letter published in the medical journal *Lancet* (October 5, 1974) in which he said that for him, personally, it seemed to help.

Curiously, he added that when he substituted magnesium alone for the nutrition program, his progress seemed to be "perhaps a little faster than when I took the entire supplement." He made the change because he noticed that some of the symptoms of magnesium deficiency were "strikingly like those I have experienced." He used 375 mg. of magnesium daily, and complete avoidance of gluten was continued. Dr. Matheson concluded his letter by noting that "The diet helps decrease the intensity of the symptoms in some cases, and the fact that dietary treatment sometimes helps suggests several lines of research."

Needless to say, Dr. Matheson was subsequently given a good going-over in print by some other doctors who accused him of promoting faddism. Dr. Matheson replied that his point was that the diet should be tested rigorously and in its complete form on a large number of people. At present, he said, "the diet described . . . is experimental only; it is not a proven treatment for multiple sclerosis."

# Music Therapy

Most of us are familiar with the relaxation and emotional refreshment that playing or listening to music can bring. But it is something else again to employ music to achieve specific health-promoting goals.

If you think about it, you'll probably recall times at which listening to music helped you untangle some particularly troublesome psychological knots, or maybe helped you get off to sleep faster.

When my daughter was an infant and indulged in one of her favorite hobbies, crying, she was invariably and quickly soothed when I would lay her down on a bed and play a majestic Beethoven symphony on the phonograph. When my son took to squalling, he was always soothed and made happy again by being walked back and forth while loud rock music blared from the radio.

But in looking through medical literature, it is surprising to find so many examples of real improvement in some rather serious clinical situations which can be achieved with music therapy. Although medical acceptance of this kind of therapy has increased dramatically over the last decade or so, there's nothing especially new about healing with music.

In the 6th century, B.C., Pythagoras regarded music and diet as the two chief means of cleansing the soul and body and maintaining the harmony and health of the whole organism. A thousand years later, in Christian Europe, medicine and music were again closely linked when the church took over the care of the sick and used the chanting of prayers as a means of therapy. And of course, music and dancing have been used as part of the healing arts of so-called primitive peoples throughout the world for no one knows how many millennia. In fact, periodic and ritualized tribal dancing is so commonplace throughout the world, with or without sickness, that its importance can hardly be overestimated. It is in fact very likely that the vigorous dancing which so many people enjoy for long hours is highly effective in working out the tightness of muscles (note the head swinging that accompanies most tribal dancing), providing valuable exercise to those who need it, inducing profound mental and physical relaxation, and binding together the participants in a tighter social unit.

## Music Therapy for Asthma

Today, it seems, most doctors are more interested in diseases than an individual's total health (much less the health of the social unit!), so logically, we find that the research into music therapy concentrates on its application to specific disease conditions. One of the most impressive recent reports comes from Dr. Meyer B. Marks, whose work has lead him to recommend that asthmatic children be encouraged to take up wind instruments when they enter junior high school. Dr. Marks, who is director of the Pediatric Allergy Clinic at the Jackson Memorial Hospital in Miami, Florida, says that playing an instrument like a clarinet or oboe improves an asthmatic child's pulmonary function and reduces the progression of the disease. A two-year study of 30 asthmatic children between the ages of 8 and 14 revealed, he says, that the 15 who were given wind instruments to play enjoyed marked clinical improvement—both physically and emotionally—over the other 15. The capacity of their lungs and other signs of pulmonary health were clearly improved. There was a visible reduction in barrel-chest deformity noted in 5 children who played their instruments diligently. A condition known as pectus carinatum ("pigeon breast"), in which the sternum is unduly prominent, disappeared almost completely in 2 boys after several years of playing. Long-term follow-up of a 12-year-old girl who had severe asthma and a depressed sternum revealed that six years later, when she became a music major at the University of Miami, she no longer had any visible deformity of the chest and her asthma was no longer considered incapacitating.

Earlier work carried out at the National Jewish Hospital in Denver, Colorado, showed that when asthmatic children partake in regular musical activities, they build endurance, develop muscle strength, and improve their posture and breath control. The younger children start out with games like patty-cake, to which the teacher introduces changing rhythms. Once they adapt to these rhythms, they're introduced to drums, xylophones, and similar instruments. Besides the health aspects of the programs, these chronically ill children are also learning that they can create, accomplish, and compete with others despite their illness.

## Music for Troubled Minds

Mental illness is probably the one medical area which has enjoyed the best results with musical therapy. Success here seems linked to the fact that music may provide the only safe and acceptable means of communication for the emotionally ill person. Because music is a nonverbal means of communication, it can help the person release feelings and emotions which have been long inhibited. Therapy may take whatever form the individual needs. He can play an instrument, analyze or discuss the music, or involve himself in physical movement such as dancing. There are numerous reports in the scientific literature of patients responding well to music therapy. Paul

Nordoff, director of music at the University of Pennsylvania's Department of Child Psychiatry, in 1965 published *Music Therapy for Handicapped Children* (Rudolf Steiner Publications, Fort Lee, N.J.) in which he outlined numerous case histories where simply encouraging disturbed children to beat on a drum while he (Nordoff) played the piano proved very helpful. Autistic and other mentally disturbed children responded well when this form of music therapy was added to their overall treatment.

Just *listening* to music can also have marked therapeutic effects. In 1964, the medical press reported that a Dutch gynecologist, Dr. T. L. A. De Bruïne, was using classical music to help nervous and frightened women overcome fear and pain during labor. After experimenting with many different types of music, Dr. De Bruïne found that classical music—the melodious and serene type—was most valuable in stimulating the patient into a fantasy world leading her out of a frightening situation. To overcome the feeling of fatigue, music with a rhythmic character is used from time to time.

Dr. De Bruïne said he had refined his repertoire to the following pieces of music: Beethoven's *Egmont* Overture and *Pastoral* Symphony; Mozart's *Eine Kleine Nachtmusik*; Chopin's polonaises, preludes, and mazurkas; Liszt's Hungarian Rhapsody no. 2; Beethoven's Symphony no. 8 (parts one and two only); and Bach's *Brandenburg* Concerto no. 2. Dr. De Bruïne said the music therapy was effective in at least four out of five cases but emphasized that the therapy is not used for every case—only in situations where women begin to cry, become restless, or feel a lot of pain. The music is then used instead of a sedative.

Curiously, there are rare cases in which music can actually *harm* a person. But the cure is also music, used in a kind of deconditioning process. In 1965, Dr. Francis M. Forster of the Department of Neurology at the University of Wisconsin Medical Center in Madison reported an interesting case of musicogenic epilepsy—a seizure brought on by music. The type of music that induces the seizure varies with each person. In the case reported by Dr. Forster, the "noxious" music was the mid-thirties type of popular sensuous music derived from C. A. Debussy and Sibelius. (Another word for this kind of music is "schmaltzy.") The patient in this case had a history over a period of 18 years of going into seizures when exposed to this kind of music. The seizures were not the full epileptic kind, but the patient would experience the pre-epileptic aura "consisting of generalized numbness and tingling, and a *déjà vu* phenomenon." Brain electrical patterns also became markedly abnormal if exposure to the music was long enough; there was sometimes "a seizure of the psycho-motor type."

In curing the patient, Dr. Forster began by playing very simple renditions of the schmaltzy song "Stardust" and proceeded to play the song in many combinations of instrumentation, gradually adding more and more of the sensuous quality which disturbed the patient. Eventually, after innumerable renditions and repetitions, the patient was completely desensitized and could listen to any music without losing control.

A more garden-variety use for music was described in an article in *Dental Abstracts* in 1965. Two groups of 20 orthodontic patients ranging in age from 10 to 22 years were studied to determine the effects of background music on their emotional tensions while being treated by the orthodontist. One group underwent treatment in the usual manner, while the other group heard background music during treatment. As measured by galvanic skin response, which measures emotional tension, the music-treated group was much more relaxed than those who heard nothing but the sound of the dentist's breathing. Low-toned, fairly monotonous music is indicated.

For information about studying to become a music therapist or where to find one in your area, contact the National Association for Music Therapy, P.O. Box 610, Lawrence, Kansas 66044, or the Music Therapy Center at 251 West Fifty-first Street, New York, New York 10019.

# Natural Healing, The Ultimate:
## How the Body Defends and Repairs Itself

**by Alan S. Bricklin, M.D.**

In order to live to reproductive age, each of us must fight off an almost continuous onslaught by disease and virulent organisms. Over the centuries we have developed an exceedingly sophisticated, complex, and effective system of defenses. Its effectiveness is attested to by the fact that we are still here, although for almost all of man's existence there was no formal medical help available.

As various life forms evolved, so did the defensive mechanisms of the organism. Even the relatively simple life forms such as amoebae and other unicellular "animals" have complicated defenses. But immunologic mechanisms, the most sophisticated protection we have, did not appear until the development of animals with back-bones, the first traces appearing in primitive marine vertebrates 400 million years ago. About 250 million years ago, a system comparable to man's appeared in higher sharks, and since then there have been additional refinements to produce the complicated, many faceted system of reptiles, birds, and finally mammals.

The methods that the human body has developed to maintain its integrity can be divided into two broad groups: those that are primarily defensive and those that are reparative.

The defensive methods can be further subdivided into those that attempt to prevent invasion by external agents such as chemicals, particles and organisms (bacteria and viruses), and those that operate once the first-line defenses have failed and our body has been "invaded."

## First-Line Defense Mechanisms

**The Epithelium** ● Of prime importance among this first line of defenses is our skin, that complex organ that, among many other functions, acts as a physical barrier between the outside world and the delicate machinery of our bodies. Its outer layer is composed of keratin, a protein formed within the surface cells of the skin. As these cells mature they become filled with keratin and finally die, leaving a nonliving layer of this tough protein. (It is large accumulations of this material that we recognize as a "callus.") Beneath the layer of keratin are the cells of the epidermis, a layer several cells thick and held together by tight intercellular connections. The innermost or basal layer of the epidermis is composed of cells which frequently divide, forming more cells which move outward as they mature, form keratin, and are finally shed to make way for new cells. In this way our skin is constantly renewing itself.

Beneath the epidermis is the dermis and together these two layers compose what we commonly call skin. The dermis contains numerous blood vessels, lymphatics, nerves, sweat glands, sebaceous glands, and hair shafts set in a background of collagen (another protein, one that is particularly tough) and elastic fibers. Together they add strength and elasticity to our skin.

The thickness of the skin varies in different parts of our bodies, depending on the stress to which it is subjected; it is very thick on the heels and soles of the feet, thin over the abdomen and face. Under normal (or rather ideal) conditions most bacteria and viruses cannot penetrate the skin, although some can. Unfortunately, there are often microscopic cracks and crevices present which will allow access of bacteria into, and in some cases, through the skin.

The skin is also impervious to many chemicals, partly due to the oily film, called sebum, which coats it and which is secreted by sebaceous glands located adjacent to hair shafts.

The sebum serves as a lubricant, helping to keep the skin smooth and pliable, as well as acting as a protective film. In addition, the fatty acids of which it is composed seem to have an inhibiting influence on certain bacteria. The acid pH of sweat acts similarly in inhibiting the growth of bacteria.

Although sebum is continually being formed, too-frequent washings with harsh soaps or immersion in water may deplete it sufficiently to cause excess drying and cracking of the skin. Vitamin A is important in the formation of epithelium, the cells that line body surfaces, either external or internal, and a deficiency tends to cause the inappropriate formation of keratin in these epithelial surfaces. The excess keratin may lead to dry flaky scales or to "toadskin." In the case of the conjunctiva and cornea, the covering or "skin" of the eye, the inappropriate formation of keratin can lead to serious visual impairment or blindness.

Sunlight, worshipped by so many people today, is potentially very harmful to the skin and our general well-being. Large amounts of sun over many years cause damage to the skin in a number of ways. The elastic tissue located in the dermis undergoes a degenerative change known as solar elastosis, leading to wrinkles and loss of natural skin tone. Dry skin is another danger of excessive exposure to sunlight. The greatest danger, however, is from the ultraviolet radiation in sunlight. This leads to an increased incidence of cancers of the skin which, although seldom life threatening, can often cause extensive disfiguring or the need for radical surgery to eliminate the tumor. For the normal person, sunlight in moderation is no danger, nor is a summer or two of sunbathing. But if you like to fish, golf, garden, etc., and expect to be doing it regularly over the years, a hat with a brim wide enough to shade the nose is a must. A shirt should also be worn. Commonly sold suntan lotions do nothing to shield the skin from the damaging ultraviolet radiation, although "sun screen" lotions are available which will effectively stop ultraviolet radiation. One of the few highly effective lotions is a solution of the vitamin PABA in ethyl alcohol; it should be reapplied about every two hours.

It is the epidermis, rather than the interior dermis, which acts primarily as a barrier. Once it has been penetrated, the rich vascular and lymphatic supply of the dermis provides access to the rest of the body. Considering the ubiquity of bacteria, and the general sterility of tissues deep in the epidermis, it can be seen that the epidermis does a rather effective job.

**Sneezing and Coughing** • The nose and the mouth provide portals of entry into the depths of the body. That portion of the nose just inside the nostrils is lined with hair which acts as a trap or screen to sift out larger invading particles and prevent their passage into the lungs. The lining or mucosa of the upper respiratory tract is composed of special cells which form the respiratory epithelium. These cells have a surface covered with numerous cilia (microscopic hairs, about $\frac{3}{1,000}$ of a millimeter long) and interspersed among these cells are numerous mucous glands which secrete a slightly sticky fluid. The combined action of the mucus and cilia traps and holds bacteria and other foreign material. A sneeze or blowing the nose may then convey these to the outside. The cilia which line the windpipe and the air passages of the lungs continually beat in such a way as to convey mucus and trapped material upward and into the back of the mouth from whence they may be expectorated or swallowed. It should be noted that cigarette smoking paralyzes this beating action of the cilia. Smokers therefore tend to accumulate more bacteria and debris in their lungs and are more prone to develop respiratory disorders. Here is a classic example of how people can weaken their natural defenses against disease.

Coughing may be voluntary or it may occur as a reflex to irritation in the tracheobronchial tree. As such it serves a protective function, helping to rid the airways of excess secretions and trapped debris.

In addition, the deep breaths that are taken between the forceful expirations that make up a cough help to insure the proper aeration of all parts of the lungs. One of the problems that develop in some people with pneumonia or painful chest injuries (such as broken ribs) is the tendency to take only shallow breaths and not to fully expand the chest. When this occurs, that part of the lung that is not being aerated tends to retain secretions, which may fill the spaces normally reserved for air, stagnate, and become a fertile growth media for bacteria. Coughing is a natural mechanism which helps to guard against this complication.

*Excessive* coughing, however, may be damaging in several ways.

The mechanics of a cough involve first the inspiration of over two quarts of air. Next the epiglottis and vocal cords close while the diaphragm and other expiratory muscles contract, building up air pressure in the lungs. The epiglottis and vocal cords then suddenly open and air rushes out, sometimes reaching velocities of 75 to 100 mph, well over hurricane force.

The physical stresses involved in coughing may damage the mucosa of the air passages or may lead to muscle damage and even broken ribs. Certain infections in the lungs may become more extensive due to coughing, as well as being spread to other people. Cardiac conditions may be aggravated by the strain of repetitive coughing and even otherwise healthy persons may lose sleep and become fatigued.

At what point does coughing become more damaging than helpful? The answer must really be individualized, but some general statements can be made. In someone who is able to clear his own secretions by voluntarily coughing, and who is bothered by excessive coughing, an antitussive (cough medicine) may be used. Someone who is *not* able to voluntarily cough up and expectorate the accumulated secretions and debris of a respiratory infection is usually better off without something to inhibit the cough reflexes. Persons who suffer from emphysema and other chronic respiratory disorders should consult their physician concerning the therapy of acute respiratory infections.

**Stomach Acidity** ● The mucosa of the mouth contain no cilia and what goes in the mouth is usually swallowed unless it is large enough for us to be aware of and expectorate. Fortunately, the contents of the stomach are normally of such a degree of acidity that most bacteria will be destroyed, although some types are able to survive and may go on to cause disease.

The acidity of a solution is indicated by its pH, a number ranging from 0 to 14 which indicates the number of free hydrogen ions in the solution. A ph of 7 is neutral, the lower numbers are more acidic, and the higher numbers are more alkaline. The scale is a logarithmic one so that the difference, for instance, between 2 and 3 represents a 10-fold difference in hydrogen ion concentration and the difference between 2 and 4, a hundred-fold difference. At rest, the pH of the fluid in the stomach is about 3, or 10,000 times more acid than neutral, and maximally may reach a pH of 1. A solution of such acidity is able to destroy most bacteria and disrupt the molecular structure of many noxious substances.

After a discussion of the acidity of the stomach, the first question which usually comes to mind is "Why doesn't the stomach digest itself?" The reasons are not entirely known but of major importance is the "mucus" secreted by certain cells of the stomach and which coats its inner surface. This mucus seems to act as a protective barrier. Continued strong acidity, however, can lead to autodigestion of the stomach with resultant ulcer formation. Caffeine and nicotine, as well as anxiety, tend to cause an increase in acidity and may contribute to the formation of ulcers in certain individuals. Such common habits as steady coffee or cola drinking and smoking may thus damage the natural protection we have against stomach acid.

In some cases bacteria secrete toxins while they grow, and when ingested may cause various gastrointestinal symptoms. In these instances, the foul smell or taste may lead to nausea and vomiting, a most definite sign of rejection by our body. Unfortunately, food contaminated by many of the more serious offenders does not appear objectionable in smell or taste and it is not until the toxins begin to take effect that nausea, vomiting, or diarrhea may intervene.

Many varied stimuli—chemical, allergic, and psychologic—may cause diarrhea. Although diarrhea may have some protective function in ridding the body of noxious substances, it seems to be more often a symptom of damage to the mucosa or of disordered bowel functions, occurring after an injury has already occurred.

**The Importance of Body Flora** ● The air and food passages of our body are guarded by yet another mechanism, and this involves the concept of "normal flora," something that applies to other areas of the body as well, including the ears, vagina, colon, skin, and parts of the urinary system. Under normal conditions these areas are populated by one or more types of bacteria. In the mouth, for instance, there are upwards of 15 types of bacteria which may be normally found and which do not indicate disease. These bacteria are considered "normal flora" for the mouth. It is important to realize that these bacteria are not weak invaders, but actually play a role in preventing disease. As unlikely as that may sound, its validity is demonstrated when the normal flora is killed off by antibiotics. When this happens there often follows an infection by a virulent (disease-producing) bacterial or fungal organism, a so-called "super-infection." The organism may have been present in small numbers in the mouth, but held in check by the normal flora.

Just how the normal flora helps prevent virulent infections is not completely understood. Part of the reason may be that bacteria need certain nutrients, and the established normal flora, by its use of available nutrients, makes it difficult for potential invaders to gain a foothold. There is also evidence that some of the bacteria indigenous to humans secrete an antibioticlike substance. In addition, the normal flora, through its waste products or secretions, may establish a milieu (for instance, a medium that is too acid) that is not conducive for the growth of other bacteria. In any case, the maintenance of normal flora is an important aspect of host defense.

The killing off of the normal flora of any region of the body is risky and may precipitate serious disease. Regular, even vigorous, scrubbing is no threat to the regular bacteria of the skin, since such actions only temporarily decrease the number, but do not eliminate the normal flora. Of more serious concern are changes due to antibiotics and variations in the internal milieu. Long-term use of antibiotics may decimate the normal population of bacteria in the bowel leading to serious diarrhea and bleeding from overgrowth of resistant organisms. *Lactobacillus acidophilus,* the bacteria present in yogurt, is the predominant bacteria present in the colons of infants. Although other types become more prevalent as we mature, some investigators have shown a protective effect of *Lactobacilli* in preventing the overgrowth of virulent organisms.

Changes in the nature of the vaginal secretions, in diabetes or pregnancy, for instance, may lead to the growth of certain fungi such as *Candida albicans* (formerly *Monilia*). In this case it is a change in the local environment that favors the fungus over the normal flora; control of the diabetes or delivery should lead to a return of the usual milieu and reestablishment of the normal flora.

## Second-Line Defense Mechanisms

So far in our discussion we have been concerned primarily with the "first-line defense mechanisms." Once these first lines have been breached, a new array of protective functions become operative—the so-called "second-line" defensive mechanisms.

**Phagocytes—Cells That 'Eat Disease' •** One of the more primitive defensive mechanisms is phagocytosis, or "eating by a cell," the process by which various types of cells ingest particles such as bacteria or pollutants. Some of the ingested particles can then be digested by enzymes in the cells and thus destroyed. Many different types of cells in the body have the ability to be phagocytic but the two most important types as far as defense is concerned are the white blood cells and the macrophages.

White blood cells are part of the formed elements of blood, as opposed to the liquid portion or plasma. There are several types of white blood cells, but the one that is most active phagocytically is the neutrophil (named so because of its appearance when stained with certain dyes). Relatively large numbers of neutrophils are present in blood, about 4,500 per cubic millimeter, the range being 2,500 to 7,000. These cells contain powerful enzymes and are able to ingest various particles (bacteria, for instance) which are considered foreign to the body. The neutrophil is active like an amoeba, and sends out extensions of its cell body to surround the material to be ingested. The particle which has been phagocytosed is encased in a saclike structure called a vacuole, formed by a part of the membrane enclosing the cytoplasm of the neutrophil. Into this vacuole the neutrophil is able to secrete enzymes which may digest the enclosed particle. Sometimes the neutrophils ingest so much material that they burst, releasing all their enzymes and digestive juices. These aid in liquefying and reducing the foreign material, and when occurring to a sufficient degree, form pus.

In areas where foreign materials, such as bacteria, are deposited, the first white cells on the scene are the neutrophils and their phagocytic activity helps dispatch the offending organisms. Normally neutrophils circulate within the blood vessels, but in areas where there is inflammation or infection they actually have the ability to migrate out of the blood vessels into the surrounding tissue in quest of foreign matter to ingest.

When there is infection in the body, the number of circulating neutrophils may increase greatly, doubling or even tripling, as the bone marrow—their site of production—releases its reserves and increases production. This increase in neutrophils is often used as an indicator of disease, more specifically infection, and is one of the parameters measured when your doctor orders a "blood count."

**How the Lymph System Cleans the Blood** • There is another group of cells which are active phagocytically but which are relatively fixed in their location and do not circulate as do the neutrophils. These cells are known by a variety of names including "macrophage," "fixed tissue macrophage," and "reticuloendothelial cell" (R-E cell); they line blood and lymph vessels and are most plentiful in the liver, spleen, and lymph nodes.

Before describing the function of the R-E cells in these locations it is necessary to give a brief account of the anatomy of the organs involved.

Lymphatics, or lymph vessels, are present throughout the body and in most internal organs. Lymph nodes (or lymph glands) are present in various locations throughout the body and tend to occur in clusters or chains, but are not present within most organs. Together they form the lymphatic system, which transports lymph fluid.

The liquid components of blood do not stay within the blood vessels but tend to leak out through the spaces between the cells that make up the walls of capillaries, the smallest blood vessels. Lymph is the fluid which filters out of the bloodstream and when present in excess amounts is known as edema. This fluid accumulates at a rapid rate and if there were no mechanism for its return to the bloodstream, we would die in about two hours from circulatory failure.

As the lymph accumulates in the tissue spaces, it enters the lymphatic channels—small, thin-walled vessels which contain one-way valves, through which the lymph is pumped by the normal contraction of nearby muscles as we go about our usual activities.

Small bits of foreign material, bacteria, etc., can also enter the lymphatics, either free or within phagocytic cells which have ingested them. These are then carried along with the flow of lymph. In the case of an uncontrolled infection, the lymphatics may act as a route of spread, providing direct access to the bloodstream, which may lead to a severe, possibly fatal sepsis (infection involving the bloodstream). The course of a spreading infection may be seen and followed with the naked eye. It is manifested by red streaks leading away from an affected area, the red streaks marking the course of lymphatic channels.

The lymphatics interconnect and merge, forming larger vessels and finally empty into the venous portion of the bloodstream near the heart and thus return the fluid to the circulatory system. But on their way back to the heart region, the lymphatics communicate with numerous lymph nodes, tiny bean-shaped glands. The interior of nodes contains many lymphocytes (a kind of white blood cell) and reticuloendothelial cells, the latter being supported by a meshlike framework. As the lymph enters the node it percolates through the meshwork and comes into intimate contact with the R-E cells. Bits of foreign material are trapped and bacteria are ingested. The lymph nodes thus act as filters protecting the bloodstream from many potential invaders.

They also serve as sentries and production factories in our immunologic system of defenses, and when they are reacting in such a way they tend to enlarge and swell, forming what we commonly know as "swollen glands." Lymph nodes which drain lymph from infected areas may also swell and become quite tender.

The liver and the spleen share certain similarities of structure with lymph nodes; they both contain an interconnecting network of channels (sinusoids) through which fluid percolates, similar to the meshwork structure of lymph nodes. In the case of the liver and spleen, however, the fluid is blood, rather than lymph, but the sinusoids are lined with R-E cells just as in the lymph nodes. In both instances, though, the R-E cells act to keep the bloodstream free of possibly injurious agents—the lymph nodes acting as primary filters and the liver and spleen as secondary filters when the lymph nodes prove inadequate or when material enters the bloodstream directly without traversing the lymphatic system.

In addition to neutrophils and R-E cells, another actively phagocytic cell is the macrophage or histiocyte, similar to an R-E cell but having the ability to move about. These cells are the scavangers of the body and usually make their appearance after the neutrophils, cleaning up the debris, including dead tissue fragments, foreign matter, and disintegrated neutrophils.

Although in general the phagocytic cells are a hardy lot, the formation of neutrophils may be paralyzed as a side effect of numerous drugs. Since neutrophils live only a few days, their numbers become rapidly depleted and we soon may be subject to very severe, life-threatening infections. Platelets (small cell fragments needed for blood clotting) are sometimes also decreased. Consequently, after starting a drug, the appearance of bleeding, easy bruisability, sudden sore throat, oral infections, or other infections should be reported to your physician immediately.

## The Amazing Immune System

In the continuous battle our bodies wage against invasion by microorganisms, be they bacteria or viruses, the strongest weapon in the arsenal is the immune system. It is part of the secondary defenses, but important enough to merit a separate section. The immune system enables the body to distinguish "self" from "nonself" and is capable of launching an attack on that which it considers nonself, and in so doing can make use of the most specific "guided missile" known to man—the antibody. Ironically, it is also capable of killing *us* in a matter of seconds and of causing many complex, serious, sometimes fatal diseases as well as numerous annoying but not serious conditions. We could not live without it, yet because of it we often endure much suffering. This two-edged sword is an exceedingly complex, sophisticated system. Physicians known as immunologists devote their entire professional lives to trying to understand it and the diseases it causes.

**The Mystery of the Mighty Antibodies ●** Antibodies are protein molecules synthesized in the body in such a way that they can react specifically against particular groupings of molecules such as those comprising portions of a bacteria or virus. This specificity is believed to be due to the *shape* of the antibody, which exactly fits into the shape of a particular area on the surface of the bacterium or virus, like one piece of a jigsaw puzzle fits into its mate.

Many different substances are capable of eliciting the formation of antibodies and such substances are called antigens. The list of potential antigens is almost endless and includes such things as bacteria, viruses, drugs, pollens, insect venoms, chemicals, foods, and foreign tissue (e.g., transplanted organs or transfused blood). When an antigen makes contact with cells of the immunologic system, a complicated and not completely understood process is initiated, leading to the formation of an antibody which is specific for the antigen which stimulated its formation.

If the antibodies were elicited by bacteria of a certain type, they will react with those bacteria but not with the hundreds of other types to which we are exposed. Certain areas of the antigen have a unique arrangement of molecules acting as antigenic determinants, and it is the spatial configuration of these areas that determines the matching configuration of the antibody elicited. The active sites on the antibody will fit neatly into the antigenic determinant sites, like a key fitting into a lock. Generally, an antibody has two active sites; that is, two areas whose shape matches that of a specific antigenic determinant; *thus it is possible for one antibody to attack and link two antigens.*

The sequence of events leading to the formation of an antibody is believed to be as follows. When an antigen enters the body, it comes in contact with a macrophage (one of the phagocytic cells described previously) which ingests it and breaks it down into smaller units. The macrophage then comes into contact with a lymphocyte (one of the white blood cells) and transfers information to it, perhaps relating to the required specificity of the antibody. The lymphocyte transforms into a plasma cell, which is well equipped for protein synthesis, and begins manufacturing antibodies of the required specificity.

Production of these antibodies occurs in the lymph nodes and other lymphoid masses, the antibodies being released into the bloodstream. These antibodies are therefore called *humoral antibodies,* since they circulate freely in the blood, one of the "humors" of older medicine.

This whole process is not a very rapid one: it is usually a matter of about a week before antibodies can be detected. However, having once formed antibodies to a particular antigen, the immune system, upon a second encounter (even years later) with the same antigen, is capable of producing antibodies at a much quicker rate—within a few days of exposure.

Humoral antibodies are the primary immune response in acute

bacterial infections and in some viral infections, but in most viral, fungal, protozoal, and in some bacterial infections, another part of the immune system is most important. It is known as cellular immunity or delayed hypersensitivity, because it involves antibodies that remain within a cell, and because the reactions involved take longer than those of humoral antibodies.

If bacteria penetrate the skin, say via a cut or open wound, and gain entrance to the circulation, antibody production is soon initiated and if we have encountered the particular species of bacterium before, the response is quite rapid. The antibody attaches to the cell wall of the bacteria and because of its ability to link with two antigens, the antibody may induce small aggregates of entrapped bacteria which are grabbed more easily by the R-E system. In addition, the antibodies with the help of substances known collectively as "complement" or the "complement system," may actually fragment and destroy the bacteria, leaving only the debris to be phagocytized by the reticuloendothelial system.

In the case of a viral infection, where the virus has entered one of our cells and humoral antibodies are not useful, cellular immunity comes into play. The virus, which at some point in its life cycle is outside the cell, stimulates production of specifically sensitized lymphocytes. These lymphocytes come into contact with the affected cells and release a variety of substances which increase the number of macrophages in the area and which—rather amazingly—impart to them the ability to directly kill cells rather than merely act as scavengers. The sensitized lymphocyte itself may also directly destroy cells.

They may also release a substance known as "transfer factor" which transfers the antibody specificity of the sensitized lymphocyte to other nearby unsensitized lymphocytes which have never come into contact with the specific antigen under attack. Transfer factor may be released by a sensitized lymphocyte as rapidly as one hour following its contact with the antigen. Once the unsensitized lymphocytes receive the transfer factor, they too can begin to manufacture the appropriate antibody and to divide. Production capacity can thus be vastly increased.

All of these possibilities do not necessarily occur during each immunologic reaction, but experimentally it is difficult to separate one from the other.

**Why Are Antibodies So 'Smart'?** • So far I have not mentioned just how an antibody comes to have a configuration that exactly complements a corresponding configuration on an antigen. The answer is far from being known and what's more, the theories are difficult to explain thoroughly without a fairly extensive background in biology, molecular biology, and biochemistry. Nonetheless, I will try to briefly present the main points of the two leading theories.

The "template" theory is the older of the two and supposes that each antibody is manufactured in response to a particular antigen which has gained access to the body. A template or mold is made of the antigenic determinant site and from this mold, the properly shaped antibody is made. The making of the mold and then of the antibody from that mold, involves complex interactions of RNA (ribose nucleic acid), amino acids, and many other cell constituents. This idea seems very appealing intellectually, but most of the experimental evidence fits in better with the second theory.

According to the "selective theory," among all of the millions of potential antibody-producing cells in the body, there is at least one with the ability to make an antibody for any antigen which we may encounter. When an antigen enters the body, it eventually comes in contact with and thus "selects" the appropriate antibody-forming cell. Once exposed to the antigen, this cell rapidly divides, forming many more cells, all with the ability to manufacture that one particular antibody. This theory requires that each cell in the body carry a vast amount of genetic information. Yet, although at first glance it seems less likely than the "template" theory, it appears to be the more probable of the two theories.

Regardless of just how the shape of an antibody is determined, once the appropriate antigen is encountered, the antibody-forming cells rapidly divide, passing on to their progeny the ability to manufacture the required antibody. In this way, a large family or "clone" of cells develops, each manufacturing the same specific antibody.

In a first encounter with a virus or other agent which stimulates delayed hypersensitivity, it is often a race between multiplication of viruses and production of antibodies in the form of sensitized lymphocytes. In the case of some viruses this is truly a life-and-death race. When a second encounter with a specific type of virus takes place, there is already a significant population of sensitized lymphocytes in the circulation and these can fairly quickly multiply so that a high level of antibodies can be reached before the virus has multiplied very much. That is the basic premise behind the practice of immunization, only that rather than using live, virulent organisms for the first encounter, killed or attenuated organisms are used. In any case, the idea is to achieve a high level of circulating antibodies before the virus has had a chance to greatly increase its numbers.

**The Immune System and Cancer** • The immune system is also believed to play a large role in protection against cancer. Scientists now generally believe that tumor cells contain antigenic determinants different from other cells in the body and hence are recognized as "nonself" by the immune system. Considering the many millions of dividing cells in the human body and the number of years we live, it seems reasonable to assume that during our lifetime more than a few cells undergo mutations (either spontaneous or induced by carcinogens) which lead to cancer. Those immunologists who believe in "immunologic surveillance" feel that once a neoplastic (cancerous) mutation takes place, the cell or cells involved are rapidly destroyed by lymphocytes. In a head-on confrontation, it takes one sensitized lymphocyte to kill one target cell.

Since people obviously do develop malignant tumors which often grow, spread, and kill, it is apparent that immunologic surveillance is not always effective. There are many theories to account for this. Some suppose simply that tumor growth is more rapid than production of sensitized lymphocytes; some suppose that the tumor cells are not sufficiently different from normal cells to stimulate a significant antibody response.

One of the more interesting theories (which, by the way, has considerable experimental evidence in its favor) envisions the presence of a special group of antibodies called "blocking antibodies." These are circulating humoral antibodies which combine with the specific antigenic determinant sites of neoplastic cells, but for reasons which are not entirely clear, they are not able to cause the destruction of the tumor cells. However, since they are occupying the antigenic sites of the tumor cells, the blocking antibodies prevent sensitized lymphocytes from combining with these sites and hence destroying the cells. As long as the antigenic determinants of the cancer cells are obscured by the blocking antibodies, the lymphocytes will not recognize them as being "nonself," and no matter how many killer lymphocytes are present, the tumor cells will be in no danger of attack from them. The cancer may then grow and spread unmolested by immunologic surveillance. In this situation, the immune system, rather than helping us combat disease, has actually fostered the development of a malignant neoplasm. Nor is this the only way in which we may be injured by our immune system.

**How the Immune System Can Hurt Us** • There are a large number of immunologic reactions which may cause more harm than good. Two worthy of mention are allergic reactions and autoimmune diseases. Most of the common allergies to foods, pollen, etc., involve a special class of antibodies known as IgE antibodies. One of the properties of IgE antibodies is their ability to attach themselves to certain cells in particular areas, such as skin or nasal mucosa, thus establishing particular organs where there is a high concentration of antibodies. When the proper antigen comes along, the antigen-antibody (Ag-Ab) reaction takes place in those areas where large numbers of antibodies have been attached—areas known as target organs. The skin and the mucosa of the nasal cavities are common target organs.

When the Ag-Ab reaction takes place between, for example, pollen and IgE, several chemical substances are released by cells in the nasal mucosa and it is these substances that lead to the common symptoms of sneezing, runny nose, etc. One of the substances released is histamine; hence the widespread use of antihistamines in treating allergic disorders.

In the case of food allergy, the Ag-Ab reaction might take place in the skin, leading to the formation of hives, or a rash. Sometimes, for reasons that are not entirely clear, an antigen (such as penicillin or insect venom) will stimulate a particularly severe allergic reaction called anaphylactic shock, in which there is a drastic fall in blood pressure and great difficulty in breathing, which may prove fatal if not treated promptly. These severe symptoms are also caused by substances released by cells in the vicinity of the Ag-Ab reaction, and can usually be effectively counteracted by epinephrine (adrenalin) and an antihistamine injected intravenously.

Quite obviously the types of antigen-antibody reactions I have just been discussing are certainly not beneficial to us and one wonders just how and why they evolved. The answer is not known. But it seems that the combination of antigens and antibodies per se is not injurious, but rather that nearby cells are injured as an unfortunate side effect, like innocent bystanders in a shoot-out between the good guys and the bad guys. This "innocent bystander" theory is also believed to account for some of the other injurious effects of allergic-type reactions. The basic reaction of Ag combining with Ab can thus still be viewed as a potentially useful mechanism, since it is "tying-up" or removing a foreign invader. Symptoms of allergic reactions, no matter how severe, are then viewed as bad side effects to a basically useful process.

Autoimmune diseases are rather complex, but basically they represent a failure of the immune system to properly distinguish "self" from "nonself," with a resultant immune reaction against the cells of our own bodies. There are several reasons for this failure, some supported by experimental evidence, others mostly by theory. We know, for example, that some bacteria commonly present in the bowel have antigenic determinants similar to or the same as certain of the blood group substances (A, B, O, etc.) of man. Exposure to these bacteria elicits antibodies that react not only with the bacteria, but also with one of the blood group substances. This accounts for us having antibodies to certain blood types, even though we may never have received a blood transfusion.

Some researchers feel a process similar to this accounts for the heart damage following certain types of infection with beta-hemolytic streptococci (strep throat). The bacteria, in this case, are antigenically similar to portions of the heart and antibodies formed against the bacteria also attack the heart, causing poststreptococcal rheumatic fever.

Another reason thought to account for some of the autoimmune diseases is damage to cells by an inflammatory process, the damage rendering the cells different in some way, and hence able to stimulate antibody formation, even though they are our own cells. Viruses are also felt to be able to cause such changes in cells. The end result of all these events is antibodies which react against our own cells, as if they were foreign bodies.

For the most part, we are unaware of the workings of the immune system, but allergic disorders, which affect most of us at some time or another, are evidence of immunity working "overtime." The large number of chemicals in the food we eat, the air we breathe, or in the various lotions, creams, and aerosol sprays we use provide a large and varied array of potential antigens. To these must be added the large numbers of naturally occurring substances to which some people are allergic. In trying to discover the cause of newly developed allergic symptoms, a good starting point is to try to discover what changes have occurred in your environment: are there new foods, new soap, new plants (pollens), new pets? The change may be in your internal environment, for it seems that emotional problems may alter our reactivity to various antigens.

## Dealing With Fever and Pain

There remain several other second-line defenses of importance. Two of them, fever and pain, although relatively "simple" in relation to the immune system, are far from well understood. Whatever their ultimate function, they cause us so much suffering that they deserve special attention.

**Why Fever?** ● Fever is one of the oldest and most generally known accompaniment of systemic illness, and although much is known about the mechanisms of its production, its purpose remains unclear. Before discussing how fever may help or hurt us, some background about heat production and regulation is needed.

Under normal circumstances the heat of our body is generated as a by-product of the many chemical reactions (metabolism) that are continuously in progress in the muscles and liver. Even when we are at rest, small portions of our muscles are contracting and relaxing, a process which generates heat. The liver is an extremely active metabolic organ, carrying on hundreds of different chemical reactions. The heat generated from these organs warms the blood passing through them and this is more than sufficient to warm our bodies to the 37°C. (98.6°F.) which is considered normal. The proper temperature is maintained by an extremely sensitive thermostat (located in the hypothalamus, a part of the brain) which controls most of the temperature regulation processes to be described.

Coarse adjustments in temperature are made by sweating or shivering. Under usual conditions, heat production is in excess, and the evaporation of sweat from the skin causes heat loss. Should a significant increase in temperature be needed, the fine contractions of muscle mentioned previously increase in amplitude and become visible—the process we know as shivering. Fine adjustments in temperature regulation are made by controlling the blood flow through the skin. The more blood that flows through the skin, the greater the heat loss as the heat dissipates into the surrounding air. Heat is conserved by restricting the blood flow to the skin and this is accomplished by contraction of the blood vessels carrying blood to the skin. Through these mechanisms, the body temperature is maintained within rather narrow limits for each individual, 96.5° to 99°F. being the range of normal values. It is usually lower in the mornings than in the afternoons, and strenuous exercise may cause a very slight elevation.

When we develop a fever, it seems that the setting of the thermostat is raised to a higher level. Initially, there may be a vasoconstriction (constriction of blood vessels), with the resultant decrease in skin temperature causing a sensation of chilling and perhaps shivering. In a neutral or cold environment, this shivering is needed to raise the body temperature to the new, higher set point of the thermostat, while in a warm environment, cessation of sweating may be sufficient to raise the body temperature.

Many different agents may cause fever, including bacteria, viruses, necrotic or dying tissue, and Ag-Ab complexes, but the final common pathway in all of these seems to be the release of pyrogens from phagocytic cells. Pyrogens are chemical substances that initiate fever production and probably exert their effect on the hypothalamus.

An antipyretic (fever-lowering drug) such as aspirin seems to "reset" the body's thermostat at a lower level, which leads to the activation of heat-loss mechanisms. This is evidenced by blood vessel dilation and sweating, following aspirin administration to feverish patients.

As mentioned before, the purpose of fever remains unexplained. Although the raised temperature is directly harmful to a few microorganisms, the vast majority are not adversely affected. Experiments designed to see if a raised temperature influenced phagocytosis or immune reactions have often produced unclear results or have shown slight, probably insignificant benefits. These experiments were generally in vitro (in "test tubes"), and it is possible that in a living organism the benefit might be of significance.

The deleterious effects of fever, as compared to its benefits, are well known. There is increased work of the heart and other organs, as well as an increased loss of fluids. The latter is often of great significance, particularly in infants and the debilitated. In addition, fever often causes generalized discomfort, with its attendant sweats and headache.

Considering all of these points, it seems that fever is of little help to the patient once it has alerted him to the fact that something is wrong. However, this latter function should not be underestimated. Fever may be the only symptom or an early symptom of a disease state which needs attention.

Having alerted us that something is amiss, does fever become a "disease" to be treated in its own right, apart from the condition that is causing the fever (assuming that the cause is known)?

The answer to this question, like many therapeutic decisions, must be individualized and depends on such factors as: the general condition and age of that patient, the cause of the fever, the height of the fever, medications already being given, and possibly other factors. In general, in an otherwise healthy individual, a fever may be treated if it causes a patient discomfort and if there is not any contraindication to the administration of an antipyretic.

Older persons, particularly those with a significant degree of cerebral atherosclerosis (hardening and blockage of the blood vessels supplying the brain), may become comatose during infections associated with fever. That is due in part to the increased metabolic demands of the brain because of the fever and the inability of the blood vessels to supply the increased amount of blood needed. Such a situation is uncommon in younger individuals. Fevers under 100°F. do not usually cause much discomfort and would not be expected to have a significant metabolic effect.

Since aspirin is the most commonly used antipyretic, those people with bleeding problems or ulcers must be somewhat cautious in their efforts to reduce fever. Fevers due to infectious processes will subside promptly once the infection is cleared up; and if this is done rapidly, antipyretics may not be needed at all.

High fever in infants may be dangerous, leading to convulsions, and it is sometimes necessary to cool the body with sponge baths or immersion in water.

In spite of the deleterious effects of fever, many feel that it must be a useful defense mechanism or it would not have survived as a generalized response of warm-blooded animals.

**Pain, the Horrible Helper** • Once the body has been invaded or has become diseased, we may also experience pain. In addition to alerting us to injury or disease, pain may serve a protective function, since it often causes us to guard or splint an injured or diseased area. This function, however, may become perverted. Complete immobility, particularly of joints, may be harmful in itself, causing pathologic stiffness even after healing. In the case of rib injuries, failure to take deep breaths because of the pain may lead to pneumonia and other pulmonary complications.

Pain is a symptom, and as such, is not damaging to the body. However, the emotional stress that it may cause, as well as lack of sleep, can cause actual physiologic damage. For this reason and others (as in the case of rib injuries mentioned above) it is often important to relieve pain. Pain is regulated in the brain and because of this it is responsive to hypnosis and other states of altered awareness, as well as to a wide variety of drugs. I might add that hypnosis may be used to induce the relaxation and pain insensitivity necessary for major surgery and that the pain relief may be continued into the postoperative period. All this with none of the potential hazards of anesthesia or pain medication! Acupuncture has received much publicity recently and is certainly worthy of much study by Western civilization.

With the exception of aspirin, no really effective analgesics can be obtained without a prescription. That is because pain is a symptom and should not be subdued until its cause is discovered and treated. Once this is done, the pain often subsides on its own. In situations where this is not the case, the discomfort of the pain must be weighed against the potential dangers of the drugs used to combat it. Since most analgesics, when used properly, have a relatively high margin of safety, alleviation of pain is a reasonable objective for the patient. The cautions that I have mentioned pertain also to the use of aspirin for minor pain, especially since much minor pain can be relieved without medication. Heat, rest, and body-relaxing techniques often do wonders.

**Coagulation—Another Vital Defense** • Coagulation or blood clotting involves a very complex series of biochemical reactions which occur rapidly once the integrity of a blood vessel is interrupted. These reactions lead to the formation of a clot, a meshwork of protein with entrapped red blood cells, white blood cells, serum, and platelets. The appearance and consistency of a fresh clot is akin to dark red Jello, and the clot serves to close up breaks in vessels preventing further loss of blood. The obvious usefulness of such a mechanism is apparent when we look at hemophiliacs, in whom the clotting procedure is defective. Before the advent of modern therapy, many hemophiliac children would bleed to death following even minor injuries.

Platelets, the small cell fragments mentioned previously, may directly plug small holes in vessels, in addition to participating in the clotting reaction. The walls of the small vessels themselves are important in preventing leaks under the normal stresses of daily activities. The cells of the walls are held together by intercellular "cement," which requires vitamin C for its production and maintenance. When vitamin C is markedly deficient, such as in scurvy, numerous small hemorrhages (petechiae) occur as blood leaks out of the millions of capillaries throughout the body.

Coagulation is only half the story of the hemostats—the natural mechanisms that control blood viscosity. Equally important is maintaining the fluidity of the blood and preventing the clotting mechanism from going too far and coagulating large quantities of blood needlessly. To accomplish this there are a series of checks and balances incorporated into the clotting mechanism, involving many activators and inhibitors. A discussion of these would be lengthy, and I mention them merely to emphasize the extreme complexity of the defensive mechanisms which have evolved to protect the uniformity of our internal environment.

There are many drugs which affect hemostasis. An anticoagulant is *intended* to hinder or inhibit coagulation, but others may do so as a side effect. Aspirin, the most commonly ingested drug (15 million pounds/year in the United States), has as one of its side effects the prolongation of clotting. In most cases this is of little importance, but sometimes it can contribute to significant bleeding, particularly in sensitive individuals.

In several studies, between 60 and 70 percent of normal subjects who ingested small doses of aspirin had slight internal bleeding from their gastrointestinal tracts. (This may have been partially due to the irritant nature of aspirin on the bowel mucosa.) Although this bleeding was slight, it was sufficient to cause mild anemia in several women. In persons with bleeding disorders, aspirin may cause significant hemorrhage.

Vitamin C is necessary for blood vessel integrity, while vitamin K is necessary for the synthesis of several of the substances participating in coagulation.

## Reparative Processes

Healing and regeneration after injury or disease are very important in the story of human survival. We would be in a sorry state if blisters and cuts never healed and broken bones never knitted.

A simple cut on the finger will illustrate the process of wound healing. Immediately following the cut, blood begins to flow from the ends of severed blood vessels, while at the same time, the clotting system is activated by substances released from the damaged cells. Soon the bleeding stops and we are left with a clot-filled defect extending through the skin and underlying tissue.

Over the next few days the cells at the cut ends of the blood vessels multiply and grow out into the defect, using the meshwork of the blood clot as a supporting framework. Fibroblasts, cells which manufacture collagen, also repopulate the defect, laying down fibrous tissue as the clot is broken down and resorbed. The basal layer of the skin grows out over the surface of the cut and regenerates new skin, while the newly formed fibrous tissue contracts somewhat, pulling the skin edges closer.

After about a week or so, healing is complete and there remains a thin layer of fibrous tissue (scar) beneath the skin as the only indication of prior trauma.

In the case of damage to an internal organ, either by disease or trauma, the process is basically the same, although differences do exist, depending on whether or not the damaged organ is able to regenerate itself. Some tissues, such as heart muscle and nerve, cannot divide and regenerate. Damaged portions of these tissues can only be replaced by fibrous tissue, which accounts in part for the seriousness of damage to these organs. On the other hand, some organs such as liver and skin are capable of replacing much of their substance if damaged.

How much of an organ can be destroyed and still leave enough working tissue to perform the necessary functions of the organ? This safety factor varies for different organs but generally is quite high.

Although we have two kidneys, one will serve us quite adequately. Close to 90 percent of the liver must be destroyed before we show signs of hepatic failure.

The processes involved in repair and regeneration require relatively large amounts of protein, vitamin C, and zinc. As the primary building material of cells, protein is especially important, while vitamin C is vital for the formation of intercellular material which helps hold the cells together and for the synthesis of collagen, one of the major supportive proteins. Zinc and vitamin A are of special importance in the healing of the skin and internal mucous membranes.

In the case of broken bones, calcium and vitamin D are the most critical nutrients for healing.

## Protecting Our Natural Protectors

In the preceding pages I have attempted to convey an idea of the many defensive and healing mechanisms that have evolved over millions of years to insure the survival of *Homo sapiens*. Although generally quite effective, these protective processes are sometimes thwarted, occasionally by their inadequacies (for nature, too, is not perfect), but more often by our own interference, however well intentioned it may be.

One of the major causes of interference with the normal actions of the human body is the effect of drugs, both singly and in combination. The use of multiple drugs is particularly complicated, since the effects of two drugs may be more than simply the sum of their individual effects. The problem of drug interaction is becoming more and more significant as the number of drugs used increases, along with the number of different specialists an individual may see. This is not to say that giving drugs in combination is bad, only that increased vigilance on the part of both the physician and patient is needed. A physician must be constantly aware of potential hazards of drug therapy, while a patient must make it his duty to inform his doctor of any medication he may be taking. In line with this, it is important to know the names of the medicines being used. You should ask your physician to instruct the pharmacist to "label as such" any medication he may prescribe.

Drugs may interfere with natural defenses in numerous ways and whole volumes have been devoted to drug effects and drug interactions. I shall mention a few examples to illustrate the wide range of potential dangers from medication. Remember, too, that I am dealing only with those effects on defensive mechanisms and neglecting other, more direct, toxic actions.

Many drugs suppress the formation of white blood cells, so vital in fighting infection. Such an action, if not promptly detected, may open the door to severe infections. The alteration of normal flora by antibiotics may also lead to severe infections. Allergic reactions to drugs may cause skin rashes with resultant fissuring and cracking of the skin, a condition which provides easy access for bacteria. Steroids, one of the most useful classes of drugs, inhibit healing and the inflammatory reaction. In patients with certain bacterial, viral, and fungal diseases, the use of steroids may prevent the body from containing and walling off the offending agent, leading to wide dissemination of disease within the body. (Vitamin A ointment applied to wounds and ulcers of patients on steroids often permits normal healing.)

In some cases the potentially harmful side effects of a drug represent a risk that must be taken because of the seriousness of the primary disease and the known effectiveness of the drug in alleviating that disease. Unfortunately, this is not always the case. Much medication is consumed when it really is not needed, and at least a portion of the blame must fall on patients. Although many illnesses are self-limiting and not a real threat to our long-term health, some patients expect to come away from the doctor's office with more than simply assurance that it will go away. They expect, if not demand, to get an often useless "shot of penicillin" for a viral cold. But physicians, too, must share the blame. In any case, the important thing to remember is that powerful medicine is not always helpful and sometimes actually harmful.

The defensive mechanisms of the body may also be damaged by many chemicals (in addition to those used as drugs). These might be in the form of poisonous pollutants, food additives, insect and animal toxins, alcohol in excess, and narcotics. Unlike drugs, however, we are often unaware that we are ingesting or breathing potentially dangerous substances, and this insidious nature makes them all the more dangerous. The ways in which these hidden chemicals may damage our natural defenses are many and varied and are beyond the scope of this discussion.

Fatigue has often been accused of causing a "lowering of

defenses" with subsequent illness, but this is difficult to evaluate scientifically. One reason is that fatigue is often associated with poor nutrition and the effects of each cannot be separated. Another reason is that fatigue may be the first symptom of disease and may then be falsely interpreted as causing the disease. However, the experience of centuries seems to suggest that adequate or extra rest is generally useful. There is also some evidence in animals that exhaustion decreases resistance to certain infections.

## Why Does the System Sometimes Fail?

As effective as the body is in fighting off disease, its defensive mechanisms may be overpowered in certain situations. One such situation is when unusually large numbers of bacteria gain access to the body—for instance, when a large area of the skin is denuded from a burn. The phagocytic and immune systems are simply not able to deal with the large numbers of bacteria at one time and a serious infection may result.

Often, people are amazed at the apparent rapidity with which disease strikes. In most cases, however, this actually represents the sudden "surfacing" of a process which was going on for some time. This silent or "subclinical" period of disease is known as the incubation period of infectious diseases. It may vary from hours (these are the few that really do have a sudden onset) to weeks. During this time the decisive battles are being waged between our defenses and the invading organisms. When the balance is tipped in favor of the invaders the disease becomes apparent, and subsides if and when medical therapy and/or our own defenses finally overpower the disease organisms.

*Numerous studies have shown that, overall, most disease is subclinical, never becoming severe enough to produce recognizable symptoms. We generally remain unaware of the battles that rage within us and this attests to the effectiveness of our natural defenses.*

A mechanism which is basically protective may, when carried to extremes, cause more harm than good. Frostbite is an example of such a process. In order to conserve heat, blood flow is shifted away from the skin, where much heat would be lost through radiation. However, the lack of blood causes pain, and if the blood flow is significantly reduced for long enough, gangrene may result from the poor circulation.

Nutrition is of course basic for all aspects of life, since it must provide the building blocks and fuel for all biological processes. Every breath we take, every thought we think, every nerve impulse which triggers a beat of our heart requires energy, and this must be provided by the food we eat. The various aspects of nutrition and healing are dealt with in detail elsewhere in this book, but at least two points deserve emphasis.

The first is that there is a renewed interest among physicians and scientists in the importance of nutrition in maintaining an optimum degree of health. I use the phrase "optimum degree of health," to emphasize that there are varying degrees of well-being and that what many people consider healthy today may in years to come prove to be less than the maximum attainable. Science and medicine are not static but continually changing, albeit slowly in some cases.

The importance of this in regard to vitamins was expressed by Drs. Perla and Marmorston over 30 years ago: "There is a growing mass of experimental evidence that the degree of saturation of the body with these important vitamin substances may affect the resistance and well-being of the host. Should this prove to be the case, a distinction will have to be made between optimum requirement of a vitamin and the minimal requirement to avoid signs of deficiency. From the point of view of preventive medicine and individual health, an abundance of vitamins in the diet, considerably in excess of present estimated minimal requirements, would probably insure a greater degree of resistance to infection and more favorable conditions for a healthier and longer life" (*Natural Resistance and Clinical Medicine,* Little, Brown & Co., Boston, 1941).

The second point is that the defensive and reparative processes are complex functions often involving many different types of tissues and enzymes. Vitamins and minerals are interwoven with many of these functions. If one link in a chain of events is weakened, the end result might fall short of expectations, even though all other aspects of the process are intact. For example, inadequate blood flow due to atherosclerosis may prevent the healing of a laceration, even though the basic mechanisms of repair are functioning properly. It thus becomes possible for seemingly remote, perhaps subtle, deficiencies to seriously affect the way in which we deal with our environment and defend ourselves against disease.

# Naturopathy

Naturopathy, or the healing of disease through natural methods, was formulated over 150 years ago, reached a certain degree of popularity in the United States during the first three decades of the 20th century, and is now all but extinct.

And that is a shame, because a really well-trained naturopath could have a great deal to offer, especially in treating minor or chronic conditions, which account for an enormous portion of medical problems and fill doctors' offices with patients who might do just as well or better being treated by a naturopath.

Naturopathy is above all the supreme eclectic medical art, drawing on everything and anything of a drugless nature to help the patient: herbs, hydrotherapy, massage, mud packs, manipulation, exercise, enemas, nutrition—whatever seems indicated for the condition *and* for the individual patient.

It is likely that the *real* practice of naturopathy has almost disappeared from the scene because of legal strictures. That is because a real naturopath *diagnoses* and *treats* disease, an occupation which is liable to result in his arrest unless he is a dentist, physician, or chiropractor. The modern practitioner of naturopathy would for his own protection have to more or less disguise himself as some sort of consultant, and even then keep his fingers crossed that the local medical monopoly does not take umbrage to his presence in the community.

I was therefore very lucky to be able to find a practicing naturopath in the person of Dr. Thomas F. Marsteller, of Sellersville, Pennsylvania, a small rural community about 40 miles north of Philadelphia. Dr. Marsteller practices by virtue of a license he holds from the state of Pennsylvania as a Drugless Therapist. Although this license is no longer conferred by the state—Dr. Marsteller's license is No. 11—those who still hold one may still legally practice any form of drugless therapy.

A tall, lanky man who perfectly fits the role of the country doctor, Dr. Marsteller is the seventh generation of his family to practice medicine ("My grandfather was a doctor until the age of 92."). He is the very model of the eclectic healer, using traditional naturopathy, manipulation, homeopathic remedies, heat treatments, commonsense psychology, and when the occasion calls for it, a little "magic."

As Dr. Marsteller took me on a tour of his offices, I noticed one room which contained a kind of vat to which some rubber hoses were connected. That, I discovered, was the colonic irrigation machine, the device I had read so much about when studying some of the literature on naturopathic medicine. I had gotten the impression from this literature that colonic irrigations are a major therapeutic technique and that a world of good is said to result from their use.

Dr. Marsteller did not change this impression, although he emphasized that he always examined patients before permitting them to undergo a colonic irrigation, to see if it was indicated. Apparently, it often is, because he has a nurse in his office who I was informed does nothing but administer these treatments.

The two hoses connected to the device merge into one channel as they approach the impressive-looking business end of the nozzle. First, a cup of water, containing some dissolved herbs and/or some sulfur or boric acid, is introduced into the rectum. After a suitable period of retention, the fluid is released, and is channeled through the second hose into the waste-receiving portion of the machine. Curiously, I noticed that there was a glass window in the return tube, and Dr. Marsteller told me it was there to permit observation of the returning material, which might reveal something of importance, such as the presence of worms. The patient is switched around to a number of positions as more water is introduced and retrieved, so that a considerable portion of the colon is flushed out.

Although constipation might seem the prime reason for such an irrigation, Dr. Marsteller believes that constipation is usually "a result of something else" and advises irrigations for a rather large number of conditions on the theory that various toxins and "sludge" are thereby removed from the system.

The next thing that drew my attention in his office was an unbelievable proliferation of small bottles, which had obviously been sitting on his shelves for many years. These, it turned out, contained the homeopathic pills which he dispenses. There were several hundreds of these bottles, some of them in his consulting office, some in a closet, and still more in a storeroom. While many of them contained only one substance, a good many contained combinations of herbs or chemicals.

Before dispensing these pills, Dr. Marsteller said he always checks his diagnosis in a book, and held up the *Pocket Manual of Homeopathic Materia Medica* by William Boerick, M.D., published by Boerick and Tafel of Philadelphia in 1927. "This is my bible," the naturopath exclaimed.

Thumbing through the volume, I was rather shocked to find belladonna, an extremely powerful herb which can cause death, described as a "great children's remedy." But then, I remembered that in homeopathic preparations this herb would be given in "triturations" which are diluted to the extent that even a tiny pill might contain only one-thousandth part of the active substance.

The idea is that "like cures like," and a very small dose of a substance which causes an ill effect in a healthy person will actually stimulate the protective reaction of the body to overcome that same ill effect in a sick person.

Thus, Dr. Marsteller said, he may give pills containing highly diluted extracts of snake venom or ground-up bee parts to a person who has been bitten by such a creature.

When I expressed some astonishment at this approach, Dr. Marsteller said testily, "I've been doing this for 44 years. It works!"

He did admit, however, that he frequently used pills or home preparations containing from six to nine ingredients because it is difficult to find the exact cause of any given symptom.

Although Dr. Marsteller sometimes uses whole herbs rather than herbal extracts in pill form ("It depends on the person's personality—some do not want to boil up a tea."), he uses them with a kind of specificity that is apparently related to the principles of homeopathy. Camomile tea, for instance, he regards as suitable only for women. If men drink it, "they will have trouble." And operating on the homeopathic principle that "like cures like," Dr. Marsteller warns that while sage is good if you have a sore throat, you ought not to drink sage tea if you are well; it may well *give* you a sore throat.

Dr. Marsteller performs various manipulations on all parts of the body. For sinus problems, for example, he will manipulate the neck and press the sinus area. For bursitis, he will probably use diathermy, or deep heat therapy. He tells patients with arthritis to avoid absolutely all white sugar, white flour, cheese, cabbage, and all dairy products unless they are fermented. He encourages consumption of raw or steamed vegetables and drinking six glasses of spring water a day.

Although from a purely logical point of view, one might imagine that people would seek drugless therapy before pharmaceuticals and surgery, this is usually not the case. Dr. Marsteller sees many patients who represent the failures of "establishment" medicine, and says with a smile—but pride, too—"They call this place the court of last resort."

Operating on the principle that whatever helps such a patient is the right therapy, Dr. Marsteller does not scorn the use of faith healing, or something akin to it, along with his other approaches. As we were talking, he suddenly told me to lay out my hands flat on the table in front of me, palms up. He then passed his right palm over mine for a few moments and asked me if I felt anything. I said my hand felt warm, which it did. He then placed his left palm over my other hand and asked what I felt. Cold, I said.

"My hands are my second eyes," the naturopath informed me. "My right hand gives power and warmth. My left hand draws out what is in the person and produces cold. This can help me in diagnosis, and diagnosis is 80 percent of the whole case."

Hmmm.

We asked Dr. Marsteller about some remedies he uses which would be of interest to readers.

"Well," he offered, "here is a kind of all-purpose salve that I use and get good results with." I sniffed it and rubbed some into my hands and it felt good. It contained eucalyptus, cayenne, althea root (marshmallow), and paraffin.

Dr. Marsteller is a great believer in the use of onions as a home remedy. For colds, he suggests eating cooked onions or making onion sandwiches. For a fever, he advises slicing some raw onions and putting them on the chest or feet. "You can make a poultice for your chest, or use white socks and hold the onions against the soles of your feet. This is a very old remedy, but I still use it."

Apple cider vinegar he regards as good for splashing on cuts or sprains. It also makes a great gargle, he says.

He then gave us what he called "an old remedy for stiffness of all kinds." To make it, "Take one grapefruit, two oranges, and three lemons, and chop them up. Put them in a blender, skin and all, with one teaspoon of cream of tartar, and then add an equal amount of spring water. Drink two shot glasses a day."

# Nausea

Vitamin B₆, or pyridoxine, is a natural specific for nausea associated with pregnancy, but only, it seems, in cases where the nausea extends past the first three months. I have no scientific or even anecdotal information to indicate that B₆ is helpful for the typical nausea which occurs during the first trimester.

Raspberry leaf tea is highly regarded for relief of morning sickness. Many herbalists recommend drinking a cup of raspberry leaf tea every day all through pregnancy. If you have some wild raspberries growing near your home, use them, because their medicinal value may be greater than the cultivated variety. This seems to be true of most herbs. One herbalist suggests mixing a decoction of raspberry leaves with cream.

Basil is another favorite. Conway claims that a cup of basil tea "will quell the most violent vomiting and nausea."

Chewing on ginger sticks or drinking ginger tea has also been recommended. Honey, nutmeg, and mace are also potentially helpful.

An 80-year-old woman told us that at the age of 77 her "tendency towards morning nausea seemed to be getting worse and was accompanied sometimes by dizziness; I had slight strokes and threatened to have more. About that time, I read somewhere that a dentist was recommending grated citrus peel to his patients and was getting results. . . . I decided to try the peel . . . as I had already discovered that bitter foods helped to relieve nausea somewhat. Ever since then, I have been grating the rind of about one-half of a lemon (or its equivalent in orange and lime peel) into my fruit salad or fruit compote once a day. It has practically cured my nausea, dizziness, and tendency toward little strokes." She added that she used a special small grater and grated a little raw carrot after the peel to catch it all.

Nutritionist Adelle Davis, speaking about vomiting in babies—which is not caused by nausea—suggests that "much throwing up can be prevented merely by adding a little magnesium oxide—one-quarter teaspoon daily—and two or three teaspoons of yeast to the formula or drinking water and/or by giving wheat germ as a cereal."

Nausea that persists without any apparent cause should be medically evaluated.

See also SEASICKNESS.

# Nutritional Therapy

Nutritional therapy has many faces. A kidney dialysis patient, for example, may be given a very carefully planned diet to follow, along with special forms of injected vitamins. Nutritional therapy for someone with lactose intolerance is much simpler, involving only the restriction of milk and other dairy products.

In this book, the emphasis is largely on simpler forms of therapy which do not require constant monitoring, intravenous feeding, or other forms of medical intervention. Neither do we devote much space to explaining dietary approaches which we feel are best followed only on the advice of a physician. Anyone who is under the nutritional guidance of a physician and has been told, for instance, to eat an extremely low-cholesterol diet, a diet very low in calcium, a salt-free diet, a diet very low in protein or certain amino acids, should consult with his or her physician before making any changes.

In many cases of illness, it is difficult to find a reliable and specific nutritional approach. Frequently, in this book, I have suggested adopting an "all-around excellent diet" or "across-the-board supplementation with a broad range of nutrients." Here, I would like to explain what I mean by those rather vague terms.

Before doing that, though, let me admit that to many scientists and some doctors, the shotgun nutritional approach lacks any therapeutic rationale. If the specific treatment is not known, their argument goes, you should not do anything at all.

It's easy to understand why some people feel that way. Traditionally, nutrition has developed around discoveries that specific substances cure specific diseases or symptoms. Vitamin C cures scurvy, niacin cures pellagra, sugar threatens the diabetic, and so forth. And the only reason to take vitamins is the appearance of these deficiency states. Recently, though, this approach to human nutrition has been rendered obsolete.

We know now that by the time the classic symptoms of deficiency disease appear, typically with roughness, cracking, bleeding, or discoloration of the skin, a good deal of "invisible" damage has been done to other organs of the body, such as the nerves and blood cells. That's because most vitamins and minerals are needed throughout the entire body, not just in the places where deficiency symptoms usually appear first.

We also know the "classic" deficiency symptoms may not appear *at all* even when deficiency is quite marked. In some people, B vitamin deficiency will show itself on the skin, while in others it will appear as fatigue or mental depression. One person with vitamin C deficiency may have bleeding gums; another normal gums but one cold after another; a third person a skin ulcer that simply refuses to heal; a fourth person aches and pains. And so forth.

It's not difficult to understand why this occurs if we realize that every individual is quite unique. *Not only do we need different amounts of nutrients to maintain the best health, but we will show the effects of less than optimal amounts in different ways.*

While that may not sound very scientific, it is nevertheless *real*istic. Look at it this way. The same dose of the same drug may cause as many as 25 different side effects (or more!) in different people. Six ounces of whiskey may leave one person unconscious, a second hyperactive, and a third barely affected. From these everyday observations, we can conclude that it is dangerously simplistic to approach the highly dynamic interface of individual nutrition and health with the expectation that everything must fit a kind of mathematical formula.

Such an approach may be very appealing to statisticians or professional researchers. In some instances, such an approach may even be appropriate. However, at the level of one person and one disease, it is clearly inappropriate and impractical. As individuals, we are not seeking Truth but Wellness.

## A Nutritional Shotgun

So much for the rhetoric. Let me now describe what I mean by a "high-nutrition diet."

First, I'm not talking about the kind of diet which might be best to follow day after day. We're assuming the presence of a health problem. And the idea is to determine if the problem can be overcome by conservative dietary measures before seeking more extreme ones—including more extreme dietary approaches. A good beginning is to rid your diet of nutritional garbage. That is easier to do at the store than it is in your kitchen, so when you go shopping, simply do not purchase any form of candy, cookies, cake, pie, soda pop, baked goods made with white flour, and foods offering little more than salt, sugar, and fat, such as pretzels, potato chips, gelatin desserts, and other such items. And don't buy anything at the deli counter.

But don't worry about going out to the parking lot with an empty shopping cart. Fill it up instead with lots of fresh fruits and vegetables. Try to buy half-a-dozen different fruits, half-a-dozen different vegetables, and half-a-dozen different salad ingredients. If you want some inspiration, buy any one of the numerous excellent natural foods cookbooks which have appeared in recent years.

The next part of the dietary approach is supplementation. Please understand that the amounts which follow are not necessarily meant to be taken on an everyday basis, nor are they a specific program for nutritional support in any given condition. They comprise nothing more than a shotgun approach (at times, shotguns can be mighty handy things to have). Keep in mind that these amounts are for adults on a daily basis, not for children.

> Vitamin A—20,000 I.U.
> Thiamine ($B_1$)—10 mg.
> Riboflavin ($B_2$)—10 mg.
> Niacin—25 to 50 mg.
> Pyridoxine ($B_6$)—10 mg.
> Pantothenic Acid—100 mg.
> PABA—100 mg.
> $B_{12}$—25 micrograms (mcg.)
> Folic Acid—400 mcg. (.4 mg.)
> Vitamin C—500 mg.
> Vitamin D—400 I.U.
> Vitamin E—400 I.U.
> Calcium—750 mg.
> Magnesium—400 mg.
> Iron—10 mg. for men; 25 mg. for women
> Zinc—30 mg.

In addition, it would make sense to take several thousand milligrams of lecithin and about a tablespoon of brewer's yeast (not food or primary yeast).

Naturally, you would want to get as many of these nutrients in a "multiple" tablet as you could. Most multiples, however, are weak when it comes to the B complex. So, you may want to take a multiple-mineral tablet for what they offer, plus a special B-complex tablet. And since I have never seen any multiple that contains more than a pittance of vitamin E, you would have to take that separately, too.

Let me emphasize again that these amounts are suggested as worthy of trial in cases where research has not developed more specific guidelines. In cases where more specific information *is* available—such as the efficacy of several thousand milligrams of vitamin C a day for hay fever—those suggestions take priority.

## Food Is More Important Than Supplements

As far as an all-around optimum diet goes, remember that supplements are just that. The person who works on a supplement program and ignores the daily diet of whole foods is like a runner who spends more time selecting a pair of track shoes than actually training.

In trying to describe an optimum diet of whole foods, we are once again talking about a very general approach that might be followed in the absence of special needs. I don't believe in urging everyone not to eat wheat or milk or egg yolks simply because a relatively small minority will develop allergies or high cholesterol levels. On the other hand, any specific information that your physician has given you, or that is in this book, takes precedence over the following guidelines.

First, let's demolish the myth of the "four food groups" and the "balanced diet." It is entirely possible to eat something from one of the four food groups at every single meal and still have a perfectly wretched diet. That is particularly true for adults. A meal consisting, for instance, of a fast-food hamburger with a bit of lettuce and tomato on it, a milkshake, and a piece of cherry pie contains meat, dairy products, fruits and vegetables, and cereal products. But at the same time, the flour in the hamburger bun and pie is about as useful for building health as sawdust is for building a house. The meat in the hamburger probably weighs less than one ounce. There is barely a trace of roughage. What's more, the meal as a whole is laced with sugar, saturated fats, salt, and additives.

A good diet has also been defined as consisting of variations on a theme of 15 to 20 percent protein, 15 to 20 percent fat, and 60 to 70 percent carbohydrates. The problem with that approach, which is favored by many dietitians, is that it is totally useless. How is one to know what percent of one's calories is coming from protein or carbohydrate? Even if you ate every meal with a table of dietary statistics in front of you, you would still have to weigh every piece of food you ate on a scale that measured in grams, and then start punching away at a calculator. You would even have to weigh things like chicken bones after you had stripped them of the edible portion. I doubt that there are more than three people in the United States who do that sort of thing; yet nutritionists blithely go on recommending that we eat certain percentages of our calories from this and that as if they were saying something meaningful.

There is a much more sensible approach to eating to improve one's health. The easiest way to begin is to start off *at least* one meal a day with a huge salad. Prepare it from the greatest variety of fresh greens and other vegetables you can find: kale, lettuce, green peppers, cucumbers, tomatoes, onions, scallions, radishes, watercress, parsley, garlic, etc. You'll be amazed how much better salads taste when you add lots of fresh crisp mixed sprouts. Use polyunsaturated oil in your dressing and use the smallest amount you can. Depend on herbs like garlic to add zest.

After eating your salad, you should feel mildly stuffed. Then, you would probably do well to eat about half of what you normally do in the way of steak, pork chops, and other meats—which all tend to be excessively high in saturated fat and even calories. If you are in the habit of drenching your vegetables with butter, cut them out altogether, because you've covered the vegetable front very nicely in your salad.

For dessert, eat an apple. After that, get out of the kitchen so you won't be tempted to nibble.

At least while you are trying to use good eating habits as a supportive measure to help overcome some health problem, you would do well to exclude *absolutely* from your diet all white sugar, all added salt, and all heavily processed snack items, ranging from gelatin desserts to potato chips.

If you are a great coffee drinker, you should at the very least change to the decaffeinated kind, and try to learn to drink it black and unsugared. Although coffee itself can be harmful to some people, it's my guess that the sugar that goes with it causes a lot more damage than the coffee itself. That is particularly true for people who become terribly tired or dizzy at various times of the day.

To the greatest extent possible, eat foods that are whole and fresh. An orange is twice as good as orange juice. An apple is about 10 times as good as apple juice if you are trying to lose weight or get your cholesterol down. A diet of whole foods and very little fat was the diet humankind depended on for 99.9 percent of its time on earth, and that is still the best diet for producing health.

To look at it in a less philosophical way, spend twice as much money as you ordinarily do in the produce section of the supermarket, half as much in the meat department, and not one cent in the canned goods or deli section.

Most people find that within a week or two after they begin to eat better, they begin to feel better.

# Obesity

**by Leonard Lear**

When Agnes Hunsberger started keeping records of her food intake, she was absolutely astonished.

"I had tried just about every diet you can think of, and none ever worked," she says today. "The amazing thing I learned in the Behavior Weight Control Program is that I was never aware before of my eating habits. Some days I was eating constantly from morning to night and *wasn't even conscious of it.*"

But Hunsberger lost 34 pounds in 20 weeks, and more importantly, she has kept it off. That is because she learned a vital principle that almost any other person can also learn and implement—that it's entirely possible to lose weight and/or maintain one's appropriate body weight without drugs, fad diets, pills, or injections.

The importance of this nirvanalike principle should be obvious. According to the U.S. Department of Public Health, over 80 million Americans are more than 20 percent overweight, and as many as 75 percent of all adult Americans may be at least 10 pounds overweight.

Our best-selling nonfiction book lists, which invariably include one or more diet books, reflect the American preoccupation with this weighty dilemma. There's the high-protein diet, the alcohol lover's diet, the water diet, the low-carbohydrate diet, the grapefruit diet, and so on ad infinitum. It would hardly be a surprise if a new diet came out next month based entirely on tangerines, elbow macaroni, and dried prunes. But while these various diets have lessened the weight of their authors' mortgage payments, they have been far less successful in permanently reducing the weight of the books' readers.

Organized or medically supervised diets may not be much better. A recent study by Dr. Albert Stunkard, who operates a behavior-modification weight control clinic at Stanford University, revealed that drop-out rates in a large variety of other diet programs ranged from 20 to 80 percent. Of those that stayed with the diet therapy, fewer than 25 percent lost 20 pounds.

"The reason these diets almost always fail is that they do not change a person's eating habits," explains Dr. Leonard Levitz, director of the Behavioral Weight Control Program at the University of Pennsylvania. "An overweight person can eat cottage cheese and celery for only so long. Eventually the dieter will feel so deprived, he'll gorge himself on all the foods he has missed and will generally gain all the lost weight back."

## Unprecedented Record of Success

The U. of P. weight control program, which was started in 1971 by Dr. Levitz, a clinical psychologist, and Dr. Henry A. Jordan, a psychiatrist, has achieved an unprecedented record of success with overweight people. The average weight loss during their 20-week sessions has been 20 pounds, and the program has achieved a remarkable keep-it-off rate of 85 percent. And the best part of all is that many of their principles can be employed by the average person in his or her own home.

"We've been successful," said Jeanette Fairorth, cotherapist with the program and instructor in preventive medicine at Jefferson Medical College in Philadelphia, "because the people who learn these principles do not have to give up ice cream, sweets, or any of the foods they're used to eating.

"We have proven conclusively that people can continue eating all the foods they enjoy and still lose weight as long as they become aware of their eating habits and make a conscious effort to change them. It's also been clearly demonstrated that the average person who is not obese can also maintain his or her proper weight by practicing these same principles."

Proof that many persons are not consciously aware of their eating habits has been provided by Dr. Stunkard, who took many overweight people from the "bird-couldn't-live-on-what-I-eat" school, hospitalized them, and fed them exactly what they claimed they ate at home. They all lost weight.

The first thing that all participants in the U. of P. program do is keep a careful record of every single instance of food intake, even if it's just a snack, a piece of candy, or a pretzel. The results are almost always quite revealing, particularly to the participants themselves.

**'I Never Realized What I Was Eating!'** • "It was amazing," declared Frances Collier. "I honestly never realized how much I was eating. By being forced to put everything down on paper, I realized that when my kids would leave food on their plates, I'd often put it in my mouth rather than throw it away. It must have become second-nature to me because I wasn't fully aware I was doing it. It probably stems from when I was a kid and my mother told me never to leave food on my plate because kids were starving in Europe."

"It's remarkable how much easier it is to change bad eating habits once the person becomes fully conscious of them," added Dr. Jordan. "You don't have to give people orders, either. Once a person becomes fully aware of his bad eating habits, he can usually figure out for himself the practical way to change them. For example, we had one woman who used to munch on snacks while she stood in the kitchen talking on the phone. After she realized what she was doing, she would always go up to the bedroom and use the extension whenever she had to use the phone. It sounds like a small thing, but when you put together a lot of these small things, you wind up saving a great many calories."

For the average person, a basic understanding of his or her own eating habits is all that's needed to eliminate the bad habits and reinforce the good ones. If you're able to answer the following questions, for example, you're well on your way to solving whatever weight problem you may have:

1. *What Other Activities Do I Engage In While Eating?*

    One woman in a U. of P. group was amazed to find that only 6 times out of 42 (21 meals and 21 snacks) in a given week did she merely sit down and eat a meal with no associated activities. In 36 cases she ate while cleaning, ironing, vacuuming, watching TV, baking, etc. "This is a very bad habit," Dr. Levitz explained, "because it means the person is not concentrating fully on his food and very often eats much more than is necessary without even being aware of it."

The obvious solution is to make eating a deliberate act with no associated activities. Furthermore, when you get up in the morning, write down a schedule for what and when you will eat that day. Set up a general time scheme and stick to it. If you've penciled in 5 P.M. for dinner, do not eat that meal before 5 even if you're hungry.

2. *Where Do I Eat?*

Many people grab something to eat almost every time they're in the kitchen. "After keeping a food-intake record," one woman said, "I suddenly became aware that I was even picking up a snack when I'd feed our dog in the kitchen. I really don't even know how long I'd been doing it because I wasn't aware I was doing it. Now I feed the dog in the cellar and keep his food down there, and I stay out of the kitchen until our mealtime."

Along these same lines, you should limit your eating to only one room in the house. Do not eat breakfast in bed, potato chips in the living room, and beer in the den. And do not eat unless you are sitting down in a chair. (You'd be surprised how much munching goes on in prone, supine, and standing positions.) The very act of sitting makes the eater more aware of his food, and awareness is the keystone of behavior modification.

3. *How Fast Do I Eat?*

This is also extremely important. Recent studies prove that people who eat fast almost invariably ingest more calories than those who eat more slowly since it takes about the same amount of time for both to feel "full."

"This is a fast-food society," stated Fairorth, "and that's one reason why so many Americans are overweight. Many Americans are literally *always* in a hurry. That's why the fast-food hamburger and chicken places have been so successful. After all, how many times have you heard a parent say to a child, 'Hurry up and finish. We don't have much time'?"

The solution here is to slow down. Before you begin to eat, sit a minute looking at the food in front of you. This will help break the habit of leaping immediately into the food and will develop a resistance to the stimulus of food. In addition, you should chew the food thoroughly and swallow each bite before taking more food into your mouth. You should also cut up your food, including fruits and vegetables, into the smallest pieces possible and eat only one piece at a time.

4. *How Available Is Food In My House?*

Obviously, if you have snacks available in plates and dishes all around your house, you're much more likely to eat them. An experiment conducted by Dr. Levitz in the U. of P. cafeteria showed that when high-calorie, low-nutrition desserts were placed at the front of the dessert counter and the low-calorie, high-nutrition desserts at the back, the former were all taken at several consecutive meals and the latter rarely taken. *When the two types were switched around at the next few meals, the exact opposite occurred.* The low-calorie foods were eaten, and the others were left.

So put your highest-calorie foods at the very back of the cupboard or refrigerator, where you're unlikely to remove all other contents to get to them. Don't leave snacks out for nibbling. Tell guests to bring flowers, not candy.

5. *Do I Use Food As a Reward Or Tranquilizer?*

This, of course, goes back to your days as a child when you were likely to be given a lollipop or ice cream cone for being a good boy or girl. Now, after a rough day at the office, you reward yourself with a martini, which also calms your nerves.

There are many other ways you can reward yourself that are not related to food. Take a hot bubblebath; listen to your stereo earphones; work on needlepoint; paint your fingernails.

Much unnecessary eating is done by housewives in the afternoon, so they should arrange their schedule to be out-of-doors as much as possible during these hours. They can do volunteer work in a hospital, school, or girl scout troop, take tennis lessons, take the dog for a walk in the park, get a part-time job, etc.

Obviously, physical exercise has to be an integral part of any weight program, and it can easily be worked into the rest of your schedule. Park your car a few blocks from the shopping center and walk the rest of the way. Get off the bus or subway one stop before your destination and walk, and so on.

You can no doubt think up a dozen or more creative suggestions yourself. The important thing is to be fully aware of all your bad eating habits and to take the appropriate steps to eliminate them. Then you can let your trash-masher put on a few pounds by eating up all your diet books.

# Orthomolecular (Megavitamin) Therapy

**Author's Note:** Orthomolecular therapy is a term coined by Dr. Linus Pauling, and it is widely misunderstood. It does not, as some people suppose, mean taking large amounts of vitamins. It means, rather, providing the body with the elements it needs to create *the correct molecular environment for optimal health.* In *some* cases this means taking large amounts of a particular vitamin. In other cases, it may mean taking only very moderate amounts to correct a deficiency or abnormality. It may also mean *eliminating* a substance from the diet, such as wheat gluten, to establish a health-promoting internal environment for a schizophrenic or someone with celiac disease.

Most often—at least so far—orthomolecular or megavitamin therapy has been associated with psychiatry. This special report is based on interviews with Dr. David Hawkins and his patients. The names of the patients, naturally, are fictitious.

**by Ruth Heyman**

Jack Burton had worked hard all his life. His father died when he was a teenager and for years he helped support his mother. In

1964, Jack was 32 years old, married, with two youngsters of his own. He was a successful hairdresser and lived comfortably with his family in the suburbs of New York. In 1964, Jack realized a dream— he left his job and opened a beauty shop of his own.

But two months after he went into business, Jack broke down. Suddenly, the man who had driven himself all his life refused to function. The man whom friends called "Smiling Jack" cried constantly, kept to his bed, and was visibly afraid of people.

"I heard voices from nowhere. With my own eyes I would sit there and watch pictures on the wall turn into monstrous figures," Jack related.

His behavior became bizarre and his humor vicious. "Could you believe that I marked up my daughter's face with shoe polish, just for fun?" At his mother's funeral, he grinned throughout the service. He hid behind trees to avoid meeting neighbors. When he drove his car, he stopped a block away from a red light because he couldn't judge the distance.

Soon Jack was in the hands of a psychiatrist and was diagnosed as schizophrenic. Kitty, his wife, sold the business and went back to work.

"He was in and out of hospitals for six years," Kitty told us. "He had shock treatment, psychotherapy, drugs . . . the works. He went from one doctor to another and they all told me he would never get well. When he was home between hospital stays, he was so heavily tranquilized that he walked around like a zombie."

In 1970, through a friend, the Burtons heard about Dr. David Hawkins and his successful treatment of schizophrenia with the use of megavitamins. In desperation, they consulted Dr. Hawkins at the North Nassau Mental Health Center in Manhasset, Long Island. The doctor advised hospitalization.

"We almost turned away. We had lost hope," said Kitty. "Then I discussed the matter with our priest who urged me to have faith. So I borrowed the money for the hospital fee, and Jack entered Brunswick Hospital in Amityville for a month's stay."

## What One Month of Treatment Accomplished

While Jack was at the hospital, he submitted to a battery of physical and psychiatric tests, including tests for altered perceptual functioning, for glucose tolerance, and for cerebral allergies to food and environmental chemicals.

Megavitamin therapy was initiated immediately with heavy doses of $B_3$ (niacin or niacinamide), $B_6$, C, and E. He was put on a high-protein, low-carbohydrate diet with caffeine and alcohol forbidden. In four weeks, he was home—happy to see his family and eager to return to work for the first time in six years.

Jack continued to consult Dr. Hawkins monthly at the clinic but these visits soon tapered off and he now sees the doctor only twice a year. He has never had a relapse but he is well aware that he will have to continue taking multiple vitamins and adhere to his diet for the rest of his life. Once or twice, he rebelled and goofed off for a few days, but when he found himself slipping into a depression, he quickly resumed his routine.

Jack is one of the thousands of schizophrenics who have been successfully treated with megavitamins at the North Nassau Mental Health Center. Patients are coming from all over the United States and as far away as Australia. What is this megavitamin therapy and why is traditional psychiatry skeptical?

## Schizophrenia—'A Genetic Biochemical Disturbance'

Dr. Hawkins, director of the clinic, discussed orthomolecular psychiatry—popularly known as megavitamin therapy—with us in his office at the suburban center.

"Orthomolecular psychiatry regards schizophrenia as a genetic biochemical disturbance. The functioning of the brain is dependent on its composition and structure, on its molecular environment," he explained. "We consider biochemical defects to be primary in causing mental illness and our emphasis is on biochemistry and nutrition. Disturbed family relations and personal conflicts may contribute to the patient's illness but psychodynamics is not our primary treatment approach. First we treat the psychosis, then we help the patient adjust to life."

Orthomolecular psychiatry believes that mental illness can result from a low concentration in the brain of any of the following vitamins: thiamine, niacin, pyridoxine, $B_{12}$, biotin, ascorbic acid, or folic acid.

But the basic biochemical defect (or defects) that causes mental illness has not yet been determined. "Scientists are working on it," said Dr. Hawkins. "Maybe we'll have the answer in 10 or 20 years.

Orthomolecular psychiatry is pragmatic, empirical. The point is—it works."

Why does the establishment resist the biochemical approach? It is understandable that specialists who have devoted a lifetime to psychodynamics will be hostile to change. Medicine has always been slow to accept new methods. The criticism leveled against orthomolecular psychiatry is that its claims have not been confirmed by controlled studies, but the megavitamin treatment regime does not lend itself to double-blind studies and the procedure would be costly. The controversy will probably continue until controlled studies weigh the efficacy of orthomolecular psychiatry against psychodynamic treatment. Although the opponents have the funding, Dr. Hawkins isn't worried.

## 'The Fact Is—It <u>Does</u> Work'

"We haven't discovered why it works, but we have clinical proof that it *does* work. Orthomolecular psychiatry is a promising branch of medicine and the public is making the decision in its favor," said Dr. Hawkins.

What is the recovery rate? "That's difficult to assess at this time," Dr. Hawkins stated. "When I first started practicing orthomolecular psychiatry in 1966, my recovery rate was double that of traditional psychiatry. Now that I'm getting difficult, chronic cases from all over the country, an estimate of the recovery rate would be inaccurate. However, we have received a modest grant from a foundation for an efficacy study and we will soon be making a detailed study of 50 cases."

Orthomolecular psychiatry developed during the 1960s when there was growing disillusionment with the psychodynamic approach, its cost in time and money and its efficacy. At the same time, there was a growing interest in the relationship between diet and mental illness. The concept of biochemical individuality was developed, pointing out the enormous difference in nutritional requirements and biochemical processes in identical siblings. Research was done on the relationship among poverty, poor diet, and mental development. The importance of detecting and treating hypoglycemia in schizophrenia was studied and work was begun on the problem of cerebral allergy to food and environmental chemicals as a cause of psychiatric symptoms.

Dr. Hawkins became interested in megavitamin treatment from members of Alcoholics Anonymous. Until 1966, the Manhasset center used traditional methods of treating schizophrenia. Bill Wilson, founder of AA, began using vitamins in treating alcoholics, especially those who were schizophrenic. Dr. Hawkins heard favorable reports, tried the vitamin therapy on his alcoholic-schizophrenic patients, and got amazing results. Subsequently, he applied the treatment to all his schizophrenic patients and dedicated himself to practicing psychiatry the orthomolecular way.

In diagnosing schizophrenia, orthomolecular psychiatrists pay particular attention to evidences of altered perceptual functioning. The use of the Hoffer-Osmond Diagnostic Test expedites appraisal of the illness far more effectively than a psychodynamic interview. It measures abnormalities of perception in sight, sound, smell, taste, and touch, and it determines thought disorders. It takes no more than 20 minutes and is self-administered. Laboratory tests include those for thyroid function, glucose tolerance, hair test analysis for trace metals, and comprehensive chemical and liver profiles. There are abnormal chemicals found in the blood or urine or tissues of schizophrenics, very much like the abnormal amount of sugar found in the blood of the diabetic.

## Nutrition and Other Therapeutic Techniques

The use of vitamins in combination and in large doses is prescribed. A typical daily dose would include four grams of niacin or niacinamide, 800 mg. of $B_6$ (pyridoxine), four grams of C, and 1,000 units of E. For the patient with low histamine level, two mg. of folic acid may be included. Zinc may be prescribed if the hair test analysis shows high copper levels. Lithium is used in treating manic-depressives. Several grams of PABA may be included if indicated. The vitamin dosage required for the individual is determined by the physician.

Are there any toxic effects in the use of megavitamins? Side effects are rare, Dr. Hawkins explained, except in the use of niacin (one form of vitamin $B_3$) which must be monitored by a physician. Niacin produces a flushing of the skin which subsides in about an hour and usually doesn't recur after the fifth or sixth dose.

Orthomolecular psychiatry is eclectic and includes many conventional psychiatric procedures. Shock treatment has multiple biochemical effects and, supported by megavitamins, the improvement is dramatic. Hormones, antidepressants, and tranquilizers are used when necessary. Phenothiazines (tranquilizers) are often prescribed, but quickly reduced to maintenance level.

Psychotherapy is not ignored. Emotional upsets affect the brain chemistry which will aggravate the biochemical problem. While the patient is psychotic, psychotherapy is merely supportive. When the patient is no longer plagued by perceptual distortions, the orthomolecular psychiatrist will help him resolve his personal problems.

## A Lifelong Illness . . . Now, At Least, Under Control

Jerry is a personable young man of 27 whose psychosis has been arrested but who continues to see Dr. Hawkins weekly for psychotherapy. He had a turbulent history of mental illness which manifested itself in early childhood with nightmares, hyperactivity, and hypersensitivity to sound. Always bright, he was at the top of his class without effort until he reached sixth grade. Then he retrogressed, couldn't concentrate on his studies, and was drawn to problem kids.

"I began to have hallucinations—the Japs were always attacking me. . . . My family spent a fortune to try to help me. For years I saw psychiatrists three times a week, while I was going in and out of different private schools. . . . I was 17 when I became involved in drugs and I would just kind of disappear for weeks at a time," Jerry says.

No psychiatrist ever told his parents that he was schizophrenic, but they always believed his illness was biochemical rather than psychogenic, since their other two children functioned well.

About five years ago, Jerry's mother heard about orthomolecular psychiatry through her rabbi and after a violent episode, Jerry was admitted to Brunswick Hospital under Dr. Hawkins's care. Megavitamin therapy was initiated and Jerry was put on a high-protein, low-carbohydrate diet. When he returned home after two months, he showed considerable improvement. He got himself a job and stayed away from drugs. However, his illness is of long standing and Jerry has deep-rooted psychological problems. While the schizophrenia is definitely under control, he still finds concentration difficult and is not employed at this time.

Is the chronic patient more difficult to help? Yes, says Dr. Hawkins. A patient who has been withdrawn for years will acquire bad habit patterns and superimposed disabilities. When the disease is caught early, the response is better.

## From Visions of Terror to a Bright Future

Lilly is an example of a schizophrenic who took ill suddenly, began orthomolecular treatment within a year, and made a dramatic recovery. Lilly, an attractive young lady with cascading dark hair and shining eyes, is now 31 years old and single.

"About six years ago," she told us, "I had a romantic breakup. It broke me up, too, and I went into a deep depression. . . . Then I began to have hallucinations. Things would seem to blow up in front of me and change colors. A white man would become black. Eerie voices were stalking me. I tried not to pay attention, but it got to the point where I couldn't concentrate, and I finally lost my job as a secretary.

"That was it . . . I panicked," said Lilly. "I went to a psychiatrist for a couple of months but psychotherapy and tranquilizers didn't help. I was so miserable, I left home. When I came back, my mother told me about megavitamin therapy and begged me to try it. She had read about it in a newspaper article."

Soon Lilly had an appointment at the clinic. Dr. Hawkins asked no psychological questions about her childhood or family. After a series of tests, he prescribed huge daily doses of vitamins $B_3$, $B_6$, C, and $B_1$, plus the high-protein, low-carbohydrate diet. In two weeks, her hallucinations ended.

Lilly went back to work and is now in "the best job I ever had." She appears confident and well integrated. She's never had a relapse and sees Dr. Hawkins only twice a year. Lilly realizes she must live with her problem all her life—like an obese person or a diabetic. She has never skipped her vitamins but when she goes off her diet, she becomes "nauseous and headachy."

Megavitamin therapy is also being successfully used in treating childhood schizophrenia, a developmental abnormality that seriously interferes with a child's functioning in all areas of his life. In the past, psychotherapy was the most common treatment and its results were questionable. The use of drugs altered the behavior disorders by sedating or tranquilizing the child, but the effect was merely stopgap. With megavitamin therapy, the improvement in children is even more impressive than in adults. Children whose treatment begins between three and nine years of age have a fine chance of recovery.

### Dannie's Doing Fine Now

Dannie, an alert 12 year old who wants to be a dentist, is a schizophrenic who has made a remarkable recovery on megavitamins. Though he always had a sleeping problem, was shy, incoordinated, and would sometimes talk to himself, his parents chalked up his growing erratic behavior to the stress of moving into a new neighborhood. They never thought there was anything wrong with him—just the usual problems of growing up. However, when he was eight years old in the second grade, his teacher noted the discrepancy between his obvious intelligence and his low I.Q. score. He was subnormal in abstract thinking.

"On the advice of the school psychologist, we consulted a pediatric psychiatrist, who suggested psychotherapy and said that a long-term treatment would probably be necessary," Dannie's mother, a nurse, told us. "We turned it down.

"Then we read a newspaper article about the North Nassau Mental Health Center, and we took Dannie there. He was immediately put on vitamins, and we noticed an improvement within a month.

"Dannie is now outgoing and relaxed," his mother continued. "He's developed a sense of humor and appears to be well accepted by his classmates. He rides a two-wheeler like the other kids on the block and, best of all, his report card is sprinkled with A's. Right now, he is taking vitamins C, $B_6$, and nicotinamide."

How often does he see the doctor?

"About nine times a year."

Readers who wish to consult an orthomolecular psychiatrist in their own area should contact the Huxley Institute for Biosocial Research at 1114 First Avenue, New York, New York 10021.

# Osteogenesis Imperfecta

Osteogenesis imperfecta is a rare metabolic disorder, which in severe cases is evident immediately at birth, when the baby emerges from the birth canal with multiple fractures. The bones are extremely fragile and will often break at the slightest touch. Deformities can develop as one break after another occurs in a child's skeleton. There is no cure for this disorder, and although many treatments have been used in an attempt to ameliorate the condition, no one treatment has been found to be completely effective.

Now, there is at least a hope that vitamin C may be of use in helping children get through the worst parts of this disease. In the July 1974 issue of *Pediatrics,* Diann Kurz and Edward J. Eyring, M.D., Ph.D., report on the results they observed in 13 patients with osteogenesis imperfecta who were given supplements of vitamin C.

The patients ranged in age from just-born to 15 years old, with symptoms ranging from severe deformities to only a few fractures. Each patient was given a daily dosage of from 1,000 to 2,000 mg. of ascorbic acid, taken in four divided doses. The infants received between 250 and 600 mg. of natural liquid vitamin C (rose hips and acerola extract) which was mixed with milk.

The children were followed for varying lengths of time ranging from 10 to 43 months. *All of them experienced a reduced number of fractures and increased physical activity during this time.*

A few examples: a six-year-old boy, during a period of a little more than three years before beginning to take vitamin C, had 32 fractures. During the same amount of time on a diet supplemented with vitamin C, he had only 10 fractures. A ten-year-old girl had suffered 14 fractures over a period of about 3½ years. During an equal period on a supplemented diet, she had only 2 new fractures. A little girl who was born with 20 bone fractures had only 2 new fractures after 17 months of supplementation with 250 mg. of rose hips vitamin C every day.

The authors of the study are quick to point out that their trials were not controlled. This means that in order for them to have true statistical significance, the children taking the vitamin C would have had to be matched very closely with other children with the same degree of illness who did not take vitamin C. Nevertheless, what they observed leads them to believe that vitamin C is probably beneficial for these children, and that larger groups should be observed to pin down the exact extent and nature of the beneficial influence.

In 1971, Clive C. Solomons, Ph.D., affiliated with the Department of Pediatrics at the University of Colorado Medical Center, reported that daily doses of magnesium oxide brought about a pronounced drop in the rate of fractures in more than half of the children with osteogenesis imperfecta which he treated. Again, there were no controls, and since many children with this disease improve with age, no definitive conclusion can be drawn. However, Dr. Solomons said there was a rough correspondence between the decrease in the fracture rate and the decrease of a blood chemical called serum pyrophosphate.

At this point, another mineral, zinc, enters the picture. In their studies with vitamin C, Dr. Eyring and Kurz noticed that the children who were given vitamin C generally experienced a lowering of zinc blood levels. They thought this was significant, or at least very odd, because ordinarily, supplementation with vitamin C enhances absorption of zinc. In any case, they *speculated* that the lowering of serum zinc may have helped matters, because zinc tends to inhibit the enzyme which breaks down serum pyrophosphate—the substance which decreased in the patients who improved on magnesium oxide.

There is another possibility, however: that the decrease in circulating zinc reflected the "taking up" of this mineral by bones, which need it for growth. In osteogenesis imperfecta, aside from the broken bones, there is frequently a stunting of growth. Growth retardation is also a characteristic of another rare disease called acrodermatitis enteropathica. And in this latter disease, it's been found that zinc supplementation restores normal growth in children who haven't yet reached the stage of prepuberty. (See ACRODERMATITIS ENTEROPATHICA earlier in this book.)

It's possible that zinc will turn out to play a major role in the therapy of osteogenesis imperfecta children.

If medical science succeeds in unlocking all the mysteries of this disease, they will have accomplished much more than giving a new lease on life to the 10,000 to 30,000 people in the United States with this condition. That's because osteogenesis imperfecta patients seem to have a significant degree of innate resistance against most forms of cancer (Solomons and Millar, *Clinical Orthopaedics and Related Research,* October 1973). And in most instances, they are "unusually cheerful individuals who seldom experience changes in mood." Even in the face of repeated surgery, they seem to maintain an optimistic outlook, and despite the ravages of the disease, many lead a very active social life and hold positions of considerable responsibility. These two apparent gifts—resistance to cancer and a cheerful, optimistic attitude—are ones that all of us want. Learning more about osteogenesis imperfecta could therefore pay enormous dividends to everyone.

The Osteogenesis Imperfecta Foundation, Inc., was founded in 1970 as a voluntary national health organization dedicated to alleviating problems associated with this disease, and sponsoring and disseminating new medical information. Write to the OIF, Inc., at 1231 May Court, Burlington, North Carolina 27215.

# Osteomyelitis

In cases of chronic osteomyelitis where the usual antibiotics and perhaps even surgery have failed to control the infection in the bone, it would be wise to call some local hospitals and find out where the nearest hyperbaric oxygen unit is located. When hyperbaric oxygen is used in addition to other approaches, the results are often most gratifying. The less the condition has been permitted to advance, the better the results that can be achieved. See also OXYGEN THERAPY, HYPERBARIC.

# Osteopathy

**by James C. McCullagh**

It happened in Kansas. One day in the 1870s, Dr. A. T. Still, a kind of "tramp" doctor who had attended a short course at the Kansas College of Physicians and Surgeons, claimed to have set 17 dislocated hips within 24 hours. How he *found* so many dislocations, let alone set them, is only one of the questions left in the wake of this medical "midwester." Later, he started an osteopathic medical college at Kirksville, Missouri, which by 1902 had 500 students. Almost overnight Kirksville became a haven for the sick and incurable.

During its century of existence, osteopathy has not escaped its share of growing pains. Some of these pains can be attributed to the founder himself, who traveled in Missouri and Kansas, working in the middle of streets adjusting joints and palpating spines. The itinerant doctor claimed to have cured every patient he treated, including those with pneumonia, asthma, and encephalitis.

Unquestionably, Dr. Still's methods of experimenting with and treating patients "in the great outdoors" were crude. But, generally speaking, medical practice was very crude indeed in the 19th century. This was the age of heroic medicine: bloodletting, blistering, leeching, cupping, sweating, and purging. There was little scientific support underlying medical practices of any kind.

Naturally, Dr. Still's claims of 100 percent medical success earned him a reputation as a quack. His students who left Kirksville without degrees to start their own osteopathic clinics gave further credence to this charge. Interestingly, Daniel Palmer, a patient of Dr. Still's, left the clinic and started a rival practice of manipulation called chiropractic.

During the first three decades of the 20th century, osteopathy— because it failed to keep abreast of scientific developments, failed to standardize licensing regulations, and failed to fully integrate manipulative therapy with a total philosophy of medicine—was considered by most to be a second-class medical profession.

## Modern Osteopaths Equal to M.D.'s

Today, all that has changed. In the last few decades, osteopathy has evolved into a respected medical profession with its members having the right to practice in all states. Osteopathic physicians (D.O.'s) have entered into the mainstream of the healing arts.

They attend medical schools comparable to those attended by M.D.'s, go through similar internship periods, and take equivalent medical exams. Both may enter any number of medical specialties after internship. According to Richard K. Snyder, D.O., Director of Medical Education at Allentown, Pennsylvania, Osteopathic Hospital, M.D.'s and osteopathic physicians regularly consult each other on patient care and medical problems.

A fundamental difference between the M.D. and the D.O. is in the practice of manipulative therapy, one of the most misunderstood tools in the osteopath's armamentarium. Dean Robert W. England, D.O., who oversees the medical curriculum at the Philadelphia College of Osteopathic Medicine, chuckles at those who believe that "all we do is crack bones." Osteopathic training "is heavy on the basic sciences," he stresses. "Our emphasis," he remarked, "is in anatomy, physiology, and neurosensory science courses." This heavy foundation allows the student "to think functionally, to consider natural immunities," and not be so pathologically oriented.

But the osteopathic medical student also spends more than 150 hours in classes and clinics learning the unique principles and practices of osteopathy. In Dr. England's words, the student "learns the body like the back of his hand." He learns to diagnose a patient's problem or complaint by feeling (palpating) certain problem areas (variously called "soft skin," osteopathic lesion, or somatic dysfunction).

After careful diagnosis—which probably would include discussion with the patient, palpation of the lesioned area, and possibly examination via X-rays—the physician may elect to apply manipulative therapy. This could be the lumbar roll for a lower back problem, the lymphatic or thoracic pump for upper respiratory complaints, or cervical traction for neck pains. And nothing has caused such misunderstanding and confusion among laypeople and doctors alike as these manipulations.

The key phrase in grasping the principles of osteopathic manipulation is "neuro-muscular-skeletal system." This refers to the dynamic interplay between nerves, the muscles (and their surrounding fibrous tissue or fascia), and the bones. Although osteopaths appreciate as well as any M.D. that there is more to the human system than this particular complex, they nevertheless find that a vast number of ailments are best approached by correcting imbalances, injuries, or tensions in the neuro-muscular-skeletal system. A classic example of a lesion or injury in this system would be low back pain, where excessive stress on the *muscles* causes abnormal movement of the *bones* or cartilage of the spine which in turn exerts pressure on the *nerves*.

### 'Manipulation' Explained

R. McFarlane Tilley, D.O., a practicing osteopathic physician, explains the function of manipulation this way: "Manipulation, carefully prescribed and related to the particular case, helps relieve acute and chronic postural and neuro-muscular-skeletal stress by reducing muscular tension, improving joint motion, relieving pressure or congestion around nerve roots, and finding or blocking myofascial [fibrous tissue surrounding muscles] trigger areas" (*Osteopathic Annals,* October 1973).

Modern osteopaths use manipulative therapy as an *adjunct* to their total practice, which might also include drugs and surgery, as well as other modalities, such as therapeutic ultrasound. Claus A. Rohweder, D.O., Associate Professor of Osteopathic Medicine, Kirksville College of Osteopathic Medicine and chairman of the Nuclear Medicine Department, told us that he "practices manipulation about 90 percent of the time." He said that manipulation helps maintain "good normal functions before organic changes appear." He also remarked that he uses manipulative therapy to some degree "to treat most infectious diseases as well as diabetes and hyperthyroidism."

Though it is probably safe to say that most people feel better after any type of manipulative therapy, it is just as safe to say that, until the last few decades, the osteopathic profession did little to support their claims about osteopathic lesions and manipulative therapy with firm scientific facts. And this was one of the primary reasons that osteopathic physicians lingered on the periphery of the medical field and probably the primary reason why people confused them with chiropractors. With good reason, osteopaths believed that they could diagnose by feeling along the spine for "lesions"; that by use of the lymphatic pump—a kind of rhythmic pressure— they could drain sinuses, and ease the painful effects of asthma by appropriate pressure to the vertebrae. But they didn't have statistical evidence that there was such a thing as an "osteopathic lesion" or that manipulative therapy was effective in providing relief.

The evidence was a long time coming. In 1941, Dr. J. S. Denslow of the Kirksville College of Osteopathic Medicine, by the use of electromyography (the insertion of a needle electrode into the muscle), showed that there existed increased electrical activity in the lesioned area.

It remained for Irvin M. Korr, Ph.D., Distinguished Professor of Physiology, Kirksville College, to put the osteopathic case beyond scientific doubt with further research. Professor Korr has provided the explanatory details of what osteopathic physicians have known intuitively all along—that there is such a thing as an "osteopathic lesion" and that manipulative therapy can work a favorable response in the critical area. Dr. Korr, a "convert" to osteopathy and a determined disciple, told us there is now a convincing neurophysiological basis for the practice of osteopathy.

## Infections Helped by Manipulation

Though many people think of manipulative therapy only in relation to lower back pains and neckaches, the practice runs far deeper. Ira C. Rumney, D.O., Professor in the Department of Osteopathic Manipulative Medicine, Kirksville College, told us that manipulation is far more than a mechanical exercise. It does, in fact, "help with any type of infection." Earlier, he had written in *Osteopathic Annals* (July 1974): "Though many antibiotics and other drugs are now available, skillfully applied manipulative therapy by the physician who knows the human anatomy, particularly muscle attachments, fascial layers, sympathetic nervous system, and lymphatic drainage, will improve the patient's chances of recovery from any infection. The basic goal of such therapy is to assist in moving body fluids."

According to Dr. Rumney, when an osteopath treats a patient with an infectious disease, the most important thing is to get the lymph moving through the lymph nodes. Lymph, a transparent, slightly yellow liquid, carries those substances—antigens—which help the body form antibodies. When an antigen passes through the lymph nodes, development of antibodies is substantially increased. In Dr. Rumney's opinion, the number of antibodies in the lymph can be increased four to seven times by passing through the nodes.

What this means to the patient suffering from a cold or sore throat is that these ailments can be effectively treated with manipulative therapy. Likewise, this is a revelation that the human body contains the seeds of its own good health.

Dr. Rumney explains further: "In the treatment of upper respiratory infections, one begins by stretching the muscles and the fascia [fibrous membranes] about the shoulder girdle and those of the thoracic cage, to mobilize the thoracic outlet, and then stretches the muscles and fascia of the neck, head, and face. After the fascia and the muscles have been stretched, any point of restricted motion between the related components of the musculoskeletal system needs to be mobilized [freed or relaxed]. This is followed by use of the lymphatic pump, a treatment designed to encourage the movement of body fluids."

According to Dr. Rumney, there is nothing exotic about this type of treatment. He remarked that it has been traditionally understood that infections such as colds, sore throats, flu, tonsillitis, and pneumonia are associated with "slowed lymphatic and venous drainage."

In order to fully understand these aspects of manipulation, we visited Dr. Snyder, who demonstrated the lymphatic pump and other osteopathic techniques.

## An Osteopath in Action

Dr. Snyder suggested that it was sound manipulative practice to first put the patient on his stomach. Then the doctor, standing to the side of the table, could, at right angles to the patient's body, provide sufficient arm pressure both to relax the patient and to snap back any vertebrae that could be out of place. (Aside from the obvious physiological benefits of such procedure, there is something basically therapeutic about the laying on of hands.)

Assuming the patient had some form of viral or bacterial infection, the doctor, after positioning the patient on his back, would move to the head of the table to work the lymphatic pump. Actually, this is a very simple maneuver. The doctor's hands are spread over the upper chest; the heels of the hands are just below the collarbone. Pressure is applied with exhalation and relaxed with inhalation at approximately 18 cycles a minute. This action is continued for approximately 10 minutes.

Apparently this was a very popular and effective type of manipulation for a variety of infections and was one of the osteopathic physician's few recourses up to the time of the massive invasion of antibiotics onto the patient-treatment scene. It was, in Dr. Snyder's words, "one of the few reliable weapons which a doctor had to fight viral infections" and he can remember spending long hours at the lymphatic pump.

No less important, manipulative therapy can bring about a feeling of well-being. When I experienced manipulative therapy at the hands of Dr. Snyder, including lumbar, pelvic, and dorsal pressures, which helped snap two vertebrae into place, I felt remarkably better and more "alive" the rest of the day.

While there exists solid clinical and laboratory evidence that manipulative therapy can be used to treat infectious diseases as well as musculoskeletal problems, "it is seldom," Dr. Snyder concedes, "that a patient asks for this type of treatment." And indications are that the average osteopathic physician himself doesn't remind his patients that there are nonchemical ways to treat most medical complaints.

To discover how the principles of osteopathy are utilized by practicing D.O.'s, we spoke to several in the field. Marvin H. Soalt, D.O., Bloomfield, New Jersey, explained that he "runs a total physical for new patients." This includes "blood and hair analysis" and "diet analysis by computer." According to Dr. Soalt, the diet analysis is "mainly used to point out the amount of sugar consumed." He acknowledged providing specific nutritional treatment for diabetes, headache, hypertension, and employing manipulation and acupuncture as parts of his practice.

## One Practitioner's Philosophy

A more typical example of osteopathic practice geared to the needs of the family is the Macungie, Pennsylvania, Medical Group, headed by William L. Bollman III, D.O.

Dr. Bollman seems in the mainstream of osteopathic medicine. He told us that he and his associates practice manipulative therapy about one-third of the time, but also admits that, occasionally, the press of time compels him to rely on drugs.

More important in his opinion is their practice of "total medicine" for the whole man. This means, first of all, "when a patient comes into my office, I bring his environment in as well as his body." Fundamental as this might sound, Dr. Bollman asserts that "we must tailor our treatment to a patient's needs; we must know when he sleeps, what he eats, where he works. Only then can we treat and prescribe."

One particular theme seems to be emphasized by most of those engaged in the teaching, practice, and scientific investigation of osteopathy: holistic medicine. This means, according to Professor Rohweder, that "we must treat the man, the whole man, with all the connotations that can be applied; we must study the man, his family, his job, his environment, his nutrition, and, yes, his structure, to determine why he reacts as he does."

There is a deep hope in osteopathic circles in America that we are entering a new age of total or holistic medicine. As Professor Korr told us, orthodox medicine is "still caught up in the Pasteur concept; find the bug and manufacture a bullet to kill it."

Although there are only about 15,000 practicing osteopaths in this country, which makes them outnumbered by their M.D. brethren better than 20 to 1, osteopaths are still in a good position to provide an alternative approach to health care for those who want it. Their heavy training in the basic physiological sciences, with emphasis on natural immunities, makes them ideally suited to stress preventive medicine, including nutritional considerations. Their unique training in manipulative therapy means that in many cases they can help the body heal itself by using their hands rather than immediately turning to painkillers, muscle relaxants, or even surgery. Their background may even make them more qualified to successfully practice some of the new drugless techniques, such as scientific relaxation therapy and acupuncture, than the average M.D. At the same time, the osteopath has first-rate medical training which other practitioners of natural healing techniques may lack.

## Profession Faces Dangers

But the dangers are just as real as the promise. Recent reports indicate that osteopathic physicians are using slightly more drugs than their medical brethren. Osteopathic physicians are not supermen: time, as Dr. Bollman acknowledged, is a factor. This might mean that eventually the D.O. will spend no more time than the M.D. on the musculoskeletal system. A lymphatic pump takes time and we might ask whether this generation of osteopathic physicians will be willing to give it. It is certainly heartening to learn that approximately 75 percent of graduating D.O.'s enter family practice to provide primary health care service. But this figure is not a reason to rejoice if, as we suspect, many D.O.'s are simply taking up where the M.D.'s left off, before they specialized themselves out of family medicine. It would be unfortunate if the osteopathic physician, who has done so much to make manipulation a vital arm of the profession, would, unwittingly, give this practice over to the chiropractor and the physical therapist.

Professor Korr, who has probably done more than any other man in America to legitimize osteopathy, leveled the following challenge at osteopaths in a recent major address: "In the course of its long struggle for recognition, the osteopathic profession appears to have forgotten why it sought recognition: to enable it to deliver and demonstrate, as widely and fully as possible, the benefits of osteopathic principles and methods. In forgetting, the profession has per mitted osteopathic manipulation to slip from its place as a key element in osteopathic practice."

The challenge has come from one of the finest voices within the profession: we can merely echo it.

# Oxygen Therapy, Hyperbaric

A young Marine who came back from Viet Nam dying of osteomyelitis of the spine presented a pathetic picture to doctors at the Long Beach, California, Naval Hospital. His weight had dropped from 160 to 80 pounds, and no treatment had been able to arrest the infection rate raging in his bones. But when he was treated with pure oxygen under high pressure (OHP), his condition swiftly turned around and he began not only to recover, but to thrive.

In London, doctors were groping for some treatment to help a 53-year-old man who had been suffering since the age of 8, when he had undergone radical mastoidectomy. Following this surgery, he had a chronic ear discharge which proved resistant to all therapy, including the surgery. Primarily because there seemed to be nothing to lose, doctors put the patient in a hyperbaric chamber with 100 percent oxygen at twice normal pressure for 90 minutes on each of four consecutive days. His ear discharge promptly ceased for the first time in 45 years.

In New York, a premature baby fought feebly for his life with an infected meningomyelocele—an abnormal protrusion of the spinal cord. Nothing was able to stop the infection until a doctor used a small portable chamber which could apply pure oxygen under pressure directly to the infected area. Two days later, the infection was cleared up and the infant was able to undergo corrective plastic surgery.

Fifteen or twenty years ago, most doctors would have laughed at such dramatic successes achieved with nothing but concentrated and pressurized oxygen. And some did more than laugh. Some of the pioneers in the field of hyperbaric oxygen were subjected to severe criticism and scorn by their colleagues, and at least one report on hyperbaric oxygen submitted to a medical journal was rejected as "absurd."

Today, hyperbaric oxygenation should still probably be regarded as in the late experimental stage. But it's undeniable that thousands of people with a variety of problems have been saved from death by the judicious use of OHP. It's considered the definitive therapy for carbon monoxide poisoning, probably the single most effective treatment for several deep-seated infections such as the gas gangrene which may develop in a limb with bad circulation, and also an extremely promising and often surprisingly effective aid in improving the mentality and behavior of people suffering "senility" caused by poor delivery of oxygenated blood to the brain.

But hyperbaric (the word simply means high pressure) oxygenation is not without its dangers. In amounts not very much greater than those used therapeutically, excess oxygen becomes toxic to certain enzyme systems and can damage eyes, lungs, and even the central nervous system. Considerable caution must be used with OHP both in selection of patients to be treated and in monitoring the heart, blood, and nerves before, after, and preferably *during* treatment. Today, as more and more hospitals install OHP units, doctors are becoming more familiar with the therapy, and an experienced practitioner should be able to reduce these risks to a very minimal level.

OHP did not become medically "respectable" until about 1970. It is no great testimony to the imagination of the medical profession that OHP is just now beginning to come into its own. Pressurized oxygen was first used medically in England three centuries ago, to treat caisson workers who developed "the bends" when they came out of the water after working in chambers pressurized with ordinary air. The pressurized pure oxygen dissolved the nitrogen bubbles which had formed in their blood and gradually restored their body chemistry to normal. Today, the same treatment is still used for diving illness and also for carbon dioxide and monoxide poisoning.

Perhaps it is a bit more difficult to understand how pure pressurized oxygen can be of help in conditions where there isn't such an obvious and immediate need to force oxygen into the system. It may help to realize that oxygen is a vitally needed nutrient, just like protein or vitamin C or calcium. But while weeks or months can go by until a deficiency of protein or vitamins can produce a life-threatening situation, oxygen deficiency symptoms develop in seconds. Irreversible brain damage and death follow in minutes. Every living cell in the body requires oxygen as its basic fuel for life processes. When oxygen starvation is localized, as it is, for example, in advanced arteriosclerosis of the legs, or frostbite, the cells in those areas grow weak and unable to perform normally, just as a motor or an engine does when it is deprived of its required amount of gasoline or electricity. Defenses against disease are vastly lowered. The reparative process becomes paralyzed. Many cells may actually die.

The result may be progressive gangrene, necessitating amputation of a limb.

## OHP Fights Harmful Bacteria

This leads us to one of the most impressive uses of OHP—and one which is relatively easy to understand: fighting infective anaerobic bacteria. These are microorganisms which can multiply and develop toxins only in the absence of oxygen. For reasons which are not at all clear, however, only certain of these organisms can be controlled by OHP. Fortunately, the organisms which are involved in a condition called gas gangrene are highly vulnerable to OHP. Gas gangrene (so-called because the bacteria actually produce gas as a metabolic by-product) usually results from an injury in an area where the circulation is poor, and destroys both muscle and skin as it grows and produces a constant wet discharge. OHP is particularly valuable here because the bacteria which cause this condition are usually highly resistant to antibiotics. A report in the *British Medical Journal* in 1965 stated that "Hyperbaric oxygen has saved both life and limb. . . . One of the most dramatic features is the almost immediate arrest of the disease and the improvement in the patient's condition. Hyperbaric treatment is combined with antibiotics, and surgery is deferred until after it is complete, when the operation can often be confined to simple procedures such as the removal of necrotic sloughs [dead tissue] and skin grafting."

Despite its success in fighting gas gangrene, OHP is almost totally ineffective against tetanus, caused by germs very closely related to the clostridium involved in gas gangrene.

Curiously, hyperbaric oxygen can also be very effective in beating down infections caused by germs which ordinarily *can* multiply in the presence of oxygen. This seems to be the case *only* when the infection is localized and imbedded in dying tissue, such as bedsores. Dr. Boguslav H. Fischer of the New York University School of

Medicine wrote in 1971 that "the main purpose of the treatment is to deliver oxygen to tissue that is suffering from relative hypoxia [oxygen starvation]." Apparently, when damaged tissue cannot utilize oxygen, it has no defense against infection. And OHP, applied *locally* to these infections, seems to turn the tide in favor of the body's natural defenses.

Dr. Fischer was the physician who reported the case of the premature baby saved from an infection with the help of locally applied OHP. He said the organism involved in that case was the bacteria known as *Aerobacter,* and added that "strep, staph, and *Klebsiella* we know are suppressed quickly."

But he also added that two other rather common infective organisms, *Pseudomonas aeruginosa* and *Candida albicans,* can actually be *stimulated* by oxygen if the pressure is not sufficiently high. "I must warn against unwarranted enthusiasm," Dr. Fischer declared. "The therapy must be applied only in properly selected cases."

One of the most experienced workers in hyperbaric oxygenation is Dr. D.J.D. Perrins of London. It was this physician who reported how OHP cleared up the ear discharge which had afflicted a patient for 45 years. And it was his work with chronic osteomyelitis which was responsible for stimulating doctors at the Long Beach Naval Hospital to try—successfully—OHP for the young Marine dying with this disease. Dr. Perrins told an international conference on OHP held in 1965 that in 17 of 24 patients with chronic osteomyelitis (an infection seated in the bones which may spread) that he treated with OHP, he obtained healing of the skin and drying up of discharges in anywhere from 4 to 32 days. He stressed, though, that one ought not to conclude that the underlying disease was influenced by OHP. He suggested rather that the extra oxygen probably stimulated the action of the body's phagocytes to wage more aggressive war against invading pathogens. He also pointed out that hyperbaric therapy for osteomyelitis is performed in conjunction with more orthodox approaches, including antibiotic therapy.

Dr. George B. Hart, who at the time of this writing was associated with the Baromedical Research Unit of the Naval Regional Medical Center in Long Beach, California, is one of the outstanding clinical researchers in the field of OHP. In the most recent report of his work (published late in 1974) Dr. Hart said that he and his colleagues had treated a total of 90 patients with osteomyelitis, all of whom had failed to improve with antibiotic or surgical therapy. In 63 out of the 90 cases, he said, hyperbaric oxygen therapy achieved complete success. All of the 27 patients who were not healed were improved, with less drainage and less bone pain.

During the course of these treatments, Dr. Hart and his colleague Dr. Robert G. Winans, discovered that the best results were achieved with patients who had the disease for a relatively shorter period of time. From this, it is reasonable to conclude that osteomyelitis patients should waste no time in talking to the doctors at an OHP clinic.

Another important finding was that treatment failures were often associated with smoking. This prompted the doctors to forbid tobacco to all patients—going so far as to drop them from therapy if they refused to quit.

Good nutrition and adequate vitamin intake were also stressed. In an article written with E. G. Mainous, D.D.S., and P. J. Boyne, D.M.D., on the use of OHP in osteomyelitis of the jawbone, Dr. Hart and colleagues said that "Vitamin E was given routinely to all patients in doses of 100 mg. per day since it has been shown experimentally to reduce the possibility of oxygen toxicity" (*Journal of the American Dental Association,* December 1973). Depending on the kind of vitamin E used, 100 mg. is equivalent to approximately 125 to 150 international units (I.U.) of vitamin E.

## Hyperbaric Oxygen Treatment in Cases of Blood Loss

Dr. Hart revealed in a 1974 report how hyperbaric oxygen can be a literal lifesaver for people such as Jehovah's Witnesses whose religious convictions forbid them from receiving a blood transfusion. He received three patients who had suffered acute blood loss for various reasons, and who all refused to have the blood transfusion that was apparently necessary to save their lives. Dr. Hart treated the patients by administering intravenous fluids, injections of iron dextran, and hyperbaric oxygen. OHP was administered at the more-or-less typical two atmospheres absolute for 60 to 90 minutes at each treatment. The number of treatments varied according to the patient. One woman required a total of 35 hours of OHP.

"Treatment with hyperbaric oxygen resulted in dramatic improvement, with reversal of the signs and symptoms of hypoxia [lack of oxygen] in all three patients," Dr. Hart reported (*Journal of the American Medical Association,* May 20, 1974).

What the treatment accomplished was to load the limited number of red blood cells which these patients had with the absolute maximum amount of oxygen, along with the iron needed to carry it. They were then able to get past the crisis stage and survive until their bodies could produce more red blood cells. For one patient out of the three, though, this didn't work. She continued to bleed from a diverticular lesion of the intestines and although she improved over her initial state, her continued loss of blood could not be overcome by the addition of extra oxygen and iron. On the fourth day of her hospitalization, her husband consented to a transfusion.

Encouraging preliminary studies suggest that hyperbaric oxygen may be a virtual "specific" in many cases of chronic dizziness. Dr. Sreedhar Nair and associates at the Norwalk Hospital in Connecticut tried a course of the treatment on seven patients with chronic vertigo which had not responded to any other treatment. Most of the patients became so dizzy simply on standing that they were unable to walk. Others could walk, but only with a staggering gait. Several of the patients were often in a confused state and two had recurrent episodes of nausea. In all but one patient, there was evidence of arteriosclerosis.

Each patient was given hyperbaric oxygen at two atmospheres absolute during a series of treatments consisting of two-hour units. The total time of treatment ranged from six hours to thirty hours.

The doctors reported that the response was "excellent" in five cases and "good" in two others. Virtually all the symptoms were either entirely cleared up or greatly reduced. A follow-up period indicated that the beneficial effect was not only temporary. Months after the treatment faltered, there were only a few scattered recurrences reported.

No one can yet say why patients with chronic vertigo are benefited by hyperbaric oxygen. However, as the researchers themselves pointed out, it seems most likely that it did the job by restoring oxygen sufficiency to centers deep in the ear or within the brain which control equilibrium. And this brings us to the most controversial—but perhaps most promising—use of hyperbaric oxygen.

## OHP and Brain Damage

The brain consumes oxygen faster than any other organ of the body. Its need for this nutrient is so great that, deprived of it for only a few minutes, it can no longer maintain consciousness. During cases of cardiac arrest, it is the brain which is in the greatest danger. While the rest of the body can get along amazingly well without oxygen for a limited time, irreversible brain damage is almost certain to occur after about seven minutes of heart stoppage.

Narrowing and hardening of the blood vessels with advancing age are believed to be a major cause of gross senility. The impairment in oxygen nutrition may also be a factor in much more subtle psychiatric changes associated with age or circulatory impairments such as a stroke. Theoretically, if oxygen sufficiency could be restored in these cases, there would be a good chance of clinical improvement. So far, the evidence seems to indicate that in some, but not all, cases of cerebral oxygen insufficiency, hyperbaric oxygen can bring about gratifying improvement.

Pioneering in this application of OHP were Eleanor A. Jacobs, Ph.D., and colleagues, all of Buffalo, New York. In 1969, they reported in the *New England Journal of Medicine* the results they achieved using OHP to treat 13 elderly male patients, all of whom had been hospitalized for many months, and in some cases for several years, because of the symptoms of senility. The patients were first given three standard tests designed to evaluate efficiency of memory, concept formation, and presence of physical brain damage. Arterial blood samples were also obtained and tested for oxygen.

Each of the 13 was treated for 90 minutes twice a day, for 15 days, with hyperbaric oxygen. At the same time, 5 other patients were used as controls, and although put in a chamber, breathed a mixture which was nearly identical to ordinary air.

When all the patients were retested, an average of 12 hours after coming out of the chamber, those who had been breathing pure oxygen showed remarkable increases in their scores, while the control patients had no significant change. In the experimental group, the mean average score on the Wechslar Memory Scale went from 76 to 103; the average score on another test went from 10 to 41; and on a third test from 25 to 49.

Blood samples taken during the tests showed a very marked increase in the amount of oxygen in the blood of those breathing the pure oxygen, while the control subjects had no increase at all. This seemed to establish a very clear relationship between increased oxygenation of the brain and mental performance in elderly senile people.

Now for the big question: Is this improvement temporary or permanent? The answer, although still not clear, is intriguing.

Dr. Jacobs and the three M.D.'s she worked with pointed out that when oxygen concentration is increased in the blood, it ordinarily diminishes very quickly, returning to normal in about 30 minutes. Oxygen levels in the brain may be normalized even sooner. But the tests which revealed improvement were given an average of 12 hours after oxygenation, which means that the improvement lasted at least 24 times longer than can be explained by the presence of extraordinary amounts of oxygen in the brain.

This classic study was carried out some years ago. In a more recent report, Dr. Jacobs said that a research team had now studied 75 "very deteriorated" persons and results continued to indicate "that improvement persists much longer than we would have expected." Although she admitted freely that she is not certain exactly how long the improvement lasts, she did venture to say that the treatment holds more promise for patients who are relatively less deteriorated. (On the other hand, she has also said three out of the five "extremely deteriorated" brain-damaged patients exhibited varying degrees of quite unexpected improvement after OHP treatments.)

Doctors at the Miami Heart Institute in Florida said in 1973 that they had been using OHP therapy with a total of 54 senile patients with generally good results—although the improvement seemed to be temporary, rather than permanent. In 1974, OHP pioneer Dr. Hart and colleague Dr. Allan E. Edwards reported gratifying results with 20 volunteers—average age 68—who complained of recent memory lapses and other signs of approaching senility. Before-and-after tests indicated the greatest improvement was achieved in the areas of short-term memory and the ability to perform complicated visual tasks. Curiously, two of the subjects reported that after treatment they had to be fitted with new glasses because their visual acuity had actually improved. Drs. Edwards and Hart also noted that following 15 OHP sessions, there was no evidence that these patients had stopped improving.

Dr. Hart has also used OHP to treat stroke patients whose improvement had "plateaued" after other therapy. His tentative conclusion in 1973 was that "there appears to be the sort of improvement that would rule out coincidence."

Dr. Edgar End, Director of the Hyperbaric Unit at Milwaukee

County General Hospital, told *Medical World News* in 1973 that he has seen "encouraging results" using OHP in a small number of brain-damaged children. Although he insisted that it was too early to draw concrete conclusions, he did note that in several cases, the improvement was so dramatic that teachers called the parents to ask them what had happened to cause the tremendous improvement in attention, cooperation, and coordination.

At least two reports have appeared in the medical literature indicating that simply breathing pure oxygen through a mask, rather than sitting in a pressurized chamber, can bring about beneficial results with senile patients. But another study indicates that oxygen without the extra pressure does not accomplish anything. All three of these studies, however, were conducted with only small groups of patients, so nothing definitive can be said at present about the beneficial psychiatric effects of breathing unpressurized oxygen.

Needless to say, research is finding out more about hyperbaric oxygen every year. Some of the research centers around relatively obscure conditions such as Fournier's disease—a kind of aggravated gangrene of the scrotum. Dr. Charles Abbott, hyperbaric chief at the St. Barnabas Medical Center in Livingston, New Jersey, has used OHP as an important tool in successfully treating 14 patients with this disease. Other research centers around much broader applications—such as the possible use of OHP in maintaining oxygen sufficiency in heart and surgery patients. Some of the early results look very promising.

# Patterning For Brain-Injured Children

The superb ability of the body to heal itself is put to no more challenging test than when confronted with serious damage to the central nervous system. A cut, a bruise, even a persistent ulcer or a broken bone is one thing. Major brain damage is something else.

The tools of medicine are not worth much in these cases, and few would even dream that the body can do anything to overcome injuries to the brain. Yet, there is a therapy—an intensive, heroic therapy—based on the conviction that with the right kind of help, the body *can* recover at least some of the functions lost to brain injury.

The name of the therapy is patterning. And this is how it works.

It's 7:30 P.M. on a Monday. A very tired Kathryn and Alan Morgan are sitting across a small desk from Arthur Sandler, top physical therapist with the Institutes for the Achievement of Human Potential.

For the past nine hours, the Morgans—including their 3½-year-old son, Karl—have been marched from one end of the Institutes's grounds to the other. Kathryn and Alan have been exhaustively questioned on every phase of young Karl's life from the time he was conceived to the rigors of the trip which brought them from their home in South Wales in the United Kingdom more than 5,000 miles to Philadelphia.

As their haggard looks prove, the day has been tough. But the hours have been tough on Karl too. He's been examined by two doctors. He's been poked and stuck all over the body with pins. He's had his feet tickled until his big toes stood straight up like thumbs. He's had brilliant lights shined directly into his eyes. He's been forced to lie on a hard board as it vibrated, while a horn blew. During the stressful day he's had three *petit mal* seizures (and will have two more before he goes to sleep).

And then, at the end of those nine hours, came Sandler's announcement. "Congratulations. Your son is brain injured."

"I never thought that I'd be happy to hear that," said Kathryn, her eyes shining with tears of happiness. "It means so much to us."

It's important that Karl Morgan is brain injured and not mentally deficient or psychotic. If he were either of the latter, he would never have been accepted into the program of the Institutes, a regimen that includes the still-controversial "patterning" program, along with megavitamin therapy.

Karl, who has the looks that make strangers say, "He's too cute to be a boy," is among an estimated 7 to 12 percent of children who are born with some form of brain damage. In his case, he was born with two strikes against him. The first strike was an undetected case of rubella that his mother contracted sometime during the first three months of pregnancy. Compounding the problem was a difficult birth that trapped his head in the birth canal for an extended time before doctors could free it, denying his brain of its critical oxygen supply.

While sitting in his mother's lap, Karl looks like any other well-developed child who's heading for his fourth birthday. But he's blind. The only thing he can do for himself is suck his thumb and roll from side to side. He says something that sounds like "Ma" when he wants his mother. His parents said that once when Karl had a coughing spell, Alan patted him on the back to soothe him. Since then, whenever he wants attention from his father, he gives a little cough.

## A Chance To Be Normal

Karl's parents believe that their son has a chance for normality, now that he's been accepted by the Institutes for treatment.

Located on over 13 acres of wooded, hilly land in the Chestnut Hill section of Philadelphia, the Institutes is known around the world for its treatment of brain-injured children through patterning techniques developed by physical therapist Dr. Glenn J. Doman and psychologist Dr. Carl H. Delacato. Through patterning—and megavitamin therapy which was introduced about two years ago—the Morgans hope to see the day when Karl can take his rightful place alongside his peers as a "normal" child.

The Institutes is actually a combination of eight different organizations under the blanket title, Institutes for the Achievement of Human Potential. Each institute is involved in a different area of interest in brain-injured children, ranging from research to teaching to rehabilitation. After a five-day evaluation and parent orientation course in Philadelphia, children are treated by their parents at home. They return to the Institutes every two months for a reevaluation and revision of their treatment program. In Karl's case, the reevaluation will be done in England, because he was one of a group of 15 children brought to the Institutes in a group. The Institutes will fly its evaluators to England where they will handle all 15 children.

The Institutes traces its beginnings back to the early 1950s when Drs. Doman and Delacato evaluated conventional treatment for brain-injured children. Much to their dismay, they found that under controlled conditions, brain-injured children who received no treatment at all were just about as well off as those who had received the accepted therapy. In fact, some who had just remained home had actually progressed more than those who were treated.

The two doctors, and Dr. Robert Doman, a physician specializing in physical medicine, and brother to Glenn Doman, virtually threw away the book and came up with an entirely new concept in treating brain-injured children. The backbone of the Doman-Delacato treatment consists of a technique they called "patterning." The technique puts into practice the theories of the late Dr. Temple Fay, a neurosurgeon who believed that when a child suffers brain damage, and loses use of critical cells, it is sometimes possible to activate the millions of surviving brain cells in such a way that they take over the functions of the dead cells.

This stimulation, which they call "neurological organization," revolves around the step-by-step development of the central nervous system. The nervous system of each new human being must go through several definite developmental stages before the brain can operate to its full potential. At birth, for example, only the lower part of the brain has been organized. The baby has only reflex actions controlled by the spinal cord and medulla. As the baby develops, the higher parts of the brain come into operation—the pons, mid-brain, and last, the cortex. The process is something like programming a blank computer. The baby "programs" his entire body through trial and error, using his senses.

A vital part of the Doman-Delacato rationale holds that if a child skips or skimps on any phase in this developmental sequence because of brain injury or lack of opportunity, there is likely to be inadequate development at higher levels.

So Drs. Doman and Delacato designed a series of patterning exercises which duplicate the early stages of the child's development. More about patterning later; right now we will only say that since the Institutes was founded some 22 years ago, more than 7,000 children have gone through the program, which boasts a success rate of about 30 percent. Success is defined as having the child competing with his peers after treatment.

## Natural Foods and Vitamins Work Wonders

While patterning has worked wonders for many children who would otherwise never have had a chance, the Institutes has come to realize that good nutrition has an important role in getting a damaged brain to function again.

"About two years ago, we had a group of kids who just didn't seem to be getting anywhere," said Dr. Roselise Wilkinson, physician in charge of the nutrition and general health programs for the Institutes. "These kids seemed to be plateauing—not getting anywhere. So we started them on a nutrition program and they started moving."

In all, there were 174 children who were put on megavitamin doses for periods of time ranging from a few days to more than a year. They received large amounts of a variety of supplements including vitamin C, the B-complex vitamins, and iron. They didn't receive vitamin E at first, but it has since been added to the program and is prescribed after the child has been in the Institutes's program for a time.

In the final results, about 25 percent of the children were helped by the therapy, according to the unpublished study which notes: "While these results cannot by any stretch be construed as 'fantastic' or a 'breakthrough', they are nevertheless in our estimation, remarkable."

Dr. Wilkinson said that as yet, there is no common denominator which will allow them to prescribe vitamin dosages across the board. For example, the Institutes regularly uses vitamin $B_6$ (pyridoxine) as one way of controlling seizures. But, she noted, "I have a few kids who seizure more on $B_6$. I find more and more that there are individual variations in the children. I can't use a blanket kind of program although we start them on a standardized dose in the beginning."

The list of supplements Karl Morgan must take indicates just how important the Institutes believes nutrition is. For example, Karl will take at least 750 mg. of vitamin C daily. It is to be given in three equal 250 mg. doses. This amount is to be doubled if Karl becomes sick. He is to be given a B-complex tablet which includes 5 mg. of vitamin $B_1$ (thiamine), $B_2$ (riboflavin), and $B_6$ every day. He is also to be given a teaspoon of cod-liver oil to supply at least 3,700 units of vitamin A and 370 units of vitamin D daily.

The Institutes also supplied Karl's parents with a list of foods to supply him with a minimum of 35 grams of protein every day, a large amount for a young child.

Besides spelling out exactly what vitamins in what dosages Karl should have, the Institutes limited his fluid intake to 20 ounces of liquid per day and eliminated all sugar along with reducing his salt intake as much as possible. The Institutes believes that restricting fluid, salt and sugar intake decreases cerebrospinal fluid production, thereby reducing cortical irritability. An injured brain, they reason, should have as little irritation as possible.

Dr. Wilkinson said that Karl could have three to four additional ounces of liquids during hot weather. She also said that there was no restriction on the amount of liquids he could take if he developed a fever.

The diet stresses natural foods and whole milk which the parent may fortify at home with supplements. Frequent meals of high-protein liver and the use of 100 percent whole grain breads and cereals are recommended, along with the serving of eggs at least once a day.     .

While telling the Morgans what they should feed Karl—as well as eat themselves—they were also told what *not* to feed him. The list includes many of the don'ts of good nutrition, especially elimination of junk foods such as potato chips and pretzels. They were also advised to avoid foods made from or containing white flour and/or refined sugar. They were told not to feed Karl bakery sweets, jams, jellies, candies, packaged mixes, frostings, prepared or packaged cereals other than granola, all hydrogenated fats or foods prepared in them, and meats containing sodium nitrate or nitrite as preservatives.

With many 3½ year olds already addicted to sugar and candies, it seems almost an impossible task to wean Karl from them. However, the Morgans are determined that Karl will have every possible chance to recover. The biggest job, however, will be for them to carry out the patterning program that Karl was given.

## Therapy Is Intensive

In the first place, the program is a time consuming one which will keep Karl, Kathryn, and Alan busy most of their waking hours. And it must be done, without fail, every day with no time off for vacations.

"If you're sick and are given medicine and don't take it, you don't expect to get well, do you?" asked Arthur Sandler. "Of course not. Karl is ill and this is his medicine."

According to the Institutes's staff, Karl has the overall function of a 5½-month-old infant even though he is partially toilet trained and can feed himself if his mother places the food on his spoon.

The program that Karl was given is designed to move him up until he reaches a mental proficiency equal to his chronological age. This is accomplished through a sequence of exercises that must be done 18 times a day along with a patterning program that must be done at least 4 times a day. The basic idea is to stimulate all of Karl's senses, reflexes, and muscles.

Brain-injured children usually have an extremely poor breathing apparatus, according to Dr. Wilkinson. Therefore, the Institutes devised a technique they call "masking" to correct the deficiency. A plastic mask with just a small breathing tube for oxygen is slipped over the face of the child. As the child continues to breathe, he ends up rebreathing carbon dioxide which is normally thrown off as a waste product. The carbon dioxide triggers a reaction in which the body automatically breathes heavier and deeper, searching for oxygen. Eventually, this forces the child to develop better breathing habits and increased pulmonary capability, resulting in more oxygen reaching the injured brain.

A negative gravity exercise to be done at least 18 times a day, calls for Karl to be held upside down. This stimulates the blood circulation in the brain.

Karl will be placed on something called the "vital stimulation machine" which is a board that vibrates and has a horn and light mounted on it. For one minute, Karl remains on the board as it vibrates. Then, a horn is sounded and a light flashed. The vibration stimulates feeling in Karl while the light should stimulate his eyes. Karl is blind but there is nothing wrong with his eyes. Therefore, the Institutes reasons, it must be caused by the brain injury. Through stimulation, the Institutes believes he can gain his sight.

The roll pattern, another part of the program, duplicates movements that normal children make when they are very small infants. Karl's legs are crossed manually from side to side while he's held on his back.

Another exercise is the trunk pattern. It calls for Karl to be held by two people. The person holding his legs then lifts them until they are far over his head, bending the trunk. This movement again duplicates one that normal children go through when they're infants but is a movement which Karl had never accomplished.

The next step in his program calls for positive gravity stimulation. This stimulates blood circulation and calls for two people to each grasp one arm and leg and swing Karl back and forth through the air.

Since Karl has never felt what it is like to move on his own, he has to be helped. This is where a small sliding board comes in. It's smooth and tilted in such a way that gravity pulls him down towards the bottom. When he moves his arms and legs, he'll find himself being propelled down the slide. As it gets easier and easier for Karl, the slide's angle will be lessened. Eventually, Karl will learn to crawl by himself.

The patterning program itself is less complicated. First, all limbs are brushed with the rough-textured pot scrubber. Then, one person turns the child's head from side to side while others move his arms and legs in a crawling motion. The patterning will take either three or five persons, depending upon how the child reacts.

Through the patterning, the Institutes hopes that Karl's uninjured brain cells will get the message that "this is what it feels like to move." Hopefully, Karl's brain cells will eventually take over the function that the people provide.

Sandler pointed out that three concepts are crucial: frequency, intensity, and duration. If the brain cells are going to be activated, they must be stimulated. And they must be stimulated often, intensely, and for a long time, if there is any hope at all for recovery.

It's a long program. It's a complicated program. It's a difficult program. And it may not work.

"We've seen profoundly hurt children recover and those mildly hurt not recover," Sandler told the Morgans. "There is no relationship to the percentage of hurt and the success of the treatment."

Though the Institutes has been forging ahead for many years with its technique, the medical profession has yet to give full approval to the technique. Though some doctors will refer patients to the Institutes, there is by no means unanimous acceptance. There have been criticisms of the program.

During the five-day orientation that parents go through with their children, the Institutes is careful to point out all the criticisms, while explaining its own point of view. In addition, the Institutes points out that its success rate is only 30 percent.

"Yes, we have failures," Dr. Glenn Doman said. "We have a lot of them. And every time we fail, it means that a child is not getting better. We wish that we'd never fail, but we do. I don't like to talk about the failures we've had or the blind alleys we've been up because that would take years. We only have a short time to tell what we know and then let you go and treat your child."

*More than one year after we wrote the above report, the Morgan family returned to Philadelphia for an evaluation by the Institutes. We talked with them and staff members to see what progress, if any, Karl had made.*

## 'We've Come a Long Way'

"It's taken us a long time but we've come a long way," Alan Morgan said reflectively. "I feel as though I now have a son. I don't know if I felt that way before all this happened. But now I really have hope that we can lick this thing."

"I don't think there's any doubt that Karl has made progress," Kathryn Morgan said firmly. "He's a different child altogether. Sometimes we look back at his pictures and that's when we discover that we have a different child."

Staff members of the Institute agree. Gretchen Kerr, one of the staff members who initially evaluated Karl, said the differences showed up in almost every aspect of Karl's deportment. "He's much more alert, has better posture, and he pays more attention to what's going on," she said.

Subjective observations aside, the Institute uses a special profile that Drs. Glenn Doman and Delacato developed to enable staff members to objectively measure progress made by patients on the program. The profile indicates that Karl has advanced to the point where he has a neurological age—or is the mental equivalent—of a child almost ten months old, compared to an age estimated at five months when he started the program over a year and a half ago.

At that time, Karl was totally blind and could only suck his thumb and roll from side to side on the floor. His communication was limited to a single guttural sound which Kathryn alone recognized as his call for her.

Since then, Karl has made great forward strides, especially with his sight. He can follow lights and distinguish some objects. He watches his patterners as they work over him and can pick out spoonsful of food when being fed.

Karl also has the ability to "turn off" his sight at will. Dr. Wilkinson says that Karl sees what he wants to see but quickly becomes bored. Then, he stops paying attention.

Karl has had no seizures for several months. Prior to that, he suffered from several *petit mal* seizures each and every day.

# Pet Therapy

**by Lois Stevenson**

Several years ago, the future looked bleak for Terry, a quiet and withdrawn seven year old. Unable to communicate verbally because of brain damage at birth, he was barely able to make his wants known.

Although doctors diagnosed his brain dysfunction as "minimal," Terry's slow progress in learning to talk led them to predict he would be dependent on his parents' care all his life.

Fortunately, Terry was placed under the skilled guidance of Mrs. Gordon Klacik of Green Brook, New Jersey, who teaches a special class for the neurologically impaired at Lincoln School in nearby New Brunswick. Klacik suggested getting Terry a dog.

"Because communication with a pet doesn't have to be on a verbal level, I felt it would relieve Terry from the tension of always struggling to be understood. At the same time, he would feel encouraged and would gain in self-confidence as he found he could communicate adequately with a living creature," she explained.

In early November, Terry's father brought home a 10-month-old collie named Duke.

"It was the turning point in Terry's life," Klacik says. "Terry blossomed out, both in the classroom and at home. He was able at last to relate personally to a living being. By the time he came back to school after Christmas vacation, the change was fantastic. He was conversing with Duke, telling him to do this and do that."

Terry went back to regular classes the next year. Now in seventh grade, he is up to grade level in every subject and is thinking about going to college.

Like Terry, thousands of children throughout the country are being led down the path to better mental health with the aid of "seeing-heart" dogs, as psychotherapists become increasingly aware of the value of pets in treating mental and emotional disorders.

Pets, in fact, are of particular help to all those who occupy a marginal position in our society—children without families, the aged, the mentally retarded, physically handicapped and inmates of correctional institutions. For those who suffer from isolation, a lack of rewarding activity, or a sense of rejection, a pet can restore a feeling of identity and self-worth.

"The animal or pet is one of the links in the golden chain leading to good mental health," declares Boris M. Levinson, Ph.D., diplomate in clinical psychology, of Elmhurst, New York.

"The possession of a pet who eagerly awaits one and responds to one's care and attention may mean the difference between maintaining contact with reality or almost total withdrawal into fantasy. Literally, a pet can occasionally represent the difference between life and death," Dr. Levinson affirms in his book, *Pet-Oriented Child Psychotherapy* (Charles C. Thomas, Springfield, Ill., 1969).

## A Psychologist Named Jingles

This text, which has become a classic in its influence on professionals who use pets in psychotherapy, is dedicated to Dr. Levinson's mixed-breed male dog, Jingles, who helped to restore many emotionally disturbed children to mental health.

"The child who comes to the therapy situation with the fear of dogs or cats and manages in the course of treatment to overcome it, has undergone tremendous emotional growth and maturity. He now may perceive his home as a friendly, tolerable place and find that his parents and peers, similarly to his pet, are friendly and well disposed toward him," Dr. Levinson says.

Just such a child is described in his book, in a case history from Mira Rothenberg, clinical director at a summer camp for emotionally disturbed youngsters. Because Dr. Levinson had loaned Jingles to the group for the summer, the boys called the dog "Levinson."

Rothenberg relates "Levinson's" experience with Andy, whom she depicts as "one of our most complicated, resistant boys." Andy was afraid of food, of walking, talking, fighting, water, air, his own shadow—and terrified of dogs. When he saw one, he screamed; if one brushed by him, he fainted.

Naturally, Andy avoided Jingles. But when the boy was crying or in one of his extremely rejective moods, Jingles always "just happened" to be sitting nearby, obviously concerned and sympathetic.

"Take him away," Andy would scream, and Jingles would quietly leave. But one day in the middle of a tantrum, as Jingles began to walk away, Andy suddenly yelled, "No, don't take him away. Andy wants 'Levinson' to stay with him."

From that point on, the friendship grew. Andy began to eat more, with extras "dropped" under the table for Jingles. He even found the courage to go swimming, after making sure that Jingles was around.

One day, very tentatively, Andy touched the tip of the dog's ear, then immediately ran away. But slowly he began to lose his fear; eventually, he was able to stroke and pat Jingles, quite openly and unafraid.

Rothenberg emphasizes the astonishing sensitivity that Jingles displayed throughout this relationship. When Andy shouted for "Levinson," the dog, no matter where he was, would suddenly appear and wait patiently at the child's side—but he never jumped up on Andy or licked his face as he did the boys who were not afraid of dogs.

## Instinctive Knowledge of Human Needs

This instinctive knowledge of each child's needs is shared by many pets used in therapy. In *Skeezer, Dog With a Mission* (Harvey House, New York, 1973), Elizabeth Yates tells the story of a friendly, intelligent, female dog of uncertain breed at the University of Michigan's Children's Psychiatric Hospital. There, Skeezer has been a trusted and beloved member of the therapy team for eight years.

Skeezer knows her job is to reach troubled children who have retreated within themselves and become resistant to human help.

Carefully trained, but responsive to each child in her own way, Skeezer offers her love to a child starved for affection, or listens attentively to a child pouring out sorrow or frustration. She will curl up on the bed to bring warm comfort to a frightened youngster on his first night at the center, or share in a boisterous game that delights her human companions.

Alice Williams, the nurse in charge of the center, tells her staff: "Take a cue from Skeezer. Watch how she feels her way into a relationship."

At the Mid-Missouri Mental Health Center on the University of Missouri-Columbia's campus, a male springer spaniel named Smudge is the children's therapist-pet. He is shared by 16 preadolescent residents aged seven to twelve, and 10 "day care" children six years old and under.

"Smudge has a very shy, retiring personality. He is not at all aggressive, which is good because we have enough overly aggressive children here," says Dr. Robert Jones, Director of Children's Services and assistant superintendent of the center. "The children respond nicely to him and enjoy having him around. The staff is enthusiastic about having him here. Having a pet helps to deinstitutionalize the place."

Pets furnish an avenue for the important emotional interchange between therapist and patient, a relationship that is essential if the patient is to be helped.

"When a child has problems serious enough to require therapy," Dr. Levinson says, "it is difficult to make contact with him and win his trust and confidence.

"Disturbed children have a strong need for physical contact, but are afraid of human contacts because they have been hurt so much and so often by people. Since the hurt is not associated with the dog, the conflict resolves itself. They will permit a dog to approach them, and they will pet the animal while telling him all about their difficulties.

"Jingles has been a great help to me in this regard. As therapy progresses, a patient will extend to me his new-found confidence and affection for my dog."

Dr. Levinson also points out that, for the therapist experienced in the use of pets, they can provide a vital source of clues and insights into human personality disturbances.

"Sometimes my cat sneaks surreptitiously into the office," he writes in *Pet-Oriented Child Psychotherapy,* "and jumps on the desk while the examination is proceeding. When the cat snuggles next to the patient, stretches her neck out, languidly lies on her back and is obviously asking to be petted, the child's response or lack of response may be symptomatic of a personality disorder.

"What is even more startling," he observes, "is the way in which the changes in a patient's relationship to a pet generally coincide with an increasing ability to handle his other problems."

### How Tom's Problem Was Discovered

Diagnosing a child's problem by observing interaction with a pet has also proved highly successful for Ethel Wolff, Ed.D., a clinical child psychologist in Philadelphia.

She describes her experience with Tom, a fourth grader who hadn't performed a single useful task since he had a tonsillectomy during his first-grade year. He simply sat in school, refusing to do anything. He was promoted solely on age, although his teachers suspected he knew the work.

His parents took him to the clinic, thinking he might be retarded. There, the psychologists concluded Tom was deeply angry, but because he repressed his inner rage and gave no indication of its cause, they were making little progress.

The breakthrough came when Dr. Wolff's collie, Chief, had an ear operation. Reluctant to leave him alone for fear he might scratch the bandage off, Dr. Wolff took the dog to her office.

Tom remembered Chief from school programs where the dog had performed magic tricks. When he saw the dog's bandaged head, Tom was immediately sympathetic. "It's too bad Chief isn't going to do any more tricks," he said.

"But why wouldn't he?" Dr. Wolff asked.

"Well, you bossy, bossy thing," the child replied, "you let those doctors and nurses touch him, you let him be operated on, you weren't there. And when he came home, you took him to his grandmother's; you didn't care what happened to him."

A few more questions, and the rest of what the psychologist needed to know poured out:

"You can tell Chief, 'Get dressed, brush your hair, go to school, eat your supper, get washed, go to bed.' You can make him do all those things, but you can never make him work again. He's going to show *you,* bossy, bossy."

This was Tom's impression of what had happened to him as a first grader, when his tonsils were removed. Dr. Wolff found he had been taken to his grandmother's so his active brothers and sisters wouldn't bother him while he recovered.

Dr. Wolff had Tom help her teach the dog a new trick, using treats as a reward for performing. The boy soon realized that Chief's motivation was his own pleasure in the reward—not to perform would be self-defeating for the dog, depriving only himself.

Tom made the connection between Chief's behavior and his own. The next time he came in, he was flourishing a paper with an "A" on it. At the end of the year, he was near the top of his class.

The first structured study of using dogs as an adjunct to psychotherapy was conducted at Ohio State University's psychiatric hospital.

There, Samuel A. Corson, Ph.D., professor of psychiatry and bio-physics, his wife Elizabeth, and psychiatrist P. H. Gwynne based their "pet-facilitated psychotherapy" on Dr. Levinson's recommenda-tion for "highly imaginative and extremely rigorous research" on the subject.

They chose 30 patients who had failed to respond favorably to traditional treatment, including individual and group psychotherapy, electroshock, drugs, and occupational and recreational therapy.

"We selected the patients who were withdrawn, self-centered, and uncommunicative; many were almost mute and psychologically bedridden. They lacked self-esteem and exhibited infantile helpless-ness and dependence," Dr. Corson noted.

Two of the 30 patients did not accept the pets at their disposal. ("Either they didn't like dogs, or they didn't like *our* dogs," Dr. Corson commented.) Results with the remaining 28 ranged from highly encouraging to dramatic. Five patients who were studied in depth exhibited "marked and sustained improvement."

## Pet Must Be Selected Carefully

But just any dog will not do, Dr. Corson emphasizes. They have to be matched carefully with the patients. "Dogs have a diversity of personalities," he says. "A reticent dog, for example, would only strengthen the negative feelings of a paranoiac patient. He might say to himself, 'See, even animals don't like me.' "

This caution is echoed by many other psychiatrists. Dr. John D. Beck, veterinarian and former director of the Ellen Prince Speyer Animal Hospital in New York City, says only an expert should select a pet for a child that is ill. "The wrong pet might make a sick person more sick and a nervous person more nervous," he asserts.

Dr. Levinson stresses this same precaution many times in his book. He states that merely assigning pets to emotionally disturbed children without psychotherapeutic supervision can be harmful. For example, playing alone with a pet may reinforce a child's withdrawal, making him solely dependent on the animal for companionship. Equally serious would be allowing a child to harm a pet, resulting in "severe guilt feelings as well as fear and anxiety" lest there be retaliation.

He also points out that placement of a pet must be done gradu-ally and with careful preparation, whether in a family undergoing

therapy or in a residential treatment center. Otherwise, "the introduction of pets may boomerang," he declares.

## Helping Education

One of the major problems in teaching disturbed children is
their lack of interest in subject matter and the difficulty of motivating
them to learn. A pet that makes education appealing to them can
be of immeasurable help.

At South Valley Elementary School in Moorestown, New Jersey,
Jeanne Rayser uses birds, snakes, and small orphaned wild animals
such as raccoons and opossums to teach her class of perceptually
impaired children.

These are youngsters of normal intelligence who have learning,
perceptual, emotional, and language problems because of minimal
brain damage. Some are unable to distinguish between left and right;
many have poor physical coordination and balance control. These
youngsters often develop severe emotional problems from the sheer
frustration of not being able to deal effectively with their physical disabilities.

Rayser recently brought an orphaned baby robin to class, where
it thrived on a diet of worms, conscientiously dug up by the children
in their yards at home, supplemented by canned dog food.

She has used the robin effectively in many ways. "If you are very
good," she tells a recalcitrant child, "you may have Robbie in your
office." The children vie for this honor, which means the robin shares
with them their quiet study period in one of the room's three cubicles
designed to mitigate distraction from the other restless children.

Rayser also used Robbie for an "experience chart story," a large
poster on which she printed Robbie's history as the children dictated
it. "When words are used in a context the children are interested in,
they are more easily recognized and remembered," she explained. At
her request, one of the boys pointed out the word "caterpillar" in the
story—a real achievement for a perceptually impaired child.

## The Lesson of Love

"Animals make such agreeable friends—they ask no questions,
they pass no criticisms," wrote the 19th century English novelist
George Eliot.

Dr. Levinson adds in *Pets and Human Development* (Charles C.
Thomas, Springfield, Ill., 1972) that animals help to satisfy deep-

rooted psychological needs in people. They bridge the gap between unfeeling, automated civilization and our need to commune with the primeval world that is part of our genetic heritage. They furnish contact comfort, make us feel needed, teach us patience and self-control, kindness and empathy.

Dr. K. Z. Lorenz says in *Man Meets Dog* (Penguin Books, Baltimore, 1965) that in having a pet "the child learns that if you want to be loved, you must love."

At the Children's Psychiatric Hospital where Skeezer is cotherapist, head nurse Williams tells her staff: "Without love, we'd only be patching up, trying to put together with adhesive tape. Love is what children need."

# Phlebitis

Phlebitis, the inflammation of a vein, usually in the leg, is one of the classic diseases of civilization, usually arising from lack of exercise or even complete immobility. Although surgery patients and other people who are confined to bed for long periods are most at risk, anyone who leads a very sedentary life is vulnerable. The danger with phlebitis is that the inflammation will produce a clot which may break loose from the vein, travel through the circulatory system, and lodge in a position where it may block the critical movement of blood. Too often, these clots wind up in the vicinity of the heart or the lungs.

If you are scheduled for surgery and you have a tendency towards phlebitis, you should discuss with the surgeon the steps he plans to take to prevent the formation of a thrombus or a clot. Probably the most common precautionary step is the use of heparin, a drug based on a normal body substance which prevents abnormal clotting. Doctors recently have been successfully experimenting with a device which applies intermittent pressure to the legs of a surgery patient to keep the blood moving, and it seems to work as well as heparin.

Following surgery, elevation and movement of the legs—preferably walking—are advisable as soon as possible. Early "ambulation," as it's called, will not only help protect against phlebitis, but against other circulatory problems and bedsores.

Besides exercise, there are dietary measures that you can take. Alton Ochsner, M.D., Emeritus Professor of Surgery at Tulane University School of Medicine, wrote in an article in the newsletter, *Executive Health,* 1974, that he discovered over a quarter of a century ago that vitamin E in the presence of calcium acts as an antithrombotic agent. "It has the advantage over other anticoagulants that it does not produce a hemorrhagic tendency and can be used safely, prophylactically."

Wilfrid Shute, M.D., one of the great pioneers in vitamin E therapy, has also reported very gratifying results with preventing and reducing phlebitis and the more serious thrombophlebitis in patients. When a patient has thrombophlebitis, Dr. Shute has found that anything less than 600 I.U. daily is inadequate. He says that with 600 I.U. or more daily, results are excellent. Smaller amounts, of course, can be used as a preventive measure or with relatively mild cases of phlebitis.

*Arizona Medicine* (16:100, 1959) carried an article by Dr. R. F. Bock, concluding that postoperative and postchildbirth thrombophlebitis responded well to 1,100 units of vitamin E per day. Usually, Dr. Bock reported, the patient feels better in 12 to 24 hours, while clinical results are apparent in 24 to 48 hours. Vitamin E therapy is also very effective for varicose ulcers, Dr. Bock added.

Many readers have told us of their experiences with vitamin E for phlebitis. One woman said that "Up until 1971 I had so much pain with phlebitis that at one time I was in bed for three months. Then a friend told me about vitamin E, and I have been taking 400 units daily, and now I walk for an hour or more every morning . . . my legs do not bother me now. I will be 70 years old soon."

Another reader, from Canada, said she had suffered for a long time with phlebitis "which eventually broke down and formed an ulcer, which would heal for a while then break open again and again. . . . I had a great area of scar tissue . . . my doctor wanted further surgery and skin graft, which I refused. I engaged a new doctor; he agreed with me that a trial with vitamin E might be of some merit. He put me on 1,600 units a day, plus application externally to the affected area. It was like magic. The ulcers healed, the scar tissue became pliable, no further breakage. The bulgy veins flattened down to normal. I stayed on vitamin E for six weeks under the doctor's supervision. Then I decreased it to 800 units per day for three months. I now continue to take 400 units each day. Never felt better in my life."

In addition to vitamin E, there is some evidence from Britain that vitamin C, in the amount of 1,000 mg. a day, may also be helpful in preventing clot formation in the legs.

# Poetry Therapy*

## by Major Judith C. Wood, USAF, NC †

Poetry therapy is, in my understanding of it, the use of poems in a group setting, to enable patients to work together in understanding and hopefully resolving some problems. Its goals are as the goals of any other group therapy experience; its approaches are unique, and, I feel, successful to a point of value and faith in the process.

The experience of poetry therapy as attempted by myself at Wright-Patterson Air Force Base Medical Center Psychiatry Service was based on the book, *Poetry Therapy* by J. J. Leedy, M.D., published by J. B. Lippincott Co., Philadelphia and Toronto, 1969. Relying on the articles, experiences, and directions included in the above book, my cotherapist and I modified the technique to apply to the Air Force psychiatric setting.

The format of the group held by myself consisted of a small number of patients—six to ten. These patients all had some element of depression as a part of their problem. The group was voluntary and no pressure was used to induce the patients either to join or to attend.

We chose the poem for its mood and tone, so that it would express what the patient might be feeling. We also selected the poem for simplicity of language. We provided one copy of the poem for each patient and therapist in the group. A therapist read the poem, giving attention to mood, rhythm, tone, and content. All of these

---

* The following essay is excerpted with permission from a longer article, "An Experience in Poetry Therapy," by Judith C. Wood, originally published in the *Journal of Psychiatric Nursing and Mental Health Services*, January-February 1975, copyright 1975 by Charles B. Slack, Thorofare, New Jersey.

† Major Judith C. Wood, USAF, NC, graduated from St. Johns School of Nursing, Pittsburgh, Pennsylvania, and at the time of this writing is assistant charge nurse of the Psychiatric Unit at the USAF Hospital, Wiesbaden, Germany.

helped to create an atmosphere in which feelings could be shared and responded to. A group discussion followed the reading of the poem. This lasted for about 45 minutes, involving all the mechanics, actions, reactions, and steady "head" work, and possibly more, which are seen in any group. The conclusion or wrap-up consisted of the patients writing at least four lines of their own, describing feelings about any aspect of the group, their problems, or anything they may formerly not have been able to say. These were then read and discussed by the group.

In the actual groups held at Wright-Patterson Medical Center Psychiatric Service, we averaged six patients per group situation. It was a strictly voluntary group and, surprisingly, no one tried to get out of it; all came faithfully and ready to work. We were two therapists, one male and one female. The age difference between therapists was about 20 years—myself 40, my cotherapist, 21. While initially I chose my cotherapist for his interest, enthusiasm, and general good rapport with all types of patients, the choice turned out to be a good one in many ways. He was able to relate better than I to the younger patients, bringing in aspects of their slang, music, and general outlook on life and the military. He, working on another ward from the one I made my headquarters, selected with much sensitivity additional patients for the group. He was also able to handle any possible physical outbursts. Then, of course, he added the male view, attitude, and feeling to the group. In all, we were able to work very harmoniously and effectively together, striving to, and succeeding in melting into the group so that our guidance was part of the experience and not labored or oppressive.

We kept the atmosphere low keyed and nonpressured, and selected the patients for their similar needs. Our poetry was selected for the depressive type of patient, with, again, the suggestions of Dr. Leedy's book for beginning the program. We later branched out on our own with lesser-known poems, poems by patients, and lyrics to popular songs. But always the poem was selected to create a mood and express what the patient might be feeling. We labored to find those poems which had an uplift, a solution—to avoid the sense of hopelessness. One example of this is "Invictus" by Henley:

> Out of the night that covers me,
>   Black as the pit from pole to pole
> I thank whatever gods there be
>   For my unconquerable soul. . . .

It matters not how strait the gate,
  How charged with punishments the scroll
I am master of my fate,
  I am the captain of my soul!

An example of a poem used in our starting group, with all new patients, is Fra Giovanni's "I Salute You":

I salute you: There is nothing I can give you which you have not got; but there is much, very much, that, while I cannot give it, you can take.

No heaven can come to us unless our hearts find rest in today. Take Heaven! No peace lies in the future which is not hidden in this present little instant. Take Peace!

The gloom of the world is but a shadow. Behind it yet within our reach, is joy. There is radiance and glory in the darkness could we but see, and to see, we have but to look. I beseech you to look.

And so, at this time, I greet you. Not quite as the world sends greetings, but with profound esteem and with prayer that for you now and forever the day breaks, and the shadows flee away.

This poem seemed to state, even in the very first lines, just how we felt about the group, and gave us a chance to get across the concept that they must work on their problems, that there was no magic.

Another poem used was "The Road Not Taken" by Robert Frost. This poem expressed to many patients indecision, or choices they might have faced and been unable to deal with. All of the poems hinted at problems not dealt with on a variety of levels and subjects.

We began the group by reading the poem, then asking the group, "How does it make you feel?" This, our favorite question to elicit response, never failed us. Always, one member would respond, opening the way for others, who all followed eventually. Very seldom did we need to prod even the most quiet, withdrawn, and hopeless feeling person in the group. This, I feel, was of great value in that these patients never got the feeling of being pushed, toyed with, or "scapegoated." The evolution of each group, and finally the whole program, was one of the most natural and least artificial of any I have experienced.

After the initial question to the group as a whole, we might receive responses such as: "It makes me feel sad," or "I get a sense of peace." Any response might be expected, depending on the mood and content of the poem. Some responses were physical, such as crying or obvious agitation shown in body movements. These, of course, had to be followed and worked out in the group. Sometimes individual sessions were held with one of the therapists and a group member after the group.

For the most part, in all our group sessions, problems of all types were able to be handled verbally. Some examples may best be shown in the writings of patients. At the end of each group, 15 minutes were allowed for each patient to write at least four lines of his own. This was also kept on a voluntary basis and not done as an assignment or something to "please the teacher."

Here again, the patients surprised us with their enthusiasm and willingness. Almost none refused to write something. After the writing each patient read his lines to the group and received comments or discussion. Again, there were no put-downs of a member's writing. At times, even the therapists became so involved in the group as to write a few lines in comment.

I would like now to give some examples of patients' writings, (for which I have received verbal permission to quote) and to point out some of the values. Most valuable was the commitment, rapport, sense of helping others, of becoming involved with others, and of working on individual problems.

> People have a bad habit
> of changing your life.
> They begin by telling you when
> to laugh, when to cry.
> Soon after, when to live and
> When to die. Where do you draw the line?
> *Mike*

This patient had much difficulty with his father, in that his life was mapped out, so to speak, for him. He wanted to please his father but had had much difficulty living up to his father's expectations. There was little communication between them, and Mike eventually ended up by taking an overdose of medication in a rather serious suicide attempt. The displacement, hostility, and frustration can be seen in his poem.

Yet, he is able to objectify it enough to put it into words. In the discussion following, he gained insight in that he realized that it was his father to whom he was directing this. He also received support from others who had felt this way. He learned that he was not alone, that hostility such as his was not so rare. He also did much more ventilating, and eventually the question came to him: "Was it really necessary to die?"

The next poem was the expression of a young girl who was beginning to realize that she was not alone in some of her feelings and problems.

### SECRETS

All men live in a world separate from mine
They have their secrets, I have mine
Hundreds of secrets new and old
Hundreds never to be told
Everyone is silent to my thoughts, as I am to theirs
But why are these secrets not to be shared?
Is it because you do not want it known
That your secrets are like my own?

*Lou Ann*

Obviously, it would be possible for me to go on and on with examples of the poetry written by patients in the group called Poetry Therapy which we conducted for about 1½ years, but hopefully, these few examples will give a small indication of the depth, scope, and functioning we were able to achieve. It must also be said that the therapists received their therapy. We also received our strokes in the process. Perhaps this little poem by Tom will demonstrate what we, the therapists, got out of it all:

I entered these walls
    weak and small
Yet I walk away
    strong and tall.

*Tom*

I feel that I cannot reiterate enough the honest, down-to-earth hard work which was done by all who participated in our poetry therapy experience. The closeness, willingness, and actual improvement of the patients was a very obvious factor in these groups. Just one more small example may serve to describe the tone of most of our groups: In seeking to help one member, several others said to him that it was as if he were in a canoe heading the wrong way, and that he must turn the canoe around and go "upstream." When he replied: "I can't do it alone." The others said: "But if we all get in the canoe, we can do it together."

It still amazes me a little that while these groups were held in the evenings, three nights a week, and were voluntary, rarely did anyone miss a group to go out on pass. What we were able to accomplish was also somewhat demonstrated by some who were discharged in the area, who asked, and were welcomed, to come back to the groups.

I feel I must again give credit and thanks to Dr. J. J. Leedy, whose book *Poetry Therapy* was, for a time, our bible. I must also credit my cotherapist, Kelly Champagne, for helping to make it work, and become a learning experience for us all, at Wright-Patterson. Then, of course, the patients, who "looked together through a new window," and saw that it worked.

> **Author's Note:** The author has asked me to include notice that the opinions in her article are hers and do not represent those of the Air Force. Protocol, you know.

# Poison Ivy

With a bad case of poison ivy, the first thing that you should do is to give a good strong laundering to any clothing that was exposed to this plant. That may include your stockings, and maybe your bed clothing and sheets as well.

The classic herbal remedy for poison ivy is jewelweed, also called touch-me-not because of the seed pods that explode when touched in the fall. This member of the *Impatiens* family has small orange flowers and leaves that gleam like mercury when held under water. Jewelweed juice squeezed on to the blisters has a soothing effect and helps the blisters dry up quickly.

One reader told us that when he crushed some of the plant and rubbed the juice all over where his granddaughter had been broken out with poison ivy, it was cleared up by the next morning. Before this, he had tried various medicines prescribed by doctors on the girl, but they had not helped much.

Another reader said that she collects large quantities of jewelweed and boils the stems, leaves, and flowers in a covered pot until the water turns a deep orange. She keeps this brew refrigerated until it's needed, and even freezes some which she says "remains potent." To use, she advises, simply swab the affected areas. The sooner you start treatment, the better it works. And it works so fast that it seems like magic, she says.

It would be good if you could buy ointments or potions of jewelweed extract, but I have yet to see them.

Washing the affected area with a baking soda solution and/or applying a baking soda poultice is another favorite remedy. The juice of the aloe vera plant, usually used to treat burns, has also been used with success to stop the itching and blistering of poison ivy. Brown soap allowed to dry on the skin and calamine lotion are two other standbys.

Vitamin E applied directly to the poison ivy may also help. It seems especially good if you have scratched the area raw.

Goldenseal, the herb, may be used, too. One reader told us of very quick and satisfactory results achieved by washing with one teaspoon of goldenseal in a pint of hot water and following up with a tea made by mixing a quarter teaspoon of the herb per cup of hot water. Take this several times a day.

Large doses of vitamin C may also be helpful, some readers have told us, apparently because of the natural antihistamine and detoxifying effects of this vitamin.

# Polyps

I am not familiar with any proven natural therapy for garden-variety nasal polyps. When these small growths begin to block breathing, the usual medical approach is to surgically remove them. One woman told us that she had severe allergies complicated by recurrent polyps which had to be removed over and over again. In her particular case, she found that going on a generally high nutrition diet, which included between 1,000 and 2,000 mg. of vitamin C daily, cleared up the allergy and the polyps. Whether this would work for anyone else, I can't say.

There is, though, some intriguing preliminary information which suggests that high doses of vitamin C can—in some instances—clear up a form of polyps in the colon which are much more serious than nasal polyps.

This information comes from Jerome J. DeCosse, M.D., Ph.D., professor and chairman of surgery at the Medical College of Wisconsin. Dr. DeCosse and his colleagues published their work in *Surgery* (November 1975), and we also interviewed Dr. DeCosse in his offices in Milwaukee.

The condition they investigated was familial polyposis, a relatively rare inherited condition in which numerous polyps erupt in the rectum. If these polyps are not periodically removed, they may become cancerous, so the condition is in some ways similar to a tumor.

Dr. DeCosse told us that his investigations were prompted by the hypothesis that human feces contain carcinogenic materials that reducing agents or antioxidants can protect against. He selected vitamin C because it is a known reducing agent.

In his study, five patients were given 3,000 mg. of vitamin C daily in time-release capsules. These capsules enable a substantial amount of vitamin C to pass through the stomach relatively intact and to come into direct contact with the walls of the intestine and fecal matter.

The results were that the rectal polyps cleared up completely in two patients, partially in two others, and increased slightly in a fifth. This suggests that vitamin C can reduce the need for repeated surgery in patients with this disease. The implications here may be even more important, since they add to the growing evidence that vitamin C can protect against cancerous or precancerous lesions.

# Prickly Heat

Prickly heat ought to be examined in medical schools as a case study of the totally unscientific nature of medical practice. For a layperson, it should be a case study of the apparent total unwillingness of medical "experts" to accept a nutritional therapy for anything other than a deficiency disease, no matter how convincing the evidence may be. Listen to this incredible story:

In the June 1943 issue of the *Journal of Laboratory and Clinical Medicine,* a report appeared in which the use of 1,000 mg. of vitamin C daily was used to clear up prickly heat so severe that pus was oozing from the inflamed areas of the skin.

In 1951, in the *Journal of the American Medical Association* (vol. 145, no. 3), Dr. Robert Stern reported his experiences with prickly heat in the humid jungles of the South Pacific during World War II. The intense itching and burning suffered by the soldiers were driving them crazy. Dr. Stern said he tried every available remedy but nothing worked until he gave soldiers 300 to 500 mg. of vitamin C daily. "The itching cleared and the rash subsided usually within half an hour . . ." he said. After the war, he added, two California doctors tested vitamin C's effectiveness on prickly heat in a hot, *dry* environment. Again, vitamin C did the job, with adults receiving 500 mg. daily and infants weighing eight pounds or less, 100 mg. daily.

Jumping ahead to the next *decade,* we have a report in *Lancet* (June 22, 1968) by Dr. T. C. Hindson, a British military dermatologist serving in Singapore. Dr. Hindson, it seems, had never heard about the previous studies concerning vitamin C and prickly heat. In fact, he admits that he stumbled on the idea when a military officer he had been treating for an intractable case of prickly heat remarked that the condition suddenly disappeared. Questioning revealed that he had been taking one gram of vitamin C a day, not for the prickly heat, of course, but to prevent colds. Dr. Hindson subsequently carried out a double-blind trial involving 30 children who had suffered from prickly heat for *at least* eight weeks. Of 15 children given vitamin C, 10 were completely cured and 4 improved after only two weeks of treatment. Among the other children, who were given dummy medication, only 2 were cured. Finally, all 30 children were then given vitamin C, and two months later, no lesions were found on *any* of the children.

Try asking your dermatologist if there's any connection at all between vitamin C and prickly heat and he or she will probably think that your *head* has been exposed to too much heat. We checked an 800-page book on tropical medicine published after the two earlier studies of vitamin C and prickly heat had been published, and there was no mention of them. In front of me now is a 2,000-page medical reference book, published four years after Dr. Hindson's study appeared in the world's leading medical journal, and the only thing recommended for severe cases of prickly heat is a course of systemic cortisone drugs.

# Prostate Problems

In men over 40, the prostate needs looking after. This may mean a yearly rectal examination. Certainly, if there are any problems with the urinary system, a urologist must be relied upon. It takes careful medical evaluation to determine whether discomfort involves an active infection, an inflammation where infection is not present, or even cancer.

The most frequent problems do not involve active infections

or progressive diseases, but rather inflammation or enlargement of the gland, which interferes with urination and intercourse. Digital massage of the gland by a doctor's gloved finger often brings temporary relief, and this must be considered a good conservative measure in many cases.

There is some evidence indicating that supplements of zinc may help prostate problems not involving infection or other serious abnormalities. The importance of zinc to the prostate is reflected in the fact that this gland contains a concentration of zinc some 10 times greater than most other organs of the body. In any event, Dr. Irving M. Bush and colleagues at the Center for the Study of Prostatic Diseases at Cook County Hospital in Chicago, and a number of other institutions, found that daily supplements of zinc ranging from 50 to 100 mg. a day improved or abolished symptoms in the majority of men complaining of chronic prostatitis (without infection) or benign prostatic enlargement. Their results, although written up in the early seventies, have not to my knowledge been published in a journal, and they must still be regarded as suggestive rather than definitive.

The use of pollen for chronic prostatitis would appear even more controversial than the use of zinc, but a substantial number of articles reporting good responses have been published, although not in American or British journals. One such report was written by Gösta Jönsson, M.D., in the *Swedish Medical Journal* (58:2487, 1961). Dr. Jönsson, of the Urological Unit of the University of Lund, Sweden, used a proprietary preparation known as Cernilton. With ten patients who were seen for at least a year, five became largely free of symptoms, and the inflammatory changes of the prostate regressed. No side effects were observed. It was also noticed that results were best when the preparation was taken daily (four tablets) without interruption.

A similar study was reported by Yutaka Saito, M.D., of the Department of Urology at the Nagasaki University School of Medicine (*Clinical and Experimental Medicine,* June 1967). Dr. Saito, using the same pollen preparation on 30 patients diagnosed as suffering from chronic prostatitis, said the treatment was "markedly effective" in 16 cases, "effective" in 13 cases, and ineffective in just one case. No drugs were given, and no side effects were observed. Dr. Saito used a dosage of six tablets a day.

Although Cernilton is basically pollen (largely timothy, maize, and rye), it also contains small amounts of a few other substances said to be microbiological extracts obtained from pollen. Whether other pollen extracts would have a similar effect, I cannot say. And Cernilton, which is manufactured in Sweden, is not to my knowledge available in the United States at present.

# Psoriasis

Thousands of years ago, the Egyptians treated psoriasis by eating an extract of a weed which grows along the Nile River and then exposing the afflicted area to the sun. As we write this, tests are being conducted on a modern version of this old technique. The final results aren't in yet, but if they turn out to be as encouraging as preliminary tests, it will be good news indeed for the millions who suffer with this skin disease.

The new treatment, developed at Harvard Medical School and Massachusetts General Hospital, involves administration of methoxsalen, a derivative of the same Nile River weed the Egyptians used. Methoxsalen is what is known as a photoactive substance, meaning that light—some specific spectrum of light—is necessary before it will do its work. The work in this case is the inhibition of the wild proliferation of skin cells which characterizes psoriasis.

In the past, methoxsalen, as well as other drugs, had been applied directly to the skin, with relatively disappointing results. Sometimes even ultraviolet light was used in conjunction with topical applications, but the results were far from sensational.

The breakthrough came when John A. Parrish, M.D., and Thomas B. Fitzpatrick, M.D., administered methoxsalen *orally* (the way the Egyptians took it) and then exposed their patients to a specially constructed ultraviolet lamp which produces wavelengths of light at the high end of the spectrum, out of the reach of ordinary ultraviolet lamps.

In all 21 persons involved in their pilot study, no more than 20 treatments over a period of three to four weeks were necessary to completely clear the wretched lesions of psoriasis. Subsequently, all of the patients who were able to continue the treatments on an outpatient basis have remained clear of lesions. Nine were unable to continue, but six of them had no recurrences for as long as six months.

A parallel study conducted by a doctor in Vienna used the same technique on 30 patients who had not responded to other therapy, and the disease was completely cleared in 29 (*New England Journal of Medicine,* December 5, 1974).

The fact that methoxsalen is a derivative of the same substance used by the Egyptians thousands of years ago is not the only link with the ancient treatment. The ultraviolet light used by Drs. Parrish and Fitzpatrick ranges in wavelength from 320 to 390 nanometers (nm.), with peak emission at 365 nm. The ultraviolet waves striking the earth in the Middle East, measured at Beersheba, Israel—less than 300 miles from the Nile River—reach peak emission at 370 nm. (*Israel Journal of Medical Sciences,* May 1975).

The fact that the Dead Sea area of Israel is rapidly becoming famous as a healing resort for psoriasis should come as no surprise. At Dead Sea resorts, patients spend weeks soaking up the same long wavelengths of ultraviolet light that ancient psoriasis sufferers enjoyed. Now doctors connected with the resorts are anticipating combining the sunshine with methoxsalen therapy as soon as the latter has been completely tested.

On the nutritional front, I don't know of anything that has been truly tested and found to reliably help psoriasis. From a number of anecdotes we've received from readers, however, it seems that vitamin E applied in ointment form and also taken orally does help some people. The ointment, if purchased commercially, should be very rich in vitamin E. Two people who used it successfully mention that the lotion contained 15,000 I.U. Lecithin taken orally has also been known to help some people.

# Psychotherapy, Natural:
## Freeing Yourself and Others From Habits That Blockade Happiness

**by Barry Bricklin, Ph.D., and Patricia M. Bricklin, Ph.D.***

Is there really such a thing as natural psychotherapy? Or, to put the question another way, is psychotherapy natural?

* Barry Bricklin, Ph.D., and Patricia M. Bricklin, Ph.D., are psychotherapists whose private practice is in Wayne, Pennsylvania, near Philadelphia. They have hosted their own TV and radio programs for several years and published a number of books, dealing primarily with learning problems and marital difficulties.

Evidence that the answer to both questions is a very positive yes comes from the animal world as well as the human.

Elephants help other troubled elephants with body contact and prolonged presence. They characteristically surround and then encourage fallen elephants to get up and join them. If the fallen elephant dies, the supportive elephants remain standing around the fallen one a very long time before moving on.

Dolphins, also, support each other with body contact.

When a monkey who seems depressed and anxious is introduced into an already existing group of monkeys, one from the group will step forward in the role of the apparent therapist. The therapist monkey will hold, caress, and soothe the anxious and depressed newcomer until the latter can join the group. (It is interesting to speculate on why only one monkey steps forward. Perhaps this is the monkey who either has the strongest nurturing or helping instinct to begin with, or else is the one best able to understand the situation. When the other monkeys see that one of their members has already taken the helping role, they do not interfere.)

What about human evidence? There is, first of all, the endocrinologic fact that chemical changes take place within a mother's body following childbirth, fostering maternal, giving responses.

There is also presumptive evidence from brain stimulation studies that the activation of certain centers of the brain leads to friendly, loving behavior. Stimulation of these centers is also thought to suppress aggressiveness.

There is further human evidence in the fact that millions of us each day help others spontaneously and without premeditation, just by general caring and "being-with" behavior.

However, just because there is apparently some deep tendency in us to help others, it is by no means assured that this tendency will always be appropriately released, or that once activated, we will do things properly. We all know how comforting some people can be at times of great stress; others seem only able to make matters worse. But you don't need a degree in counseling or psychology to be able to improve tremendously your ability to help others heal their psychic hurts. With some honest effort, you will not only become much more effective in giving natural therapy at times of great stress but more effective at helping other people break out of chronic, day after day hang-ups that may be making their lives miserable or, at least, crippling their ability to enjoy personal freedom and happiness.

## What Is Psychotherapy All About?

Before giving some guidelines on how to best utilize your innate capacity to help others who are troubled, let's sketch in a picture of what the kind of psychotherapy we're referring to is all about.

Words, just simple, everyday words, are prime therapeutic tools. Words can make you smile, cry, blush, sweat, shiver, feel ecstatic or quake in your boots. Words, in short, affect your emotional state profoundly.

Psychological therapies promote mental health by combining just-right words with exceptionally honest person-to-person relationships.

A shorthand definition of psychological health is "growth-potential." The capacity to grow or change psychologically is a core skill in maintaining mental health, for this is the only way one can avoid crippling impasse situations. Chronic arguments with the spouse, extreme tension, depressive moods, perpetual unhappiness, the use of violence—all of these conditions represent impasse or *blockade points*. The person engaging in such behaviors cannot get beyond them. He or she cannot find new and creative ways to advance past these sticky points and hence cannot find new satisfactions and freedom from tensions.

Mental health is *not* finding "final answers," or the "ultimate" in advice. It is rather gaining the ability to see things in new and rational lights—the capacity to expand awareness across a range of situations.

Good mental health is *not* something that descends from outside. It is not something that mysteriously follows from magical advice given by a psychologist or psychiatrist. *It is something we win for ourselves, learning to make decisions that, for us, are right and on-target.*

The professionally trained therapist uses talk, relationship, massage, and a host of other behavior-changing strategies to help people expand their awarenesses and thereby gain the feedback information they need to make decisions that will be right for them.

Natural psychotherapy occurs when any of us, spontaneously and without thought of immediate personal gain, behave toward another individual in a way that promotes this kind of awareness-expanding growth.

When we are in the presence of naturally therapeutic people, we experience the expansive feelings born of true confidence, true because they are based on what we are *really* thinking and feeling, not on some mask we fearfully wear for the world at large. The true guru makes us whole by returning to us parts of ourselves we had previously disowned. The disowned part may have been assertiveness, liveliness, curiosity, sexual feelings, or any other quality. The natural therapist, then, puts us more in tune with our deep-down, real selves.

When your psyche and your biology are working at their best, you will find it natural and easy to be a good listener, to be supportive and understanding—all without demanding immediate reciprocation or imposing yourself on the recipient of your therapy—i.e., you will not try to pass off preaching, lecturing, advising, or glory seeking as true, giving, listening empathy. *True giving* is very different from the way the French writer Balzac described friendship—a pact whereby someone gives a little in return for which he expects a lot.

To be able to give and to be naturally therapeutic, three conditions must be satisfied. All three involve a harmonious relationship between one's biology and psyche. The giving individual must be relaxed and nondefensive; have her or his own needs satisfied; and have proper vitality.

## Learning to Relax and 'Give'

A feeling of fulfillment is the result of having these conditions met, and only a fulfilled person can truly give. Others may *seem* to give, but there is always some catch or gimmick or demand or unconscious blackmail behind the "giving." In fact, a lot of what is seen in the world as giving is really *manipulation*.

Myra's behavior is a perfect illustration. She makes a big fuss over her husband when he comes home. But in truth, she can hardly wait for him to sit down and listen to her gripes and complaints. She hardly hears what her husband says about his day. Her show of warmth is in reality a demand that he devote hours listening to her. The proof is that on those days when he is unable to reciprocate immediately, she becomes blaming and hostile.

To realize a state of relaxation and the associated position of being nondefensive, *we must learn to air our deep hurts*. This helps us to achieve a psychological state in which we begin to know what we really want and what we want to avoid.

Sometimes our deep hurts need only be voiced and known to ourselves. Sometimes, though, especially if they involve chronic hurting behavior on the part of someone else, they must be voiced to this other person. *The great trick of success here is to learn to avoid blaming the other person when you do air your hurts.*

Remember, you are not retaliating, not settling the score, and not blaming the other person in any way for your hurt—even if you feel sure that he is responsible for it. If you blame him, he is not going to listen to you anyway. He'll immediately go on the defensive. Think of it this way: your aim is to *inform* others so they are *aware* of what's going on. You aren't hurling blame.

If your spouse does not seem to pay attention to you, instead of saying something like: "You selfish person, you never care about me," say, "I feel so alone when you seem distant."

Notice how you focus on *your* feelings, not your mate's actions. In both cases you are *airing* your hurt, but when you do it the second way, you are going to find yourself an audience rather than an opponent!

To really rid yourself of frozen hurts, it is necessary to get beyond the layer of surface anger which so often dominates overt behavior. Behind all surface anger, there are deeper hurts and disappointments.

Take Jack's case. He came to see us because he found himself perpetually angry with his son, Glenn. Glenn, 11 years old, was a nonaggressive youngster who lived in a neighborhood of toughies. When the lad backed away from a fight, Jack became enraged:

"You damn sissy. Get out there and defend yourself or don't come home!"

Jack's wife convinced him he was hurting Glenn and should seek help.

**The Technique of 'Inner Shouting'** ● We taught Jack the trick of "inner shouting." Inner shouting is a process whereby you spontaneously and without prior thought shout to yourself (inside your own head; if you do it out loud you might be carted away). The process works best when combined with body relaxation.

This strategy recognizes the fact that deliberate thinking, e.g., "Now let's see, why do I yell at Glenn?" is the poorest way to expand awareness. If we truly want to find out what we are thinking and feeling at a deep level, we must act spontaneously; we must blurt things out rather than just say them. We have to sneak up on our deep-down feelings, because we have learned to deny them access to awareness. *And we must focus on our hurts or pains or humiliations more than on our angers.* The anger is only the symptom—we want to get at the underlying cause of the problem.

Jack tried this. Here is how he reported his experience:

"The first time I tried it I was stiff, awkward. I yelled, 'I can't stand it, Glenn, when you back away from a fight! You're a sissy!'

"The next time I did it I could begin to see what you were driving at. I could see more of my own fears showing up. I yelled something like, 'Can't you see, Glenn, that everybody will *see* you're a sissy. And don't you realize how people will take advantage of you?'

"But it was the third time I screamed to myself that I started to get down to the real guts of my personality. In fact, I almost began crying at one point. I shouted, 'When you back away it hurts me. I don't want you to have to settle for less in life like I did. I don't want you to be unhappy and cowardly . . . like I was. I love you so much. I can't stand to see you humiliated.' This is where I cried— when I realized how much I loved Glenn and how much I couldn't stand his humiliation.

"On other occasions when I've shouted to myself I recognized how much *I* fear being humiliated, and how much *I* fear I'm really weak. Also, that having a weak son may be evidence I'm weak. That's one of the main reasons I can't stand seeing Glenn back down."

We taught Jack that it would be helpful not only to air these hurts to himself but also to Glenn. He proceeded to tell Glenn how his yelling came from his deep fears and embarrassments and, most importantly from his love. This, of course, helped Glenn enormously.

## Learn What You Really Want

The second step in achieving a state of fulfillment and therefore the ability to give in a therapeutic way involves having your own needs satisfied. This means you must first recognize what you truly want. Again, deep body relaxation and feeling-talk or inner shouting can help. The more you pinpoint what you want, the more you can go after it. What we want is not always obvious.

Larry's experience is revealing. Even as a youngster, he was interested in art. Early in his career he fell under the spell of a famous teacher who impressed him tremendously. Without realizing it, Larry swallowed all his teacher's ideas on the subject, even though many of them were quite different from his own. Larry had liked the arts of all lands, the classical styles of early Greece and the Renaissance, the gingerbread, goblins-and-elves style of parts of Germany, the excitements and colors of the impressionists, the bizarre doodads of the surrealists. His famous teacher liked classical forms only and taught that all else was distortion and fraud.

For years, Larry tried to live his teacher's way. He would tell his friends that only early Greek and certain Renaissance artists were worthwhile, that his friends were wasting their time visiting countries or museums not richly endowed with the "classics." At the same time, Larry denied himself the rich banquet table of selections the world had to offer in the realm of art and architecture.

His veneration for the famous teacher, coupled with an intense desire to be liked by this teacher, had blinded him to his true, deep-down feelings.

Larry consulted us because of stomach pains for which no medical treatment was effective. As things turned out, they represented his psychophysiologic reaction to trying to "swallow" a group of ideas wrong for him. (The body will frequently act out mental conflicts in this way.)

Helped to be more free, open, and confident with body relaxation and inner shouting, Larry perceived that he had been living a lie. Once he realized he did not need the loving adoration of his teacher, and that he was trying to live, feel, and think in a way he couldn't digest, not only did his stomach pains clear up, but he rediscovered his own true desires—that he wanted to enjoy the contributions of all artists and countries, not just a few.

Larry's case illustrates how discovering what we want can be a gradual process. But it is also—or should be—a process that goes on as long as we live, since our interests and values may constantly change. The healthier we are, the more easily we know that which we seek. Ideal health implies almost immediate awareness of likes and dislikes, loves and hates, what's good for us and what's bad for us. An ideally healthy person would not have sought to be completely loyal to a teacher by swallowing ideas wrong for himself, and hence would not have gotten into Larry's position. He would have recognized right away that famous or not, some of the teacher's ideas were indigestible.

Let us emphasize that when we say an ideally healthy person

knows what he wants, we do not mean he or she will necessarily want some certain thing forever. We mean that the healthy person, *at any given point in time,* will more or less know what is wanted. And even more importantly, we do not mean that everything the healthy person wants will necessarily be good for him. No one, healthy or not, can be right all the time. Truth, in the sense of knowing what you want, is learned gradually.

The healthy person does not vow to be right—*he vows rather to remain open and responsive to feedback information as it accumulates, so he can gradually focus in on what's right, keeping what's good, and getting rid of what's bad.* When the healthy person gets something originally wanted but ultimately not right, he tries over again, until things feel on-target.

**Frustration Is Not Automatic** ● Let us assume, then, that you are learning how to pinpoint what you deeply and truly want. Two possibilities now exist. Either you will get what you desire and your feelings of fulfillment will increase, or you will not. In the latter case, you must decide if you can change the situation by pursuing your goals more vigorously. If not, if that which you want is really beyond your reach, then you must flexibly change your goals and settle for something else. You can aid this process by learning not to build unfulfilled desires into catastrophes. *Remember, frustration is not automatic. We talk ourselves into feeling frustrated by inward catastrophizing.*

Take the man who does not get the seats he requested for a sporting event. This particular fellow ends up feeling frustrated and angry. As psychologist Albert Ellis reminds us, such feelings do not follow automatically upon the happening of an external event, but rather from what we quickly and persistently (and, usually unknowingly) tell ourselves *after* the event. In the case of our man who did not get the tickets he wanted, the messages that flashed through his mind were: "I can't stand it when I don't get what I want. I *should* get what I want. I deserve what I want!" He thus "catastrophizes" himself into a snit and denies himself the flexibility of readjusting his goals.

People who over their lives have already accumulated a collection of irrational, "I-demand-to-have" beliefs, will be more prone to frustrate themselves over unfulfilled desires than will others. A person who deep down inside harbors beliefs similar to those that follow would be a likely candidate for both a low boiling point and an inability to flexibly shift goals:

"Nothing good ever happens to me."

"I'm never good at getting things done."

"I *should* get what I want so long as I'm nice to people."

"I should be able to please others if I try hard enough."

"I never should really say 'no' to anyone."

"No one should every really say 'no' to me."

When you think over whether or not you have such beliefs, go slowly—for these are deep-down attitudes which rarely focus squarely in the center of awareness. Take a long hard look not only at your feelings as you know them, but look also at your typical actions, to see if they have the flavor of these beliefs.

The irrational beliefs would be working behind the scenes, pulling the strings of your feelings and actions, but not showing themselves in any up-front, direct way. If you frustrate easily, chances are you harbor attitudes similar to those listed.

People whose personalities are riddled with such beliefs go around unconsciously making bitter demands on themselves as well as on others. They are perpetually frustrated, because reality so frequently cannot deliver that which they *think* they need.

## You Must Have Adequate Vitality

The third step toward fulfillment and the ability to give involves having proper vitality. This factor is overlooked not only among laypeople, but also among physicians and psychologists. A person who lacks vitality feels frequently depressed and drained. A person who feels "down" is certainly not going to have much to give to others.

In our opinions, a good many of the people currently receiving psychological help only, are in fact suffering from a host of subtle problems involving poor nutrition and a lack of exercise and rest. The trouble is that "depletion" conditions are often only noticed at extremes; their roles at intermediate levels go undiagnosed and untreated. For example, if an individual has chronic and severe low blood sugar (most cases of which can be controlled by proper diet), his ailing state will be obvious. In addition to suffering a host of minor complaints, he is apt to feel exceedingly tired and depressed.

But what about the individual whose blood sugar level varies only occasionally and never really drops tremendously low? She or he is apt to feel "blue" rather than severely depressed, mildly tense rather than panicky, tired rather than extremely fatigued, put-off by people rather than enraged by them. This person—and her or his physician—are *not* likely to think of low blood sugar as the cause of the difficulties. She or he is more likely to be labeled "neurotic" or "nervous." Too bad, because proper nutrition would be as helpful, if not more helpful, than psychological help alone.

At any rate, proper vitality is a necessary condition to feeling fulfilled and hence of being in the mood to give to others. Pay attention to your diet, to exercise, and to getting adequate rest. If you neglect these factors you are paying a much higher price than you realize (and probably attributing your difficulties to "nerves").

Hopefully, you have now scaled the three steps that will release your capacity to act therapeutically. By engaging in spontaneous feeling talk, and by choosing your external environments, including foods, wisely, you have learned how better to relax and be non-defensive, satisfy your own needs, and increase your vitality.

Feeling more fulfilled, you are prepared to act therapeutically toward others. Another way of saying this is that once you have discovered how to be good to yourself, you are ready to be good to others.

## Two Basic Skills in Therapy

There are two core therapeutic skills: effective listening and reflective communication. In order to listen, one must overcome a number of rather powerful desires—and the more one feels unfulfilled, the more intense these desires will be.

(Most of the people who *think* they are listening in fact are interrupting, preaching, moralizing, bragging, giving superficial reassurances, and/or otherwise dispensing Earnest Advice. The troubled person, on the other hand, really needs to be *listened to*, and none of these activities has anything to do with listening. When we should be listening, we are often preparing our next statements. The majority of conversations are really double monologues. Person B waits for A to pause for breath, and when she does, B relaunches his own thing.)

Reflective communication is any talk or gesture or attitude that helps another person clarify what he is really thinking and feeling at a given moment, in the depths of his guts.

Listening and reflective communication both foster independence, as they offer a symbolic hand-on-the-shoulder closeness and support. They aid the recipient to clarify, in stages, his or her own thoughts and feelings, and hence expand awareness and grow.

**How to Be an Effective Listener** • Listening, though seemingly simple, is one of the most beneficially powerful things one human can do for another. The sad thing is that so few of us do it well.

The most common mistakes we make when people tell us their troubles are (1) to assume *we* should solve them; (2) to tell what *we* would do under the same circumstances; and/or (3) to pooh-pooh the problem, by saying, for example, "Oh, that's not so bad, wait till you hear what happened to me!"

Troubled people do not really want *your* solutions, even though they may often think they do, nor do they really care what *you* would do in a similar case. And they certainly don't want to be told that their problems are nothing while yours are stupendously worse.

What they really require is empathy—the knowledge that you care—and a good sounding board against which they can work out their own solutions.

It is tremendously helpful for a person to feel she or he is being understood. We should never underestimate the psychological healing power in this. When you listen to someone you are doing a number of important things for that person. You are, first of all, showing that you care. You, so to speak, have a hand on his shoulder and are encouraging him to face up to the problem secure in the knowledge that he has a supporter behind him, someone who not only cares but who has faith that the problem will be solved. You are helping him to feel less lonely, less isolated. He is not facing the stress all by himself.

**An Example of Therapeutic Listening** • Many years ago, when the oldest of our four children, Brian, was 1½ years old, we found ourselves in the midst of a serious encephalitis epidemic in which many people died. The initial warning symptom was a rapid elevation in body temperature. One day Brian's temperature shot up to 105°F. We were alarmed. An accurate but exceedingly unhelpful and nonpsychologically oriented general practitioner came to examine him. His great words of wisdom, said sarcastically, were "What are you so worried about? Statistically speaking it's probably not encephalitis."

He was telling us we were stupid to be concerned (and making, by the way, error number 3, pooh-poohing someone else's worries). Additionally, he was making error numbers 1 and 2, implying that if we were he, we would not be worried.

Scientifically, this doctor was doing nothing wrong or unethical. There was no way (within the realm of reason) he could make a more positive diagnosis. And his statistics were right: encephalitis was a long shot. There was nothing of much scientific value that he could tell us at that point. Other friends and relatives in the house at the time agreed with him; don't worry, it's not encephalitis.

But from a grandfather we were to learn that day something that would not only help us at the time, but would provide the groundwork for our later understanding of the tremendous healing powers in empathy, understanding, and good listening.

He let us talk to him of our fear and worry. He said nothing. He did not pooh-pooh our fear. He did not tell us, "What are you worried about?" He did not tell us what he had done under similar circumstances (he had nursed two of his six children through deadly epidemics, all without modern antibiotics). He did not seek to console us with superficial reassurances.

When we were talked out, he simply put his hands on our shoulders and quietly said: "Sometimes it's very hard to be a parent."

We immediately felt a good bit better. Why? He didn't help Brian (who, luckily, did not have encephalitis). He did not really solve anything. He gave no advice. But he did something the importance of which we were to understand formally only years later, as more mature psychologists: he let us know that he understood and cared about the pain and fear we were experiencing. He did not use the occasion as an opportunity to glorify himself (by telling us how he acted on a similar occasion), he did not make us feel even more inferior (by pointing out that he had nursed extremely ill children through far worse crises), and he did not try to dismiss the problem (by the old what-are-you-worrying-about trick). He verbally and physically put his hands on our shoulders and showed us that he shared our pain, that he understood what we were going through.

**Helping Others Heal Themselves With Reflective Communication** ●
You are engaging in reflective communication any time you do or say something in such a way as to afford someone else a chance to look at his or her own behavior in a gentle, neutral way, just as a

mirror would. The communication may be an understanding grunt, a shaking of the head in an I-understand-what-you're-saying way, or, what is probably best, a simple restating of what the other person has just said.

Reflective communication (a) encourages personal responsibility, but at the same time makes responsibilities and decisions, by its implicit hand-on-the-shoulder emotional tone, seem less threatening; (b) shows the other person you trust her to solve her own problems; (c) facilitates the ability to see things in new lights; and (d) because of its mirrorlike nature, promotes insight into self-defeating behavior patterns.

Reflective communication takes advantage of the fact that even though people often act as though they want advice and will frequently seem to take it, in reality they usually only change their behavior *permanently* when they have discovered or come upon the altered thinking or acting on their own.

In instances where people solve problems by taking the advice of others, they lose more than they gain. They are merely increasing their infantile dependence; that is, convincing themselves ever anew that safety and security reside in being able to manipulate others into taking over.

The technique of reflective communication may be summed up as follows: when someone passes the psychological buck to you, you gently and neutrally pass it back.

Sally (irritably): "My husband never picks up after himself."
Here are some "wrong" responses:

"I would never let my husband get away with that!"
"Why don't you yell at him!"
"Men are jerks anyhow!"
"Oh, isn't that a shame."

The first response is a brag; the second, useless advice in which the giver assumes she is better able than Sally to know how to handle things; the third, a senseless unhelpful remark in which the speaker, instead of helping, merely reveals her *own* problems; and the fourth, a patronizing put-down.

The "right" response would be a reflective communication:

"It's very annoying when your husband won't pick up after himself."

This seemingly innocuous, almost simpleminded reflection of

the verbal content and emotional tone of Sally's complaint contains much more healing potential than you might realize. In fact, we're certain that when you just read what we considered the "right" response, you said to yourself, "How can merely repeating someone's words help?"

The answer is that such a response addresses itself in a powerful way to the other person's personality.

If stated sincerely, it shows you care.

It shows respect for this other individual's independence and brains.

Its I'm-with-you tone reduces feelings of isolation.

Perhaps most importantly, *it encourages a person to carry his or her thinking one step forward.*

Since it's not a piece of advice, a self-seeking complaint, a brag, a put-down or whatever, *it's open ended. It therefore encourages further confident, self-directed thinking.*

In our example, Sally can now say:

"Yes, and I don't know what to do."

The reflective communicator could then say (as a statement, not a question):

"You feel you've tried *everything* you can think of to solve this problem."

Sally can now really ponder what she has, for one reason or another, refused to deal with:

"Gee, have I in fact really tried *everything?*"

Chances are she hasn't. Perhaps she is merely afraid of assertion. Perhaps she has never learned to consider alternatives. Or perhaps she is severely neurotic and inhibited. Actually, it makes no difference what her problem is. The important thing is that the reflective communicator is encouraging Sally to recognize with full clarity what she may only have dimly perceived—that she has options. *In this way, the impasse is broken and growth allowed to go on.* Further, by bringing the whole problem out into the open, Sally will be gently pushed to actually *try* other solutions.

"But wouldn't it," you ask, "have been more helpful to have offered Sally a solution? For example, suppose one of the other people had the experience of having said to her similarly behaving husband, 'Look, you bum, you never pick up after yourself and I'm not cooking you any more meals until you do!' And suppose this worked. Wouldn't it have been more helpful for her to share this advice with Sally rather than merely to have reflected Sally's own thoughts back to her?"

The answer can be given simply: No.

**Troubled People Don't Want Your Advice** ● First, Sally, like almost all complainers or even active advice seekers, *needs confidence more than information.* This can be proven in that if she had had the confidence, she undoubtedly not only would have come across the suggested plan on her own, but would already have either ruled it out as wrong for her or have put it into operation.

Advice giving does not raise, it lowers, confidence.

Second, what works in one family situation can rarely be simplistically transplanted to another. The history of each family and each relationship is unique. What a simple annoyed look does in one situation may do nothing in another. Yelling in one relationship may get results—at least in the short run—but in another, breed bitter retaliatory hostility.

Third, and this is a subtle but extremely important point, people caught in impasse situations can only grow or progress from exactly where they are hung up. Most people fail to help themselves change psychologically because they try to act from where they would *like* to be, rather than from where they are.

To illustrate, Sally is not ready to take a firm stand with her husband. *If she were, she would have. She has not even been able to envision this as a workable possibility.* In fact, Sally has not really recognized that she has *any* options. Here is the exact impasse point. Here is where she is hung up. Here is the point from which she must begin her growth process, no other.

When the reflective communicator leads Sally to the point where she can think to herself, "Gee, have I in fact really tried everything?" Sally is out of her trap. She is moving. And she is starting her journey from the only point she could start from, the true blockade point.

A reflective communication is the behavior pattern with the highest chance of helping a person to grow from his exact impasse point. A reflective communication does this because it allows a person to grope around long enough to *find* the blockade point. By not *imposing* a solution, it avoids the risk of asking an individual to start the growth process at point five when the hang-up is at point one.

Advice usually demands that a person do something wrong for him, or that he do something still one or two steps out of his psychological reach.

**Tips on Using Reflective Communication** ● Never phrase them as questions. Suppose a husband, after being informed that some acquaintances, Joe and Margaret Palmer, were coming to dinner, said:
"I can't stand the Palmers!"

The wife thinks she is making a reflective communication by saying (in a true questioning tone):
"You say you can't stand the Palmers?"

If reflective communications are phrased as simple questions, the other person, the husband in this case, would think his wife was either dense or had a hearing loss. He would, of course, not think about what had been reflected. He would either look at his wife as though she was crazy or else merely repeat his initial statement.
"That's right, I can't stand the Palmers!"

In this instance, a useful reflective communication (and the subsequent conversation) might go something like this:
"There's something about the Palmers that is very irritating to you."
"I can't put my finger on it, but I know that I'm uncomfortable when I'm with them."

Notice how the husband is now on his way to discovering what it is about the Palmers that causes him to react negatively.

Notice especially how much more effective the wife's communication has been than if she had responded oh-so typically, "What do you mean you can't stand the Palmers!? They're perfectly nice people!" or "Well, I don't care what you can't stand! I happen to like them, and besides we owe them a dinner!"

In either instance all that would have resulted would have been an argument. By *not* challenging her husband, and by *not* putting forth her own opinion, she allows the conversation, and *her husband's thinking,* to go forward. She ignores the judgmental, angry tone in her husband's voice, and reflects the essence of his sentiment:
"There's something about the Palmers that is very irritating to you."

Because his reaction has not been angrily attacked, the husband is freed of any need to justify himself, which would only have entrenched him even more firmly in his negative position. Because a reflective communication is in essence an invitation to continue one's thinking, the husband can begin pinpointing the cause of his aversion:

"I can't put my finger on it, but I know that I'm uncomfortable when I'm with them."

Note how the husband, with only one reflective communication, has taken a step forward in his thinking. He recognizes that to say he can't stand the Palmers is an excessive, too-inclusive remark. He sees now that there is something about them that makes him *uncomfortable*. This is already a horse of another color, for now he does not have to justify why he cannot stand them, but can—realistically and hence effectively—figure out what it is about them that makes him *uncomfortable*.

The wife continues her reflective communication. Notice how she rephrases her husband's feelings in a way that expands his view of the situation:

"There's something about the Palmers, maybe something in what they typically say or do, that upsets you."

"Yeah. It's more him than her. I don't know, the conversation just doesn't flow with him. Talking to him is an effort. I'm not relaxed when I talk to him."

"When you talk to Joe Palmer you can't be yourself."

"Yes, that's it. I can't be myself. Wait! I have it! It's the way he exaggerates. He embellishes his stories in ways I know are not truthful. And we're supposed to sit there and not blow the whistle on him. And some of what he says, boy, what whoppers. You can't relax and be yourself when you have to hold back your spontaneous reactions. And my reaction is really to say, 'Look Joe, come off it.' And there's also, now that I think about it, subtle prejudices always creeping into his remarks. Nothing blatant, but they're there. It's an effort not to respond to them."

**Where Does It Lead?**  ● Here then, we are almost at the end of a very constructive interchange. The husband, because his wife did not challenge him but instead reflected his thoughts, understands quite clearly what he only dimly perceived before. The wife, too, has profited by the exchange, because she now understands that behind her husband's initial negativism was more than arbitrary grouchiness.

Our husband and wife are at this point free to conclude the episode in a number of ways.

One psychologically legitimate ending might go like this:

Wife: "I understand now why you're uncomfortable with the Palmers. But let me suggest that much of your problem would resolve itself if you *didn't* hold back on your spontaneous feelings. Say what's really on your mind after Joe speaks. Tell him you would appreciate his stories just as much without the exaggerations, and let him know you don't share his prejudices. Not only would this freedom relieve you of the uptight feeling you have when you're with him, but would force the two of you to decide if you could tolerate an honest relationship. If Joe doesn't like you when you're honest, then that's it, the end of your getting together."

Or, she could say:

"Now I appreciate and understand your feelings. Please go along with me this one time, since I like Margaret Palmer so much, and in the future I'll meet her in ways that won't involve you with Joe."

Remember, anything that enables the other individual to see himself in a gentle, emotionally neutral, reflective light will be helpful. Pay strict attention to what is said to you, and try to rephrase it in a way that pinpoints *both* its emotional and verbal content.

For another example, let's go back to the situation of Jack and his son Glenn, the youngster who is fearful of fighting. Previously, his father would yell and blame when Glenn retreated. Later, after learning the technique of spontaneous inner shouting, he was able to pinpoint how his own hurts and fears crippled his ability to "give" to Glenn at these crisis points. Freed of his blockades, he was able to master the art of reflective communication. Here is how it would go.

Glenn comes in the house; he just walked away from a fight. He is silent.

Jack (reflecting Glenn's emotional status and likely thinking): "It's hard and embarrassing to have to walk away from a fight."

Glenn, a little stunned by his father's understanding, still says nothing.

At this point, the interchange, for the time being, is over.

A few weeks later, the same kind of thing happens.

Glenn comes in crying:

"I can't stand these kids around here!"

Before, Dad would have yelled for Glenn to get out there and fight back. Now, realizing his anger was caused by his pain and humiliation and love for Glenn, he was able to say:

"It must be agitating inside when part of you wants so much to hit back but part is still scared."

Note the understanding in the tone of the communications. Note the emphasis, and here is the heart of the matter, on *pinpointing the exact feelings Glenn is experiencing at the moment.* For here is the point from which Glenn must start any journey to increase his confidence.

Jack and Glenn's case is instructive (they are real people). Before long, Glenn, feeling that at last someone understood and accepted him, began to feel more confident. In a few months, although by no means an aggressive toughie, he stood up for himself frequently, and more importantly, could walk away from fights he judged himself unable to win without feeling like a disgusting failure.

**More Tactical Tips** • Continue reflective communications as long as they seem feasible. It the dialogue bogs down, try to figure out what is causing this to happen. The reflective communicator tries to stay exactly where the other person is. If the focus of interest switches from a central theme to something else, the reflective communicator also switches. In the following illustration, the important theme eventually becomes not the original item Amy started out to talk about, but rather her fear of revealing herself.

Amy: "I get nervous when people compliment me."

(Think now of all the wrong things it would be so simple to say here, like "Gee, that's funny." Or, "Hell, I love to get compliments!" Or, patronizingly: "You shouldn't, because you really deserve compliments.")

Instead, the good reflective communicator, let's call her Betty, will say (matter-of-factly):

"You feel uncomfortable when people compliment you."

Amy: "Yes, there's something about them that makes me uncomfortable."

Betty: "You just can't seem to put your finger on what it is, but you know that there is something about them that makes you feel ill at ease."

Amy (beginning to carry her thinking forward, and hence dent the impasse): "I think it has something to do with obligations. Somehow, when people give me compliments, I feel obligated."

Betty: "The feeling of being obligated makes you uptight in some way."

Amy: "Yes, it reminds me of . . ." (her voice trails off at this point).

There is a pause in the conversation. The reflective communicator now says:

"It's hard for you to continue."

Amy: "Yes, a thought just popped into my mind, but I really am embarrassed to say it. I was reminded of another situation in which I didn't know how to handle obligations. But I'm embarrassed to talk about it."

Betty: "Sometimes it's very difficult to share things with other people. We're afraid we'll be rejected or laughed at."

Notice how Betty has abandoned the attempt to track down Amy's feelings about obligations, and instead has switched to the new impasse point, Amy's fear of revealing herself.

This, then, is what the reflective communicator does. He or she tries to stay in step with the friend, holding up a gentle, neutral, I'm-with-you mirror.

Combine this with effective listening and you've put together a one-two therapy that promotes growth and happiness in a mighty powerful way.

## Summary

1. Learn to *air* your hurts in a neutral way. Don't *accuse* or blame the other person; focus exclusively on your own honest feelings. E.g., *don't* say, "You come home late because you can't stand being with me!" Instead say: "When you come home late, it makes me depressed and angry. I feel like you don't love me any more." This opens the door to communication while an angry outburst slams it closed.

2. When you feel terribly angry, use the technique of inner shouting to get in touch with deep-down emotions. Try to relax and spontaneously blurt out what you feel is hurting you. Forget about your anger for the moment; focus on what's *hurting* you.

3. Seek to learn what *you* really want in life, with the help of relaxation and inner shouting.

4. Disappointments are natural; learn not to build them up into catastrophes.
5. Pay attention to diet, exercise, and rest. Physical vitality is essential to psychological health.
6. To help others, first learn to be an effective listener.
7. Then master the powerful technique of reflective communication, to help others grow past a psychological impasse.

# Radiation Poisoning

In the event that you would be exposed to fallout from a nuclear accident, run, do not walk, to the nearest jug of sodium alginate or algin. This natural extract from sea kelp is amazingly effective in ridding the body of radioactive strontium 90.

It isn't that the algin circulates through the body and picks off particles of this radioactive mineral. On the contrary, algin is completely indigestible and never leaves the intestinal tract. What happens is that the strontium 90 circulates through the bloodstream and even in and out of the GI tract. But once it hits the GI tract, the alginate grabs hold of it, binds it, and excretes it with the body wastes.

The research on which these statements is based was carried out at the Gastrointestinal Research Laboratories of McGill University in Montreal, supported by a grant from the Bureau of Radiological Health of the United States Public Health Service. That research was done on mice, not humans, but it was established that algin is from 50 to 80 percent protective against the strontium 90. According to a letter we have from the office of the Division of Biomedical and Environmental Research of the Atomic Energy Commission, maximum protection against radioactive poisoning for humans means a *minimum* intake of 10 grams of alginate a day. That's only about one-third of an ounce, but alginate is very powdery and light so we are talking about several tablespoons. In a real crunch, it would seem advisable to take two generous tablespoons four times a day to insure that there is always an ample amount in all portions of the GI tract. Algin must be taken mixed with sufficient fluids to get it down. Some kind of thick soup is best. If you're using tablets, which usually weigh only half a gram, chew up six to eight and swallow with milk four times a day.

Pectin, which occurs bountifully in apples and certain other fruits, also has a propensity to bind radioactive strontium and carry it out of the system. If you cannot get alginate, use a lot of pectin. If you have access to apples, grate or mash two or three of them and eat three or four times a day. If using pectin tablets, chew up and swallow a dozen of them three or four times daily.

In the absence of either algin or pectin, chew up three or four calcium or dolomite (calcium plus magnesium) tablets about four times a day. Calcium and magnesium, like algin and pectin, tend to bind strontium 90 and remove it from the system.

Finally, generous amounts of brewer's yeast should be taken.

## Help for the Radiation Patient

There is another kind of radiation poisoning, which follows therapeutic X-ray treatment. Until very recently, it was believed by many doctors that when a tumor is being treated by X-rays, the patient should be more or less starved. The theory was that a tumor, because of its rapid growth rate, required more nutrients than other parts of the body. So starve the body and you starve the tumor. Unfortunately, it's now been shown that the typical result of this approach is that many patients become so malnourished that they rapidly succumb from massive infections. The evidence also sharply contradicts the theory that good nutrition for the patient with cancer will cause increased growth of the tumor. Dr. Edward M. Copeland and Dr. Stanley J. Dudrick, both of Houston, told the 1975 Clinical Congress of the American College of Surgeons held in San Francisco that running the full range of nutrients into a cancer patient's blood does *not* stimulate the growth of the cancer but rather makes the patient stronger and better able to recover. Even in cases where the patient is beyond help, the better nutrition makes his last days more comfortable.

It appears there may be a number of nutrients that can specifically help the patient who has been rendered weak and nauseous by repeated doses of radiation. At least, there is evidence of this in animals. Dr. Boris Sokoloff and associates at the Florida Southern College at Lakeland, Florida, tested various vitamin P (bioflavonoid) compounds on rats and found that death resulting from X-ray was reduced to 10 percent in the group of rats receiving the vitamin P, as against a death rate of 80 percent in other rats. The authors suggested in the *Journal of Clinical Investigation* (April 1951) that the vitamin seems to help by protecting the capillaries and intercellular cement.

Pantothenic acid, the B vitamin so important in all states of stress, may also be helpful. Dr. I. Szorady of Hungary reported in *Acta Paediatrica* (IV:1, 1963) that mice who are given pantothenate and then exposed to heavy radiation had a survival time twice as long as those who weren't supplemented before exposure.

H. Mattie and associates wrote in the *British Medical Journal* (July 1967) that giving vitamin $B_6$ to patients suffering loss of appetite, nausea, and a general feeling of sickness after exposure to therapeutic radiation was remarkably effective in reducing symptoms.

The most recent study I have come across was published in a German medical journal concerned with therapeutic radiation and indicates that bee pollen may be quite helpful in reducing side effects. The article was published in *Strahlentherapie* [Radiotherapy] (150, 5:500-506, 1975), written by P. Hernuss and colleagues, who are associated with several radiological clinics and universities in Germany.

The patients were 25 women with inoperable cancer of the uterine neck, who were given a combined radium and cobalt 60 therapy. Ten of the patients served as a control group, receiving only radiation, while 15 others were also given 20 grams (about three-quarters of an ounce) of pollen three times a day throughout the duration of the radiotherapy. The authors note that the pollen came from France and was collected in pollen traps which removed the material from the rear legs of bees.

A number of blood tests calculated to measure the various indices of general health revealed that the women who took the pollen were considerably better off. There was, for instance, an increase in whole blood cells, serum protein, and gamma globulins.

Subjectively, the patients were also helped. Compared to the women who did not receive the pollen, those who did experienced only half as much nausea, less than one-fifth as much poor appetite, half as many sleep disorders, less than half as much inflammation in the urinary and rectal areas, and just one-third as much worsening of general condition.

"The function and the mechanism of action of pollen is essentially unexplained up to the present," the authors state (we had the article translated from the German), but also declare that "In summary, a good tolerance and favorable influence of the pollen diet as an adjuvant to radiotherapy in female genital carcinoma was found. According to the present results, there is a justification to use this therapy and to look for further clarification of the mechanism of action of this natural curative agent."

For physicians who may be interested, the source of the pollen was the company of E. Hagen, Freilassing, Federal Republic of Germany.

# Reflexology (Zone Therapy)

Reflexology is a very specialized form of massage which, its advocates claim, is able to restore normalcy of function and give relief from pain to virtually any part of the body. Little or no attention has been paid to this therapy by serious investigators, but lately there has been some interest in it, due entirely to the growing popularity of the related therapy of acupuncture.

The two basic modes of this therapy are foot reflexology, which is probably the best known, and hand reflexology. Together, they are also known as zone therapy. This art has had a rather strange history, the term zone therapy having been coined by Edwin F. Bowers, M.D., some 75 years ago. Shortly thereafter, it was further popularized and systematized by William H. FitzGerald, M.D. In the twenties and thirties, it seems to have been taken up with some eagerness by naturopaths, although these practitioners had so many different modes of therapy at their disposal, ranging from phyto-therapy (herbs) to heliotherapy (sunshine) that they do not seem to have been particularly excited about reflexology.

The art was then taken up by a masseuse, Eunice Ingham, who developed what she called the Ingham Reflex Method of Compression Massage, whose principles she elucidated in a number of privately printed books. Her students and followers set themselves up as "foot reflexologists" and a handful of them still practice in relative obscurity.

The peculiar thing about reflexology is not that it might work, but that there is no good reason why it should *not* work. At least, anyone who has read the numerous reports on ear acupuncture would probably feel this way.

In ear acupuncture, or auriculotherapy, there is the assumption that on the outer surface of the ear there exist points which are connected to many other points on and *in* the human body. In fact, these points on the ear are distributed in a pattern which reflects the shape of the human *fetus in situ*. In other words, the lobe of the ear approximately represents the head. As you move up the ear, you reach points of the body which are closer to the feet. However peculiar this may sound, the fact is that top Oriental and Western practitioners of acupuncture have used ear acupuncture with what they claim to be gratifying success.

In reflexology, or zone therapy, the bottom of the feet, rather than the ears, is believed to contain points connected to all other parts of the body.

Imagine that someone is lying on a table in front of you, face up, with his feet together. As you look at his feet, imagine that both of them, put together, are a "map" of the body in which the toes represent the head area, the ball of the feet the solar plexus area, the arch of the feet the intestines, and so on. You are now seeing things the way a zone therapist does.

Let's say you have a headache. The thing to do is vigorously massage the fleshy underpart of the big toe. Do you have an earache? Move over to the third toe, drop down an inch, and rub like the dickens. (If it's your right ear that hurts, rub your right foot.) Backache? The inner part of the arch on both feet represents the spine, so massage there, a few inches up from the heel. Very basically, this is how a reflexologist goes about his business.

I have heard one or two doctors say that they have been able to achieve some success using foot reflexology, but that is not much to go by. I personally don't know anyone who has been treated by a reflexologist, although in a newspaper account which I read sometime ago, the writer did admit that one definite result of treatment was that his feet were very sore. This would not bother practitioners, however, since they believe a sore point on the foot is only an indication that some other part of your body is ill. In fact, one method of locating the right point to massage is to apply strong pressure to various portions of your foot until you find a point that hurts. You are then supposed to begin rubbing and "work out the tenderness."

## Do You Know What You're Rubbing?

Although it may sound paradoxical to apply strong pressure to a point on your foot that hurts, that is exactly what the usual home treatment is for ordinary aching feet. And this is also, in my opinion, why it is extraordinarily difficult to prove or disprove anything about reflexology on your own. What I mean is this:

Let's say you come home after a tiring day and the ball of your foot, the metatarsal area, aches. Most of us would assume that the ache is there because the way shoes are constructed, particularly shoes with high heels, tremendous pressure is exerted on the ball of the foot with every step you take. So you rub this area—or even better, get someone else to rub it—and gradually, the tightness and the aching are relieved as muscles and other structures are stretched, relaxed, and bathed with a brisk flow of blood. Soon, your whole body feels much better.

But a reflexologist would take a completely different view of what you've done. After a hectic day, he or she would say, your heart is tired, your nerves are frazzled, and perhaps from smoking or pollution, your lungs also need help. And these are exactly the organs you stimulate when massaging the ball of your foot!

Maybe the arches of your feet ache when you come home, so you rub them. The reflexologist would say that it isn't so much that you are wearing improper shoes which cause arch strain, but that your intestines aren't working very well, and by massaging the arch area, you gradually feel better because your bowels feel better.

In any case, with personal experimentation and the experiences of acquaintances, I cannot say that I have found any of the principles of foot reflexology to be helpful to any specific body part. On the other hand, I must admit that, personally, I find nothing so totally relaxing and invigorating as a brisk massage of the *entire* foot.

Until just recently, most of the books that were available on reflexology were not very helpful and amounted to little more than glorification of the author. Now, I know of two books which at least explain reflexology sufficiently so that if you want to give it a try, you will be able to understand just how to go about it. One is a paperback book, *Zone Therapy,* by Anika Bergson and Vladimir Tuchack (Pinnacle Books, New York, 1974) and another is *Hand Reflexology* by Mildred Carter (Parker, West Nyack, New York,

1975). I should mention that in the Carter book a technique is described whereby clamps are affixed to the fingers to maintain pressure, and this technique, it seems to me, could have very deleterious effects on someone with poor peripheral circulation.

# Relaxation Therapy

Have you worried about a recurrent abdominal pain, had it checked by your doctor and been told it's not appendicitis, not cancer, not diverticulitis, but probably a spastic colon?

Do you wonder why your jaw or face muscles hurt? And perhaps your ears and neck as well?

Are you troubled by diarrhea for which neither you nor your doctor can find a cause or cure?

On a busy day with many obligations, do you feel your head begin to pound as tensions pile up?

Do thoughts of your daily obligations and omissions dart around in your mind when you go to bed, make you restless, tight, and weary but not sleepy?

These and many other conditions—including pain originally misdiagnosed as arthritis—are now yielding to drugless therapy at the Pain Control Center at the University of Pennsylvania in Philadelphia. There, Dr. Arnold Gessel told us, both physicians and patients have learned that many of the aches, pains, and discomforts of living can be caused by unconscious, chronic muscle tensing. More important, by learning how to relax in a scientific manner, many people are finding that when they learn how to turn off their unconscious "tension switch," their symptoms are also turned off. And they're doing it without painkillers, drugs, surgery, or psychotherapy.

The preventive implications are even more striking. Serious diseases which are believed to be caused by or related to tension include high blood pressure, heart attacks, gastric ulcers, and back muscle deterioration—the kind that can lead to "slipped disk" and spinal fusion operations. Learning how to be untense is a health measure to forestall such developments.

A typical case history: A patient came to Dr. Gessel complaining that his jaws ached so much he could not even comfortably chew his food. (This condition, known as masticatory pain dysfunction syndrome, or MPD, afflicts an estimated two million Americans, Dr. Gessel said. If left untreated, it can force a patient to go on a liquid diet, with serious weight loss occurring after a time.) But this patient, *typically,* had a number of other problems—seemingly unrelated to the muscle ache in his jaw. Alternating constipation and diarrhea were so severe they left him with pus in the lower abdomen. Although he had sought medical help for these problems, his prescribed medication had not given him much relief.

Dr. Gessel treated the patient mainly for the clenched jaw condition, but simultaneously with relaxation in this area, the man's colon symptoms also subsided, and disappeared eventually.

This was no coincidence, either, because Dr. Gessel has repeatedly observed that when muscles in one area are trained to relax, muscles in other areas also relax at the same time. So the time and effort that it takes to overcome one particular problem can pay surprising dividends.

"When a patient takes control of his own body and teaches it how to relax," Dr. Gessel says, "he's putting his physiological money in the bank."

Professional guidance and remarkable new monitoring equipment such as psychiatrist Gessel provides his patients, are a tremendous help in learning this art of relaxation for health. But they are not essential. With or without professional help, relaxation training is essentially a do-it-yourself proposition. You yourself must be highly motivated to put in the time required for regular practice. While you are learning, Dr. Gessel says, the *minimum* requirement is close to an hour's practice four days a week.

The technique he teaches, which involves learning muscle-by-muscle how to consciously sense the smallest contraction and its subsequent release, is not a new discovery. The "father" of this therapy, Dr. Edmund Jacobson (still an active practitioner), published his first medical paper on the subject in 1910. Though the Jacobson method has been around a long time, until recent years it has not been taken very seriously by the medical profession. Some even thought his work smacked of quackery—an all too familiar epithet for prophets in the field of health!

## Learning to Engineer Your Own Muscles

Today's revived interest in the technique, Dr. Gessel told us, stems from a new approach in psychiatry. In recent years, a growing number of psychiatrists have concentrated on treating the patient's behavior problem in and of itself—be it muscle tension, stuttering, fear of leaving the house, alcoholism, or whatever. This is the reverse of what we think of as the classic psychiatric approach of searching first for the original source of behavior problems—primarily in early childhood traumas.

In the medical specialty of psychiatry, the behavior therapy school advanced tremendously with the coming of sophisticated electronic equipment for measuring and recording bodily processes, Dr. Gessel explained. Using biofeedback equipment (machines that "feed back" information about biological happenings within the body), the patient can monitor his own progress as he attempts to change a behavior pattern.

Specifically, in relaxation training, the machine gives a reading of electrical volts emitted by the muscle group to which it is connected by electrodes placed on the surface of the arm, face, leg, or other portions of the body. The voltage, which is visually displayed, is a measure of the muscle's tension.

If the patient believes he has relaxed a particular muscle group but the voltage shows otherwise, then he knows he's doing something wrong and tries again for a better performance. As he learns to relax a muscle group completely, the biofeedback machine shows him he has dropped the voltage down to near zero.

Dr. Gessel, who several years ago took time off from his duties at U. of P. to study under Dr. Jacobson, uses a custom-made biofeedback apparatus. Through earphones the patient hears a tone that rises in pitch as muscle activity increases and diminishes as the activity subsides. At the same time, the machine gives a precise readout of voltage strength.

Dr. Gessel noted that most biofeedback equipment available to the public is too crude to be useful in evaluating muscle relaxation. "These machines will show you high voltage in deliberate contraction and low voltage in deliberate relaxation," he explains. "But they're no help in the crucial area—which is how to eliminate the *unconscious residual tensions*. Mail-order biofeedback machines can't discern these minute electrical impulses." But don't feel too bad about that, because you can do yourself a lot of good without access to a highly sensitive biofeedback machine.

## How to Relax at Home

The first thing you have to do in getting started is to set aside necessary *undisturbed* time. If there are kids in the household, plan to have someone else in charge while you retire for your self-teaching session. Turn off the phone or get out of earshot.

Even though you have located a pain which you think is tension-caused, this is *not* the place to begin your relaxation training.

"*Trying* to relax a painful muscle area," Dr. Gessel says, "causes tension in itself."

The Jacobson training method begins with muscle tension sensing and relaxing in the arm. Lie on your back, feet uncrossed, arms at your side, eyes open, for three or four minutes. Don't look at the clock; just make a guess when you think the time has passed. Now close your eyes very slowly and keep them gently closed until the session is over.

After another few minutes, you're ready to make your first exploration of sensing muscle tension in one arm. Bend your hand up at the wrist and hold it steadily in that position. You will note a sensation in the active muscles in the forearm and recognize that this "feeling" differs from other sensations caused by contact with clothing, the pressure of the mattress or couch, etc. The sensation, you recognize, is caused by contraction of the muscle. After a few minutes, you discontinue wrist bending and note the disappearance of the sensation. You "go negative," as Dr. Jacobson puts it.

If you follow the Jacobson method faithfully, you will repeat this single arm muscle practice again after three or four minutes, then a third time after another brief interval, and thereafter "go negative" for the rest of the hour-long session.

Other arm muscle sensations are perceived (and relaxed) in subsequent sessions, until you get to practice "progressive tension and relaxation" of the whole arm. Then you move on to the other arm, legs, abdomen, back, chest, shoulders, neck, and finally to the muscles of the eyes and speech region.

This exact sequence and speed of progress do not have to be rigidly followed in every case. With patients being treated for facial pain, for example, Dr. Gessel begins with arm muscles, then moves on to contractions in the neck and shoulders, and finally to the muscle tensions involved in teeth clamping and grinding.

It's worthwhile to note that unconscious abuse of the muscles apparently has no age limits. A 12-year-old girl came to Dr. Gessel specifically for a painful jaw condition, but she had also been diagnosed as having arthritis because of the aches and pains she suffered throughout her body. Shy and sensitive, this girl was markedly round shouldered. Dr. Gessel determined she was an "over-achiever" who drove herself to accomplishment to overcome feelings of inferiority.

After only a few sessions this bright girl learned to master her emotions by disciplined relaxation of her body muscles. All of her symptoms of arthritis and muscle spasms disappeared. Her mother reported that her daughter's posture also improved "100 percent." And the ever-present fatigue which had bothered the girl also vanished, even though she remained just as involved in school activities as before. In other words, she was accomplishing just as much, but now she was in control of her own body.

Dr. Gessel has been especially impressed with the success he has had in enabling his patients to overcome insomnia and get a good night's sleep. In fact, sleep improvement is one of the first things patients usually report, regardless of what they are being treated for. Dr. Gessel explains that human beings are the only living creatures known to be able to carry images inside their heads when they are not actually looking at them. So we lie sleepless by the hour, reproducing images of terror, unhappiness, or joy, by calling these visions to mind. While we cannot necessarily control all our thoughts, Dr. Gessel says, we *can* control our muscles. And because there is a unity between muscles and mentality, it often happens that when the muscles relax, the mind also unwinds.

How long does it take such patients to become "cured"? Judging from Dr. Gessel's report in the journal *Psychosomatics* (September/October 1971), remission of facial pain can occur following a single session with the doctor and four days of home practice—or, at the other extreme, only after five years and 27 clinical visits. Ingrained habits are the hardest to break, and Dr. Gessel has found that the earlier the tension habit is detected the speedier will be the relief gained from treatment.

Each practice session with muscle relaxation, Dr. Gessel informed us, gives you *cumulative* benefits.  Because there's constant back-and-forth communication between the brain and nerve cells that stimulate muscle fibers, when you succeed in deeply relaxing a single muscle group you also promote a lessening of muscular tension all over the body.

### Practice Four Times a Week

This overall reduced tension is not fleeting but continues for as long as 48 hours.  That's why Dr. Gessel says four times a week is a minimum requirement for practice sessions (he recommends daily practice).  After 48 hours you lose the accumulated benefit of previous practice and your muscles are as slow to learn as if you were just starting.

For those who want to learn this technique of relaxation, Dr. Gessel recommends Dr. Jacobson's popular paperback book, *You Must Relax* (McGraw-Hill Book Co., New York, 1957).  This volume includes detailed instructions for day-to-day practice.  There is also a brief how-to booklet by Dr. Jacobson, designed for patient use along with a text for physicians.  This is available from J. B. Lippincott Co. (New York) and entitled *Self-Operations Control*. It's not for sale as a single copy though; you have to pay $4.00 for ten copies.

So impressive are the results of Dr. Gessel's work that one of the school systems in the Philadelphia area is considering muscle relaxation training for their problem children.  For the average person who is reasonably healthy but just beginning to experience tension-related ailments, Dr. Gessel suggests that learning this method of relaxation could help prevent the development of more serious symptoms.

See also BIOFEEDBACK.

# Rumination

Rumination is normal in cows who chew their cud.  In children, it is a strange and very dangerous behavioral disorder.  Actually, children who ruminate don't exactly rechew their food: they simply bring it up and let it slowly dribble out of their mouth.  There is no vomiting or nausea or even disgust involved; apparently it is a purely voluntary act.

It seems probable, if not likely, that children displaying this bizarre behavior may be psychologically troubled. But the behavior itself must first be brought under control. Infants who ruminate derive very little nourishment from their food and suffer from malnutrition, poor resistance to disease, and dehydration, all too frequently leading to an early death.

Electric shock treatment has been used to condition children against ruminating; a cruel cure indeed. Now, it seems there is a much more humane way of teaching these children not to bring up their food. Sajwaj and colleagues at the University of Mississippi Medical Center found that the conditioning process could be carried out with plain, unsweetened lemon juice. They first tried it on one child, squirting the juice into her mouth whenever she was seen to be ruminating. Results came swiftly. The child all but stopped ruminating after just two days and began gaining weight. The cure is generally completely effective within a month or two, the researchers say.

Lemon juice packaged in a squeezable container seems to be the most convenient way of shooting the juice to a ruminating child.

# Schizophrenia

The classic nutritional approach to schizophrenia and other psychoses is described under our entry for ORTHOMOLECULAR (MEGAVITAMIN) THERAPY.

One important additional therapeutic dimension for schizophrenia is the elimination from the diet of every trace of gluten-containing cereal—which means primarily wheat, but also rye, barley, and oats. Under the entry on CELIAC DISEASE, you will read of the pioneering work of Dr. F. Curtis Dohan. Dr. Dohan told us that he first suspected a connection between celiac disease and schizophrenia when he observed that certain substances excreted in the urine of schizophrenics were also in the urine of celiacs. In a series of experiments, he put a number of schizophrenia patients on a diet which completely excluded not only gluten, but milk and other dairy products as well. Milk was excluded because some celiacs will not improve unless gluten *and* milk are eliminated. The results of these experiments strongly suggested that patients who were put on the gluten-free, milk-free diet improved much more rapidly than those who were not.

Nevertheless, doctors in general did not act upon these findings, probably because they had not been duplicated and—equally important—because of the general reluctance of doctors to afford dietary factors an important place in the treatment of mental disease. Just as we completed this book, however, Dr. Dohan's work *was* confirmed, in a study carried out by Drs. Man Mohan Singh and Stanley R. Kay of the Clinical Psychopharmacology Unit of the Bronx Psychiatric Center, and published in *Science* (January 30, 1976).

Drs. Singh and Kay put schizophrenic patients on a diet which excluded all cereal grains and milk, while giving them one of the standard medications used for schizophrenia. They found that when wheat gluten was "sneaked" into their diet, the improvement in their condition was sharply halted or reversed. The study was constructed in a scientifically elegant manner which excluded the possibility that the results observed were due to chance, psychological suggestion, or the bias of the doctors.

While it is not necessarily true that gluten is the *cause* of all schizophrenia, or that all schizophrenics will greatly improve when taken off gluten, the doctors conclude that "how wheat gluten may contribute to the schizophrenic process is a matter of speculation at this stage, but it does seem to be an important exogenous [i.e., dietary] factor which, when combined with genetic predisposition to schizophrenia, promotes the development of this condition."

# Seasickness

A bad toothache can drive you crazy and an ear infection can be agonizing. But a good case of seasickness can make you feel like committing suicide. Those who have never been seasick cannot even imagine what a horrible sensation it is. So I am sorry to say that I don't have any surefire preventive or remedy; I have known many people who got seasick even after taking Dramamine.

An old remedy for seasickness is to suck a lemon at the very first sign of nausea. How effective that is, I hope I never discover, as I long ago determined to never again put myself in the situation where I could get seasick.

If you want to do some ocean fishing and you are susceptible to this unholy malady, I suggest that the one maneuver you should avoid at all costs is anchoring the boat in swells. Generally, as long as the boat keeps moving at a good clip, there is no trouble. But the big swells you encounter on an ocean liner are something else again.

# Senility

From a medical or physiological point of view, the statement that someone is suffering from senility is about as meaningful as saying that someone is suffering from pimples. Senility is merely a catchall phrase which implies a deterioration in mental function associated with age. And that deterioration—change is a more accurate word—may be caused by a great variety of factors, including, among others, cholesterol-clogged blood vessels, a major stroke, a series of minor strokes, physical injury, a tumor, depression, and any one of a variety of nutritional deficiencies. It may also involve atrophy, or wasting away of the brain cells, with the presence of plaques in the brain tangled with nerve fibers, the cause of which is still a mystery, but which only accounts for a small fraction of the psychiatric problems which occur in older people. For many of the other causes, there are therapeutic steps which can be taken to arrest or reverse the damage, so it is wrong—very wrong—to look upon senility as inevitable.

From a nutritional point of view, my study of the available literature leads me to believe that the wisest approach is a general one, designed to insure adequacy of all required elements. In some cases, it may be difficult or impossible to reform the whole food diet of the patient, and in these cases broad-spectrum supplementation with vitamins and minerals, and perhaps even protein, is advisable. There are so many studies showing that psychiatric symptoms such as confusion, agitation, depression, irritability, and so forth can be caused by nutritional deficiencies, that from a practical point of view, it is not necessary to dwell on them individually. Further, it is highly impractical to try to determine that a particular patient is deficient, for instance, in vitamin $B_6$, but not in niacin. The appropriate approach, as I said, is a broad one, using reasonably generous amounts of all vitamins and all minerals. A multivitamin, multimineral preparation would be very useful here. However, few multimineral preparations contain much zinc, and since several studies have associated zinc deficiency with mental problems, it would be wise to include 15 to 30 mg. of zinc in the daily diet.

Recently, herbalists have become interested in the medical finding that vincamine, a substance found in the familiar ground cover periwinkle or creeping myrtle (*Vinca minor*), is said to improve the mental condition of some patients with senility caused by poor circulation. A press release from the American Chemical Society dated May 29, 1974, refers to vincamine as "an antisenility chemical," and quotes one university pharmacology expert as saying that "people in Europe and France who have been selling vincamine as a drug said that research has shown beneficial effects on some forms of senility by increasing the oxygen transport to the brain. They claim some dramatic results."

# Shiatsu

Shiatsu, which in Japanese means "finger pressure," may be thought of as a cross between acupuncture and massage. The art was developed in Japan over the last 40 years by Tokujiro Namikoshi, who claims to have treated more than 100,000 patients for a wide variety of illnesses. It seems to be just catching on in the United States, but so far it has not been used by medical acupuncturists with anywhere near the enthusiasm they have shown for the more traditional form of acupuncture, using needles.

Shiatsu is similar to massage in that it stresses the importance of deeply relaxing tense or exhausted muscles. By loosening the muscles, blood flow is improved and the accumulation of lactic acid, usually blamed for muscle aches, is swiftly reduced. It differs from massage in that pressure is applied much more vigorously, usually with the ball of the thumb, and sometimes even with the thumbnail.

With acupuncture, it shares the concept that there are points on the body (which may be far removed from the part that hurts) which when stimulated, bring about beneficial results. Thus, pressure to the plantar arch of the foot is not only recommended for aching feet, but to eliminate weariness throughout the body, and even relieve ailments of the kidneys, with which organ, according to Shiatsu principles, the plantar arch is closely related.

Usually, the bulb (not the tip) of the thumb is used to apply pressure. The pressure should be firm, and the force used will vary from patient to patient and from one part of the body to another. In general, according to Namikoshi, the pressure should be "sufficient to cause a sensation midway between pleasure and pain." The application of the pressure should last from five to seven seconds—no more. It may be repeated three or four times. A Shiatsu treatment from a professional may last 30 minutes or more, but for self-treatment, several minutes at a time, a few times a day, is typical.

Even though the amateur cannot hope to duplicate the finesse of the professional (who, in Japan, has probably graduated from the Nippon Shiatsu School), the individual is actually urged to practice Shiatsu on himself daily. There are two reasons for this. First, the Shiatsu theory holds that the fingers are closely related to key organs of the body, while the entire left hand is closely related to the heart. By practicing Shiatsu, you strengthen your fingers, and therefore strengthen your whole body.

In a much more general sense, it's felt that generous applications of Shiatsu all over the body improve the total health and circulation, and help prevent disease.

### Shiatsu for the Flu and Other Ailments

If you want to give Shiatsu a try, a good time to do so would be when you have a cold or the flu, accompanied by a sore throat, fever, and perhaps diarrhea. To reduce the pain of sore throat by Shiatsu principles, grasp your left thumb with your right hand. At the bottom corner of the U around the thumbnail, on the side facing towards your body, there is a point located a scant one-tenth of an inch in from the corner. Instead of using the pressure of the bulb of your thumb, place the thumbnail of your right hand directly over the target point on your left thumb and press vigorously. Hold the pressure about seven seconds and then release it. There should be a mark in your skin when you release the pressure. Repeat three times. Then switch hands and apply pressure to the inside corner of your right-hand thumb with your left thumbnail.

To relieve fever and diarrhea according to Shiatsu techniques, move to the index finger. Here, locate the same point you are using on your thumb, which you will find just a tiny fraction of an inch from the corner of the nail, on the side facing your thumb. Again, use the thumbnail of the opposite hand and apply pressure for five to seven seconds, repeating three times on both hands.

A number of rather easy-to-perform Shiatsu techniques are given by Pedro Chan in his *Finger Acupressure* (Price, Stern, Sloan Publishers, Los Angeles, 1974). For a headache, place the thumb of one hand into the angle where the thumb bone of the other hand meets the bone of the index finger (on the upper side of the hand). Massage in a small circular movement for about one minute, and repeat as many times as you want on each hand. Preferably, you should get someone else to apply the treatment to you, rubbing both hands at the same time. Two other headache points are located just below the occipital bone or the base of your skull, and about 1½ inches to the side of the midline of the head. Sit down, bend your head forward, place your fingers on your scalp, your thumbs on the headache points, and massage vigorously.

To treat the pain of a toothache, first use the headache points on your hands, as above. Then, if the toothache is in the upper jaw, hold your thumb over the middle of your ear and move it forward until it reaches the depression under the bone about an inch in front of your ear. Sit down or lie down, and press hard. If the toothache is in the lower jaw, place the thumb on your jawbone at the point where it angles toward the front of your head, and massage vigorously.

Chan recommends two points to treat dizziness. First, use the thumb and index finger to pinch hard just between your eyebrows. Another point for dizziness is located between the first and second metatarsal bones, located about two inches in from the angle where your big toe meets your second toe. Use the thumbnail to press hard.

For drowsiness, bite the tip of your tongue and then swallow the saliva, Chan recommends. For bed-wetting, use the nail of the thumb to press hard in the joint crease that's closest to the tip of your little finger. If this doesn't do the trick, Chan suggests, move down to the second crease, closer to the hand, and press hard there. Repeat often on both hands.

## Shiatsu and Sex

Practiced by a man and woman, Shiatsu can be used to overcome sexual problems and enhance the enjoyment of sexual relations, according to Namikoshi. To help the male partner, the woman should press lightly on various points along the base of his spine, from the coccyx or "tailbone" up to the waist level. At each point, she should press for three seconds and give 10 applications. Also recommended is pressing with three fingers into a point located directly on the midline of the abdomen and just an inch or two under the breastbone. This is said to promote sexual energy. Still another place suitable for relatively gentle pressure is located at the top border of the pubic hair. Finally, firm pressure first around the anus and then on the perineal area, between the anus and the genitals, is also said to stimulate response.

All this may sound rather exotic to a Westerner, but apparently it doesn't grab the Japanese that way. According to Namikoshi, "Squeezing the testicles firmly—a Japanese proverb says once for every year of your life—proves particularly invigorating as one grows older."

For the woman, the man should apply firm but gentle palm pressure to the area where the woman's leg joins the hip. Pressure along the sacrum, or the very foundation of the spine, between the buttocks, is also recommended.

To learn more about this Japanese art, read *Shiatsu* by Tokujiro Namikoshi (Japan Publications, San Francisco). The first American edition appeared in 1972.

A much smaller book is Pedro Chan's *Finger Acupressure,* mentioned earlier.

A Shiatsu wall chart and other educational materials may be available from the Shiatsu Dojo of New York at 1 Sherman Square, New York, New York 10023. Shiatsu is also taught at the Dojo.

A chiropractic approach to acupressure and massage is presented in *Touch for Health* by John F. Thie, D.C. (DeVorss & Co., Santa Monica, 1973).

# Shingles

Shingles, or herpes zoster, occurs when major sensory nerves are infected with the herpes zoster virus. Blisters appear on the skin and the area surrounding the inflamed nerve—usually the chest. Itching and pain may be unbelievably severe. Even after the infection has subsided and the blisters have disappeared, the pain may linger on. Doctors call this postherpetic neuralgia, and believe it is caused by scarring and excess fiber on the damaged nerve. The pain is most likely to linger when the victim is 40 years old or more.

Two Los Angeles dermatologists, Samuel Ayres, Jr., M.D., and Richard Mihan, M.D., believe they have found a natural substance which in many cases can relieve this postherpetic pain: vitamin E.

Over a period of four years, they treated 13 patients with vitamin E, administered both orally and directly to the lesions. The oral doses varied from 400 to 1,600 units daily, taken before meals. The results were reported in the December 1973 issue of the *Archives of Dermatology*.

Eleven of the patients had experienced moderate to severe pain for more than six months. Seven of these had suffered for over one year; one for 13 years; and one for 19 years. After taking vitamin E, nine of the thirteen patients reported complete or almost complete control of pain. The two patients who had neuralgia the longest were in this group. Of the remaining four patients, two were moderately improved, and two were only slightly helped.

One patient, a 67-year-old woman, had suffered terrible pain in her left thigh and leg for nine months after being hospitalized with an acute attack of herpes zoster. She was taking codeine twice a day or aspirin six to ten times a day in an effort to make life bearable. The doctors started her out with 100 I.U. of vitamin E daily, which was gradually stepped up over the next several months to 1,200 I.U. In addition, the woman was given a vitamin E cream to apply directly to her skin. Some improvement was noted within a few weeks, and after seven months her postherpes pain was gone completely.

Although the number of patients was limited, and the study was not controlled with a placebo group, Drs. Ayres and Mihan suggest that the relief achieved with vitamin E may have been real: ". . . In view of its long duration in many of our cases, we do not believe it is coincidence."

Another doctor who tried this regimen on some patients reported that it failed to bring about relief, but writing in the March 1975 issue of the *Archives of Dermatology,* Drs. Ayres and Mihan emphasized the importance of taking enough vitamin E—from 1,200 to 1,600 I.U. daily. It is also necessary, they say, to keep the treatment for six months or more before results can be judged, because of ronic deep-seated nature of the pain.

anything other than drugs or surgery help shingles while

it is in the "active" stage? Perhaps. One reader informs us of very good results in turning off attacks of shingles by taking a lot of liver pills. Another reader, a nurse, said that she healed the lesions of shingles on her husband's chest by applying vitamin E squeezed from a capsule directly to the rash three times a day.

# Sickle Cell Anemia

As we write this, a two-year controlled study of supplemental zinc therapy for sickle cell anemia patients is underway. We learned this from George J. Brewer, M.D., of the Department of Human Genetics at the University of Michigan in Ann Arbor. Dr. Brewer and his colleagues have already conducted preliminary trials of zinc therapy among a small number of sickle cell anemia victims. The results they've seen are very encouraging.

One young man had been hospitalized seven times in six months with crippling attacks of severe abdominal pain and vomiting, called crises. Doctors feared for his life during one especially long crisis. And when he wasn't in the hospital, roaming chest and back pains tortured him.

As a volunteer in a clinical trial, he began taking zinc supplements. During the first six months of treatment, he had only two relatively mild crises which required hospitalization. Then, his doctors found that many common foods, especially bread, tend to inhibit absorption of zinc. With this young man, as with subsequent patients, they divided the daily supplement of 267 mg. of zinc into six doses administered *between* meals to aid absorption. At the time of this report, he had gone three months without a crisis. He also had a steady job and a greatly expanded social life.

Another young victim of sickle cell anemia had an average of four crises a year before taking zinc. During 13 months of zinc therapy he had only two crises—both triggered by strenuous activities. He is now attending school regularly for the first time in years.

Sickle cell anemia affects mostly black people in the United States, but is incorrectly assumed to affect *only* black people. As many as 142,000 white Americans may be carrying the hereditary trait, which can produce a child with the disease if the carrier marries another carrier.

Dr. Ananda S. Prasad, Professor of Medicine, Wayne State University School of Medicine, has found that blood levels of zinc are significantly lower in sickle cell anemia patients than in healthy people. He and Dr. Brewer theorize that zinc prevents red blood cells from bending or sickling. When the cells become sickled, they cannot release oxygen to the surrounding tissue. The result is stunted growth, poor healing, and pain.

# Skin Cracks

When cracks appear around the lips, they are often, but not always, a sign of B-vitamin deficiency. The tongue may also look peculiar. It is difficult to differentially diagnose separate B-vitamin deficiencies, so the practical course is to take generous supplements of the entire B complex.

We received two rather unusual letters involving cracks in the *fingers*. In one case, a reader said that she was having tiny splits in the skin adjacent to the tips of her nails. Her doctor recommended that she take extra vitamin C and the condition rapidly cleared up.

In another case, a reader suffered for 10 years with what her doctors termed a virus on her fingers "which continually spread and worsened. Around my nails the skin became crusty, dry, cracked, bleeding, and looked like warts. Typing, playing piano, and everything else was becoming agonizing. I had them burned off three times by different doctors. They still returned bigger and better, and my fingers were numb about one-eighth of an inch in. As a last resort and completely frustrated, I quadrupled my vitamin A and D intake. That very night my numb fingers started tingling. Within a week the encrustations peeled off and bright new pink skin was there. I couldn't believe it at first. However, I continued the high intake of vitamins A and D and my skin is still very healthy."

# Skin, Dry

Dry skin is one of the first signs of a vitamin A deficiency. It doesn't mean that you are necessarily deficient in vitamin A, but the first thing you should do is to check your diet. This is particularly true if you have gooseflesh on your legs or arms that does not go away. If you do have these bumps (check particularly the outside of your thighs), the appropriate action is to take 25,000 to 50,000 units of vitamin A every day for one or two weeks, and then go to a maintenance level of 10,000 to 20,000 units daily.

Cod-liver oil, which is naturally rich both in vitamins A and D, can also be applied topically. One woman who had dry flaking skin for many years—despite trying every lotion and oil imaginable—literally solved her problem overnight by applying some of the cod-liver oil to her legs and taking a teaspoonful by mouth.

If your diet seems to be sufficient in vitamin A—which means that you eat foods like carrots, sweet potatoes, tomatoes, and liver—your dry skin problem may be a result of inadequate unsaturated oils. Try adding two tablespoons of some good polyunsaturated salad oil, such as corn, safflower, or sunflower, to your daily salad. You can also rub such oils on your skin, and a good amount of them will actually be directly absorbed.

Dry, rough, etched skin may respond well to vitamin E. Some, of course, should be taken internally, but applying it directly to the skin will produce faster results. Creams and lotions claiming to contain vitamin E ordinarily do not have a rich concentration of this vitamin. Wheat germ oil is a good source, or you may simply open a vitamin E capsule and squeeze the contents on your skin. A surprisingly large number of people have told us that vitamin E seems to do wonders for dry, rough skin.

The wife of a beekeeper told us that she noticed that during the collection season, her husband's hands were incredibly soft and smooth. So she started giving herself honey facials every day. Soon her skin, too, she said, became very soft, and no wrinkles have developed. To give herself the honey facial, she would tie her hair back, smooth pure raw liquid honey all over her face and neck, let it set for 15 minutes, and then wipe it off with a damp cloth.

Dry rough hands are extremely common, and in the overwhelming number of cases, the culprit is soap or detergents. Recent evidence I've seen shows that soap is even worse for your hands than had previously been suspected, and that even a small amount sufficiently upsets the natural chemistry of the skin to invite trouble. Therefore, before anything else, I would recommend wearing gloves whenever you do the dishes or handle wet laundry.

There are several excellent herbal treatments for dry hands. A reader passed along this one:

> Soak whole or cracked flaxseed (linseed), three rounded tablespoons, overnight in one pint of warm water. Then boil and strain to remove as much gel as possible. The gel is what you want. Discard the seeds. Then add a little less than a pint of clear vinegar to the brew, along with two or three ounces of glycerin, which you can buy at the drugstore. Heat the mixture to boiling, remove from heat, and then beat with an eggbeater for one minute to keep the glycerin from separating. Then bottle it. It will last for a long time. When you want to use it, simply dampen your hands with the solution, rub it in, and let it dry.

This reader thoughtfully added the caution that when you are boiling the seeds, don't go away, because the kettle boils over very easily.

Gayelord Hauser, the popular health and beauty writer, recommends this lotion for dry scaly scalp or skin:

> Put two heaping tablespoons of dried peppermint leaves into a pint of water. Let come to a boil and simmer for three minutes. Put through a fine strainer and then add a pint of pure cider vinegar. Apply with cotton. The vinegar helps restore the acid mantle.

# Skin, Oily

Washing your face frequently with soap can do more harm than good if you have oily skin. The more you wash, the more oil your skin will secrete. It's better to wash your face only with water, unless it is really dirty, when a very mild soap can be used.

One thing that seems to help oily skin is a periodic facial mask made with brewer's yeast. Mix one teaspoon of yeast with enough water or skim milk to make a loose liquid paste. Apply to freshly cleansed skin that has been rinsed with water containing a few drops of apple cider vinegar. Pat the yeast mixture into all areas of the face and allow it to dry completely before rinsing away with warm and then cool water. Blot dry.

Conway, the British herbalist, says that an infusion or tea made from marigold petals "provides the ideal balance" for an over-oily skin.

# Smell, Lost Sense Of

Although it has been medically reported that zinc supplements can sometimes restore a lost or distorted sense of taste, I am not familiar with any reports in medical literature about zinc for a poor sense of smell. Nonetheless, two readers told us that they were astounded to discover that zinc supplements did the trick for them. One was a college student who said he had a very poor sense of smell, and when he increased his zinc intake to 45 mg. a day, he noticed in three weeks that "I was being rewarded with an uncanny sense of smell."

Another reader told us that "My sinus-wracked husband, who has been unable to smell for over 10 years, is sniffing with joy once again. He can't believe it!" The amount of zinc he was taking was 30 mg. a day. Curiously, results were noticed after the same period of time mentioned by the college student—three weeks.

# Sore Throat

The herbs most valued for use as a gargle and/or tea to ease the pain of a sore throat are sage (especially red sage), eucalyptus, horehound, fenugreek, and marshmallow. Don't skimp on the honey when drinking these teas for sore throat.

Meyer, the herbalist, recommended horehound tea with honey, a pinch of cayenne, and one teaspoon of vinegar, to be taken hot at bedtime.

For hoarseness, Hutchens recommends making a syrup of grated horseradish, honey, and water, and taking one teaspoon every hour.

If you have a "strep" throat you usually know it because the pain is very severe. In these cases, or when the soreness persists, see a physician.

# Spa Therapy

A spa is a place where nature has decided to bring forth a spring whose water is either hot or has an unusually high mineral content (preferably both), and where human beings have done their part by erecting buildings and other structures to make the benefits of this water easily accessible to the public.

Each year, hundreds of thousands of people all over the world visit such spas for anywhere from a few days to a few months, and most go away feeling much better than they did when they came there. It's difficult, though, to put your finger on exactly what it is about spas in general that make them effective restorers—at least temporarily—of health and tranquility.

Consider first the spa water. In nearly every case, it is the water peculiar to that particular spa which makes or breaks its reputation. Typically, the chief minerals in spa water are sodium, calcium, magnesium, bicarbonate, and sulfate. Many springs are actually radioactive, although not to the point that they are dangerous— unless you were to drink the water every day for months or years. The consensus is that the mild degree of radioactivity, like the mineral matter which so often gives spa water a disagreeable taste or strong odor, is part of the therapeutic essence of spa treatment.

The way in which a spa visitor interacts with the water is limited only by the imagination. Depending upon which spa you go to, you may be encouraged to drink it, swim in it, soak in it, exercise in it, be hosed down with it, shower in it, inhale its vapors, or have it introduced into any one of the body orifices.

The theory behind all these forms of hydrotherapy is that the minerals (and possibly the radioactivity) of the water will, in very small amounts, actually enter your system by way of the skin or mucous membranes and help restore your entire system to a healthier state.

In Germany, the mineral content of spa water is considered so important that detailed scientific analyses are published for each spa and will be sent to you on request. For example, when we wrote to a spa at Wiesbaden, in West Germany, we received a report listing precisely how much of some twenty different minerals and five compounds are in the water (e.g., sodium, 2,633 mg./kg.; calcium, 342.3 mg./kg.; zinc, .014 mg./kg.; etc.). We also received a letter declaring that "The waters of our 26 hot springs with a natural temperature of 154° F. emanate from a depth of about 6,000 feet. The healing effect comprises rheumatic complaints and other motor disturbances such as intervertebral disk troubles, post-traumatic injuries following accidents, and others. In these cases the water is used for bathing, underwater massage, and underwater medical gymnastics. In form of drinking and inhalation treatments, it is applied to catarrhs of the respiratory organs."

## A Spa Should Teach, Not Cure

Today, though, there's more brewing in some German spas than hot sulfury water. Health leaders are beginning to ask more of spas. It isn't enough, they say, to only make someone feel better for a few weeks. The goal should be to *educate* the spa visitor to be able to feel better all the time by living a more healthful life.

As is so often the case with important social changes, this change is prompted in large part by economic considerations. In Germany, as in Italy and France, spa treatment is covered by government health insurance. And the economy being what it is today, German health leaders who have ties with spas now believe that the available money provided by health insurance should be used "as rationally as possible."

An article by Loni Skulima of the *Frankfurter Rundschau,* translated in the *German Tribune* (November 7, 1974), explains that "some patients treated suffer disorders caused by risk factors that can only be reduced by radically changing their mode of life in the long term. This applies to nutrition, exercise, and leisure-time activities." And obviously, a few weeks at a spa, no matter how helpful, aren't going to change a person's lifestyle. The only thing that will do the trick is a process of intensive education and motivation.

And the spa, which is directed and supervised by doctors, but maintains an atmosphere of relaxation and comfort, in contrast to the atmosphere of anxiety which hangs over most hospitals, could be just the right place to carry out such a program.

Professor W. Schulenberg, head of Germany's Hanover College of Education, explains a few of the new ideas he wants to see put into practice at German spas.

First, no medicines or treatments should be prescribed at spas "without an explanation of the purpose of the treatment, its actual nature, its probable consequences, and its relevance to the patient's biological condition."

Further, "the patient will no longer undergo treatment with blind obedience towards the doctor but will realize that he has to assume an active role."

I imagine those are welcome words to all those Americans who have too often found that blind obedience not only to doctors, but to nurses and even clerks, is a nearly mandatory condition of receiving attention in a hospital. But the Germans aren't changing things just to give people more civil liberties. The idea, says Professor Schulenberg, is to teach the patient to see his health as a complicated interrelationship of various factors, running the gamut from his heredity to his eating and drinking habits and even the way he behaves at work and at home.

At Bad Nauheim, a well-known German spa, the preventive approach to health has already begun. In the old days, someone who was addicted to cigarettes, alcohol, or excessive eating would probably be subjected to a "cure" which would leave him healthier for a couple of weeks at most. Today, spa guests with such habits are given group and behavioral therapy at which they learn how to permanently change their habits, and thereby help themselves to better health on a life-long basis. Although each patient consults with a physician, most of the therapy is carried out in groups, so it turns out to be much less expensive than getting the same kind of help at a doctor's office or in a traditional hospital.

At the Hohenried spa, the chef and his assistants give actual cooking courses to the patient and his family so that they know how to prepare tasty dishes that are good for their health. Other spas are now emphasizing sports. The idea is not simply to give a patient exercise while he's at the spa, but to teach him better ways of using his leisure time once he's left the spa and returned home. Hopefully, a new kind of professional facility will emerge, where the emphasis is almost entirely on maintaining health, rather than curing sickness.

Dr. Theo Kleinschmidt, head physician at a small cluster of spa clinics, wants to see the kind of approach that will "place patients in the center of attention instead of relying more on technology." In practice, Dr. Kleinschmidt says, this means the spa of the future should employ lectures, free-wheeling discussions, films, libraries, and every other communication resource to educate the patient. Nor would this education be only medical or nutritional in nature. Psychologists, educators, spiritual advisors, sex counsellors, and perhaps even artists and craftsmen could be profitably employed in teaching people how to lead a more relaxed, enjoyable, and healthier life.

**Author's Note:**   To learn something about spas closer to home, I asked a writer who frequents spas for her impressions. Her reply follows.

## Two Spas: Worlds Apart, Both Wonderful

### by Grace Halsell

Two of my favorite spas, Palm Aire in Pompano Beach, Florida, and Rancho La Puerta, just below San Diego, California, in Tecate, Mexico, are worlds apart—in more ways than one.

Palm Aire is all luxury. You work hard, but you get plenty of pampering, too. When you enter, you walk on marble floors, move on to plush carpeting. You are surrounded by soft pastels, soft music. There's always an attendant, so that you never want for a toga or a towel or talented hands to soothe ruffled, urban nerves or massage away sore muscles.

Checking into Palm Aire is like going aboard a great ocean liner—first class. You quickly forget problems at home. It's a well-run ship. You turn yourself over to activities that were planned by pros.

By contrast, Rancho La Puerta stresses outdoor living. Its environment is more rustic, and it features do-it-yourself routines. Going there, I felt as I did at 16 on my first camping expedition, where I met friends who lasted forever.

Just being in Mexico gives it a special flavor. You are housed in small, separate *casas* scattered over the spacious ranch grounds, and a good hiking distance from any place you want to go, such as the *casa* for your meals or the swimming pool or the yoga class.

I waked each morning before six, without an alarm, to be with the early risers who hiked up and down a mountain before breakfast. At nine, I watched spa director Helene Eberle run with a gazelle's speed across the grounds and ring a large bell announcing the first exercise class. Helene, a beautiful, blonde native of Brooklyn, not only "teaches" you how to move faster and with more rhythm, but she is so glowingly alive that she inspires you to keep moving, even when you feel awkward and lumbering. She's singing, shouting, exulting—her entire being a big hurrah for life.

**Emphasis on Good Nutrition** • Both at Rancho La Puerta and Palm Aire, I find a great emphasis on good nutrition. Spa directors remind you: You are what you eat. When you sit down for breakfast at Palm Aire, you see vitamins in front of your plate. The staff will tell you: "A proper diet is essential to good health and a sound mind. If you are on a very low caloric intake you can protect yourself with extra vitamins."

At Rancho La Puerta you eat organically grown fruits and vegetables from the ranch gardens. You will be tempted each day by Rancho La Puerta's homemade whole wheat bread (not for dieters), and you will be urged to drink acidophilus (cultured) milk, introduced at Rancho La Puerta by its founder, the European writer and philosopher, Dr. Edmond Bordeaux Szekely.

At either spa, the low-calorie, appetizing, and well-planned meals make it easy for you to lose weight.

Palm Aire's director, Mourad Khaireldin, says, "Men lose much easier than women, probably because eons ago, woman, the child-bearer, was built so that as a protective measure, she stored fat more easily. A man may lose five pounds in a day or two, but it generally takes a woman a week or longer.

"We don't encourage 'crash diet' programs so much as we encourage you to get motivated, to work toward the figure you want to attain. It does not actually matter *when* you attain it but what is important is for you to always work toward your goal, and once you've reached it, to maintain it."

At five feet, three inches, I checked into Palm Aire weighing 132 pounds and after 10 days I checked out weighing 122 pounds.

Next time I hope to lose about five more pounds, and then maintain it.

**A Daily Program** • Checking into the spa, you first get a doctor's examination. If you want to lose weight and your health is good, he says it's all right for you to go on the 600-calories-a-day diet. Each day, you choose your own menu, high in protein, low in fat, and well balanced. You also get a card each day, with a full schedule of activities. A typical day runs like this:

| | |
|---|---|
| 9:10 A.M. | Warm-Up Class (supervised) |
| 9:40 | Special Spa Conditioning Class |
| 10:20 | Whirlpool |
| 11:00 | Water Exercise Class (supervised) |

| 11:40 | Body Massage |
| 12:20 P.M. | Time for Sun and Relaxation |
| 1:00 | Lunch (Spa Dining Room) |
| 2:40 | Loofa Bath and Salt Glo |
| 3:20 | Herbal Wrap |
| 4:00 | Yoga Instruction |
| 4:40 | Facial Treatment |

(Supervised classes in jogging, walking, and advanced calisthenics can also be included in your program, if you so desire.)

In the warm-up class, I found myself exercising with 30 other women. Sans makeup, in our yellow sweat suits, we were a special "sisterhood." We found it easy to introduce ourselves, to relate common battles against our bulges and our modern adventures to regain our once svelte past. One woman told me she had just lost a breast in surgery, another woman said her husband had left her for a younger woman. While being steamed, saunaed, rubbed, scrubbed, exercised, sunned, and wrapped in herbs, the way Cleopatra was, the clientele also benefited from a form of group therapy. It is a place where the widowed, divorced, or single woman can come alone—and easily find companions. Or, a wife may come with her husband and they can play tennis, swim, and golf together, as well as benefit from the spa's other activities.

If you go to either spa, you can, with proper motivation, lose weight and come out in better shape than you went in.

**Why We Seem to Need the Spa** ● In the days of our parents, no one, perhaps, needed to go to a spa. Their jobs of plowing fields, maintaining big farmhouses, or walking to and from town, were "natural" exercise.

Since the days of our forefathers, we have advanced technologically, and because of our modern sanitation, we aren't likely to die of some quick, acute illness. Yet health is still a very personal matter, an individual responsibility.

When I walk into Palm Aire, I know that I am in the hands of true professionals, dedicated to the health of their clients. Spa Director Khaireldin, a native of Egypt, who has run European spas, studied yoga in India, and devoted a lifetime to his profession of good health, takes clients jogging each morning.

But he says, "You don't need to come here and pay me to run with you. You can do it at home, every morning. What I can teach you are some good habits. And to remind you of some that you once knew, but might have forgotten."

A busy New York lawyer says: "I get all tensed up. I don't take 'vacations', I go down to the spa. I play water volleyball and forget all about my problems. I get in shape, and I stay that way for about six months. Then I know it's time for reorientation, so I go back to the spa. It saves me going to a psychiatrist, and to M.D.'s. The spa is cheaper than any hospital."

Spas have always been a way of life in Europe. I have visited spas in such well-known resorts as Baden-Baden and Wiesbaden, Germany, as well as in Austria, France, and Spain. Many Europeans check their bodies into spas with the regularity that we Americans put our automobiles through inspection. For as long as memory, European men and women have gone "to take the baths," to drink mineral waters, and get massages. And many of the Old World ideas about spas are coming here.

I saw a sign at Palm Aire:  You've only one life, and it pays to live it with good health.

I hope to remember that.

# Tachycardia
# (Rapid Heartbeat)

People who are subject to intermittent attacks of an abnormally fast heartbeat are said to have paroxysmal tachycardia. If you have this condition, it's possible that you are already on drugs to help control it; in any case, before doing anything, you should carefully discuss it with your doctor.

Several recent reports in *Lancet* indicate that there is a very simple way that patients can be taught to return their racing pulse to normal without using drugs. The technique consists of nothing but plunging your face into a basin of cool water.

That must sound ridiculous, almost medieval, but doctors call the body's reaction to submersion of the face in water the "diving reflex." It almost seems that we have some built-in defense mechanism that, sensing that we may be drowning, swiftly slows down the heart to conserve oxygen.

Dr. N. G. Hunt and colleagues of Britain wrote in *Lancet* (March 8, 1975) that when the face is immersed in 65-degree water (cool, but not ice cold), there is a dramatic reduction in heart rate. Curiously, very warm water produces no change at all, and if a person merely holds his breath without plunging his face into water, the change is insignificant. The British doctors add that while very cold water will also reduce the heart rate, it is not as effective as mildly cold water and may also be dangerous because of the shock.

Before attempting this therapy, discuss it with your physician. You may refer him to the article by Dr. Hunt, and to an earlier article, also in *Lancet* (January 4, 1975), by Dr. Kern Wildenthal and colleagues. The reason for caution is that there are different kinds of tachycardia and several conditions which may make using this technique unwise. When patients are properly selected and taught the technique, however, it does offer great potential benefits for those with paroxysmal atrial tachycardia. In some cases, patients who do not respond to drugs or a special massage *do* respond to the "diving reflex" after 20 to 30 seconds of immersion.

# Tai-Chi

**by Walter B. Dudley**

Tai-Chi Chuan, a unique system of exercise developed hundreds of years ago in China by Taoist monks, has recently been attracting the attention of American medical personnel and physical educators. In hospital tests this exotic exercise has favorably impressed cardiologists as a form of activity that has potential in the treatment of heart patients. According to the Chinese, who have a much longer experience than Americans with Tai-Chi, its practice for 20 minutes a day over a period of years can prolong youthful vigor and rejuvenate the body.

The 108 basic moves or forms of Tai-Chi use every part of the body. Hands, elbows, fists, legs, shoulders, head, buttocks, feet, toes, sides of feet—even the eyes—are all brought into play in a pattern of continually flowing movement. The exercise is performed in a slow, almost leisurely manner, without any special muscular effort. And because it isn't strenuous, anyone from eight to eighty can practice Tai-Chi at no risk to himself and with the promise of renewed vitality and longer life.

In China, Tai-Chi is viewed with great respect, and many Chinese claim that it has been known to lower high blood pressure and to alleviate joint diseases and gastric disturbances. For most of its long history, the exercise was a jealously guarded secret of the Chinese elite, and the Communists, who took over all of the Chinese mainland in 1949, viewed it with suspicion. In their efforts to bring revolutionary thinking to the fore, they discouraged Tai-Chi explaining that it was too traditional. Later, however, they had second thoughts, and in recognition of its therapeutic value, they began to encourage its regular practice.

Now Tai-Chi is part of the routine of millions of people in China, a fact that is illustrated by numerous documentary films. In the newsreels of President Nixon's visit there in 1972, for example, several of the films show solo and mass demonstrations of the art of Tai-Chi. Not only China, but the Soviet Union as well, has found value in this once elitist calisthenic. After a Soviet delegation to China saw and was impressed by Tai-Chi, it was carried back to the Soviet Union where training classes have opened and several books on the subject have been published with the sanction of the government.

Tai-Chi began to catch on in the United States in the 1960s. Although it was practiced secretly in Chinatowns over the country before that time, few, if any, of the practitioners were interested in sharing their knowledge outside their own group. In fact, they often resented the activities of the Chinese Tai-Chi masters—mostly recent immigrants from Taiwan and Hong Kong—when they started classes that were open to non-Chinese pupils. Like the Chinese aristocrats of centuries past, they believed that knowledge of the exercise should be reserved for a limited group.

In spite of such reservations, Tai-Chi began to attract devotees among non-Chinese Americans. At first, the Tai-Chi schools were limited to the East and West Coasts, but they soon began to spread inland across the country. Now, along with acupuncture, the art of Tai-Chi is getting official attention from the medical community, and thousands of Americans are discovering this easy, "effortless" way to lasting health and long life.

## Doesn't Strain the Heart

One test of Tai-Chi's effect on the heart was made recently at Montefiore Hospital in New York City. Doctor Lenore Zoeman, chief of physical therapy, took an electrocardiogram on a well-known Tai-Chi teacher, Sophia Delza, the foremost woman instructor of Tai-Chi in the Western world. Although it is normally the case that exercise increases the heart rate, the cardiogram on Delza indicated that her heart rate was not changed when she practiced Tai-Chi. While lay-people might not be impressed, doctors appreciate the rare value of an activity that does not put stress on the heart and they are alert to its therapeutic possibilities. According to Dr. Louis Brinberg, a cardiologist at New York's Mount Sinai Hospital, "It will be interesting to see what can be done with Tai-Chi when used as an adjunct to the usual therapy of cardiac patients."

The value of Tai-Chi seems to stem as much from its psychological as from its physiological effects. The fact that modern medicine is finding more and more connections between mental attitudes and physical health may indeed help to explain the value of Tai-Chi, which is designed to have a calming effect on the mind and nervous system. Comparing it to exercises more familiar to us, Dr. Isabel Wright, a New York psychiatrist, commented, "Western calisthenics, with their mindless 1-2-3 repetitions, don't really get to the heart of the matter. In fact, they often do more harm than good. What is needed is a total exercise, one that encompasses both *mind and body*. I've recommended the practice of Tai-Chi to many of my patients."

## A Natural Tranquilizer

It has been quite conclusively demonstrated that Tai-Chi has a tranquilizing effect on the emotions. The overburdened executive, the harassed housewife, the uptight student, the anxious clerk—all might discover that a 10-minute break for a round of Tai-Chi can put them in a better frame of mind and help them to bear the pressures of everyday living without ulcers or nervous breakdowns.

Remarking on this aspect of Tai-Chi, Dr. Herman Ziffer, a New York endocrinologist, said, "In this urban life we lead, most people don't exercise enough. Tai-Chi certainly, especially since it is done slowly and gently, is excellent physical therapy. I heartily recommend it to people of all ages."

Probably the most difficult Tai-Chi principle for a beginner to follow is the one of complete relaxation. Most Westerners attack daily exercise as though they were wrestling with a bear. They don't really enjoy doing it. Up and down, puff, puff, back and forth.

By contrast, Tai-Chi requires that you relax your facial muscles, shoulders, abdomen, thighs, and follow the shifting pattern of movements with a light, calm mind. Eventually you will experience a sensation almost as though you were floating.

By their very nature, all of the movements of Tai-Chi are geared to encourage relaxation. The weight of the body shifts continuously from one foot to the other and the movements are performed in circles, arcs, and spirals. The end of each movement becomes the beginning of the next one, which conserves energy and produces a feeling of tranquility and emotional security.

In order to perform the exercise properly, the body must move as a unit, and this principle of unity-in-movement is one of the ways in which it contrasts most basically to Western calisthenics, which use various parts of the body independently. Dr. Robert J. Rogers, a Chappaqua, New York, psychologist and Tai-Chi practitioner, believes that Tai-Chi "practiced correctly over a long period of time, creates a kind of protective psychological shield that helps a person combat stress, which is one of the main causes of disease."

## The Mystery of 'Chi'

At the heart of Tai-Chi is the Chinese concept of *chi,* a word of many meanings—air, vitality, spirit, breath, atmosphere, and circulation. It is hard to define *chi.* One Tai-Chi expert calls it "biophysical energy generated by respiratory rhythm." Perhaps the best English equivalent is "intrinsic energy," or "vital force." Whatever *chi* is, doctors of Chinese medicine say it can be cultivated through practice of the exercise and stored in a spot called the *tan-t'ien,* located exactly three inches below the navel. Once stored, the *chi* can be circulated by the mind throughout the body. In an ancient Chinese treatise on Tai-Chi, the author states, "The mind directs the *chi,* which sinks deeply and permeates the bones. The *chi* circulates freely, mobilizing the body so that it heeds the direction of the mind. If the *chi* is correctly cultivated, your spirit of vitality will rise and you will feel as though your head were suspended by a string from above." It is this "vital energy," as manifested through the Tai-Chi exercise, that accounts for the prolongation and rejuvenation of life.

Master William C. C. Chen, of the Tai-Chi School in New York City, was asked about the mystery of *chi* and replied: "It is certainly a mystery, but it works. Look at acupuncture; it has cured apparently incurable diseases, even though it is not yet clear how it works. All I can say is, if you practice Tai-Chi every day, you will eventually build up this inner strength or *chi*."

At a demonstration in Madison Square Garden's Forum, Master Chen demonstrated the proof of his *chi*. Four hefty volunteers, astride a motorcycle—weighing a total of more than 1,000 pounds—rode over Chen's stomach as he lay on the floor. Later these same volunteers took turns punching him repeatedly in the abdomen using full force. After several minutes the punchers became tired and gave up, but Master Chen just smiled.

The Tai-Chi postures which follow are just a few of the many which may be practiced.

## BEGINNING OF TAI-CHI

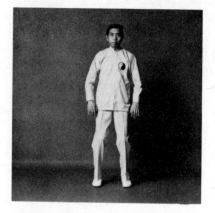

**1.** Stand *relaxed.* Elbows and knees slightly bent.

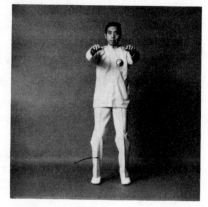

**2.** Raise arms *slowly* to shoulder height.

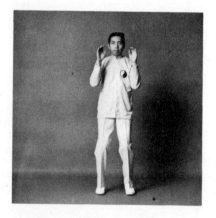

**3.** Draw back your arms by bending your elbows.

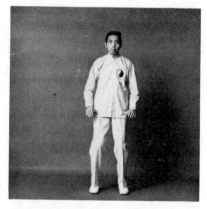

**4.** Let your arms sink *gently* to your sides. You are again in the beginning position.

**Note:**
Do not exert force, but let your arms rise as though they were floating up from water to the surface. In the same way, let them fall to your sides again without strain. Concentrate on total relaxation.

# WARD OFF WITH YOUR LEFT HAND

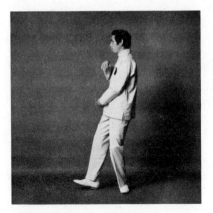

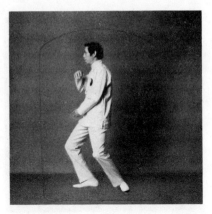

**1.** This movement follows "Beginning of Tai-Chi." Shift your weight to your left foot, turn on your right heel, toes raised slightly, to your right.

**2.** Now shift your weight to your right foot. Left leg is relaxed.

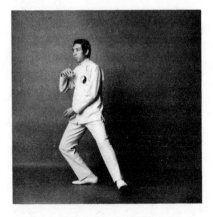

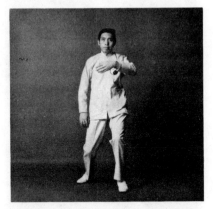

**3.** Step out with your left foot, heel touching floor slightly.

**4.** Shift your weight to your left foot and pivot to front. As you do, left arm rises, palm turned in, to chest height while right arm sinks gently to side. Follow by pivoting slightly to left and perform similar movements to "ward off with right hand."

**Note:**
Remember to move the body in one unit. This rule applies to all movements in Tai-Chi.

## SQUATTING DOWN

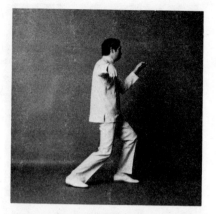

**1.** Stand with body weight on left foot, right leg relaxed, left arm, palm out and bent at elbow, as in photo 1.

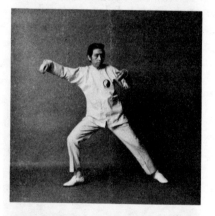

**2.** Pivot to right, shifting weight onto right foot; arms and body move in one unit.

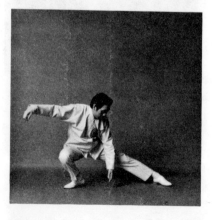

**3.** Squat down, left arm dropping gently in front of you, right arm extended with wrist limp.

**Note:**
Try to relax the left leg as you go down, so that it is not stretched taut. Once again, move slowly, softly, without any visible effort.

# GOLDEN COCK STANDS ON ONE LEG

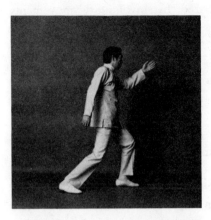

**1.** This posture follows "Squatting Down." From a squatting position, the weight shifts forward to left foot, body rising, with left arm, slightly bent, extending, as in photo 1.

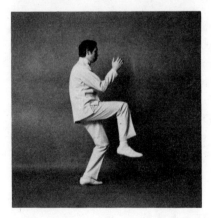

**2.** Lift right knee to waist height; right arm, with elbow bent, lifts upward in an arc, while right arm falls to side. Notice how left knee is slightly curved.

**Note:**
Don't raise the knee too high or you will begin to feel tension. Let your eyes follow your hand. And remember to move slowly!

# Tardive Dyskinesia

This condition is characterized by involuntary movements, typically of the mouth area, and is most often (perhaps always) seen as a side effect of drugs given for psychiatric problems. Antihistamines have also been blamed.

The condition is not easy to treat on a permanent basis, but there has been one promising study which shows a role for the vitamin choline.

When choline was given to a patient with tardive dyskinesia, who in the course of a typical minute would make 31 tongue protrusions, 32 complete jaw-chewing motions, and 24 lip-puckering movements, he improved to the point where he had only 4 tongue protrusions, 12 chewing motions, and no lip-puckering movements. This effect was not seen until his dose of choline chloride was raised to 16 grams a day.

During this treatment, increased sweating and salivation were observed. When the choline therapy was discontinued, the movements returned to the previous frequency in just three days.

If you wish to discuss this with your physician, you may direct him or her to the *New England Journal of Medicine,* July 17, 1975, page 152, "Choline for Tardive Dyskinesia," a letter from Kenneth L. Davis, M.D., and colleagues from the Stanford University School of Medicine.

# Taste, Lost Sense Of

The relatively sudden loss of one's sense of taste is sufficient reason for a visit to a doctor, preferably a neurologist. Once it has been determined that the reduction, distortion, or loss of the sense of taste is not due to nerve damage or abnormality, zinc supplements can be tried. Robert I. Henkin, M.D., of Georgetown University Hospital in Washington, D.C., pioneered in this field and was able to cure a surprisingly large number of people (taste disturbances aren't nearly as rare as you might suppose) with zinc.

Probably 50 mg. of zinc a day continued for several weeks

would be sufficient to determine if this mineral will help. If taste is then normalized, the amount of zinc could probably be cut in half.

In one case, reported in the *Journal of the American Medical Association* (January 5, 1976), it was noted that a patient with this problem was sent by his physician to a neurosurgeon, whose findings were negative. "The patient subsequently read an article on loss of taste and zinc deficiency in a lay publication. A pharmacist supplied him with a zinc-containing vitamin preparation, and after taking it for several weeks, the patient claimed complete recovery," the editors of the journal wrote.

# Thrush

Thrush is a fungal infection of the mouth and is characterized by small, white patches. It's caused by *Candida albicans,* the same organism responsible for most of the so-called yeast infections of the vagina.

It will usually respond well to B-complex supplementation and supplements of *Lactobacillus acidophilus,* the beneficial bacteria which occur in some strains of yogurt. The most dependable form of this latter preparation is sold in many drugstores, where it is kept refrigerated to insure viability of the organisms. We know of one recent case where thrush in an infant, which had resisted medical treatment for many weeks, cleared up swiftly when the nursing mother boosted her intake of B vitamins and fed the child about one-third teaspoon of the acidophilus (in powder form) mixed with water three times a day.

# Tic Douloureux

Tic douloureux, or trigeminal neuralgia, can be exquisitely painful and may require constant drug use or even nerve block surgery in the facial area.

Many acupuncturists have reported very gratifying results with tic douloureux patients. Acupuncture is certainly a logical alternative in any severe case.

Purely on some anecdotal information, it might be a good idea to try a gram of calcium a day plus 400 I.U. of vitamin D. One woman who said that she had severe neuritis in her lower left jaw reported that she obtained complete relief after taking several teaspoons a day of brewer's yeast fortified with vitamin $B_{12}$. If it's difficult for you to take brewer's yeast, take a B-complex supplement that has all the B factors in it, including $B_{12}$.

# Tooth Grinding

Tooth grinding or bruxism occurs during sleep and seems to be more frequent in children than adults. Before taking the child (or yourself) to a psychologist or beginning a program of systematic relaxation, try chewing up a few calcium or bone meal tablets before going to sleep. Just as calcium frequently helps cramps, it seems to also reduce contractions of the jaw muscles.

Typical report: A four-year-old girl had been grinding her teeth for over a year. When her mother asked the dentist what could be done for her, he said nothing until her permanent teeth came in. She then began grinding up two bone meal tablets and putting them in a tablespoon of wheat germ, all of which she mixed up in some buckwheat pancake batter to make a pancake for her daughter. "The results were immediate. The very first night she did not grind her teeth and hasn't since, except for two days we were away from home and I didn't give her the bone meal and wheat germ."

# Tooth Loss

## A New Way of Brushing to Save Your Teeth
**by Stephen M. Feldman, D.D.S., M.S. Ed.***

To a medical doctor, Anna would have appeared to be a perfectly healthy young woman: about 20 years old, rather slender and

* Dr. Stephen M. Feldman is Assistant Professor of Periodontics and Coordinator of Preventive Dentistry Programs at the College of Medicine and Dentistry of New Jersey, New Jersey Dental School, Jersey City.

attractive. But as a periodontist, or gum specialist, I was struck by the fact that her gums were red, swollen, and puffy. She told me that they not only bled when she brushed them, but also when she ate anything hard or fibrous like corn on the cob, apples, or almost any other type of firm fruit. She had been suffering from this problem for several years, she admitted.

Anna was not very concerned about the problem because like most people, she thought of oral health in terms of cavities, and she was proud of the fact that she brushed her teeth several times a day in the up-and-down manner she'd been taught, and very rarely needed a filling. But the condition of Anna's mouth told me that before too long she would develop dental problems far more serious than cavities and would probably wind up needing a dental prosthesis, which is the polite name for false teeth.

In people past the age of about 35, I explained to her, by far the greatest cause of tooth loss is gums that bleed, recede, and eventually become so weak and incompetent that they can no longer protect the bone that holds the teeth firmly in place. I also explained that if she followed a new technique of brushing which I showed her, she could heal her gums and tremendously reduce the chances that she would need a prosthesis in the future.

When I saw her about five days later, I noticed that her gums had stopped bleeding almost completely. Within a matter of weeks, her gum color changed from unhealthy red to a healthy pink. This particular patient's gums haven't bled and have remained healthy for the past six years. I know this for a fact because I wound up marrying that young patient and I see her gums almost every day.

The technique which I demonstrated to Anna is called the Bass brushing technique, and learning how to use it daily will pay anyone handsome dividends in terms of a cleaner mouth, fresher breath, healthier gums, and teeth that stay where they're supposed to.

Before explaining the Bass technique, though, I'd like to say a few words about brushing in general. Here is a statement recently made by the American Society for Preventive Dentistry: "Even if you brush your teeth twice a day and see your dentist twice a year, this would not be enough to stop dental disease."

But what's wrong with brushing twice a day? Is more frequent brushing necessary? Well, it really doesn't matter if you brush your teeth 50 times a day—you could still get dental problems. Brushing, just *any* kind of brushing, does not necessarily remove *plaque,* and it is plaque that is the major cause of both periodontal or gum disease and tooth decay as well.

Plaque is an invisible, sticky, harmful bacterial deposit that continually forms on your teeth. Its accumulation cannot readily be prevented. But if plaque is removed effectively at least once a day, it will rarely be able to damage your teeth and gums. So when we talk about better mouth health, we should be talking about plaque removal, rather than just brushing.

## Don't Brush Your Gums Off Your Teeth

Brushing certainly can get rid of plaque but only if it is done correctly. Many conscientious people follow the advice of a jingle that goes: "Brush your teeth the way they grow, down from above and up from below." This is a good rhyme but a poor way to brush your teeth.

Perhaps you use a medium or hard toothbrush and scrub the daylights out of your teeth, using a back-and-forth motion. *A medium or hard brush is likely to scrub your gums right off your teeth,* leaving you with gum recession, notches on your teeth, and tooth sensitivity. Many people I have examined, including young people, already have one or more of these problems because of a brush that is too hard.

This takes us to the work of Dr. Charles C. Bass, Dean Emeritus of Tulane University Medical School in New Orleans, who back in 1948 developed the technique that we are teaching today to dental students as well as patients.

Curiously, Dr. Bass was a physician, not a dentist. He became interested in preventive dentistry for one reason—which is probably the same reason you are reading this article—he had personal dental problems. Although he was brushing his teeth twice a day and seeing his dentist regularly, he was still getting cavities and his gums bled occasionally when he brushed them.

As a physician, he realized that bleeding from the epithelium is neither normal nor healthy. The fact that his gums were bleeding meant that the epithelium was broken and that germs could enter his system and infect the bone that supports the teeth.

Dr. Bass wondered if the toothbrush he was using had anything to do with his dental problems. Having several lenses around, he casually began looking at the bristles of his toothbrush under magnification. He suddenly realized that something was definitely wrong with conventional toothbrushes. Looking at the magnified bristle ends, he noticed they had "sharp, rough corners." The points of the bristles looked to him just like miniature knives! No wonder his mouth was bleeding.

## Soft, Flexible Brush Needed to Dislodge Plaque

Dr. Bass knew enough about dentistry to realize that germs that cause gum damage are lodged in the plaque at the gum line where the teeth and gums meet, and within the gum crevice—the shallow space between the gums and teeth. But when those sharp bristles were used to remove plaque from the gum line, they tended to scratch the delicate gum tissue or even puncture it, creating small holes. Furthermore, he discovered that it's difficult to push the thick bristles of a hard toothbrush into the gum crevice, which is normally a very narrow space.

Dr. Bass concluded that the right kind of toothbrush should have thin, flexible bristles that would be easy to put into the gum crevice to clean out plaque. The thinner bristles needed to be rounded off and polished at their ends, so that the filament tip would be smooth and not sharp. Dr. Bass's modifications resulted in a new brush head that was soft and flexible enough to bend when pressed against the gums. To top it off, the bristles reached further into the crevices of the teeth and the biting surfaces as well, where many cavities begin.

After using such a brush, Dr. Bass declared: "The author maintains his own teeth and gums free from active dental disease. No hemorrhage occurs from his gums" (*Dental Items of Interest,* 70:697, 1948).

Most of my patients who have learned Bass's method could also make that statement, and so could I. Could you?

If you would like to, let's get started. The first thing you will need is a proper toothbrush.

Dr. Bass recommended a toothbrush which has a plain, straight handle and is about six inches long. The brush head should be small in size, about an inch or less, with the bristles arranged straight in a line.

The toothbrush is one case in which something synthetic (nylon) is better than something natural. When a natural bristle is cut in the manufacturing process, it breaks off leaving a rough or sharp-angle surface that is not easily rounded and polished, as is the case with nylon filaments. Nylon bristles also soften up under warm water, which is not true of natural bristles. So your toothbrush should have soft, nylon bristles which are rounded and polished. For children, the same basic design is used but the brush is smaller.

Dr. Bass created a brush himself which is still being made today and goes by the name of "Bass" Right-kind/Sub-G. The "Sub-G" stands for sub-gum. This is not a Chinese delicacy—it refers to the fact that the small brush head is designed to reach under the gum line and into the gum crevice.

While Dr. Bass was somewhat insistent on the use of one particular brush, most dentists today teaching disease control are more flexible on this issue. There are many brushes on the market that are soft and have rounded, polished bristles, and are therefore useful and safe for removing plaque. The key words to remember are "soft," "rounded," and either "polished" or "satinized." I have been in supermarkets where every brush was the wrong kind, including the soft ones, so look carefully at any brush you buy. Drugstores generally seem to have a better selection of brushes than supermarkets.

**Toothpaste** ● What about toothpaste? Toothpaste is not actually necessary for removing plaque and preventing gum disease, but it may help remove stain, which is a brown material that forms around your teeth, especially if you drink coffee, tea, or smoke tobacco. It won't do any good on stain that has accumulated over the months, but it will remove stain as it forms on a daily basis. However, I would avoid using any highly abrasive toothpaste, such as those heavily advertised as being good for getting teeth their whitest. Teeth are not white; they are various shades of yellow. The use of abrasive toothpaste can lead to very annoying tooth sensitivity.

On the positive side, there is an effervescence that occurs when using toothpaste which can aid in removing plaque.

## How to Brush the Bass Way

To brush the Bass way, put the ends of the toothbrush bristles directly into the crevice where your teeth meet your gums, pushing them in as far as possible, at about a 45 degree angle to the long way of the teeth. Use firm pressure and wiggle the brush back and forth with short strokes. The base of the brush head will be moving much more than the tips of the bristles, which will remain nearly stationary. This action helps dislodge plaque, which is the whole point of the procedure.

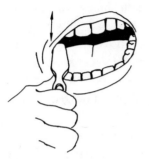

*To dislodge plaque, wiggle the brush back and forth right in the crevice where your teeth meet your gums.*

Your gums may bleed when you first try this. If they do, it is either a sign that your gums are unhealthy or that you picked an improper toothbrush. If you continue to brush correctly with a proper brush, the bleeding should go away within five days, and your gums will toughen up. Once this happens, even vigorous brushing will not cause bleeding, except for ulcerated areas which may not have healed.

To brush the biting surfaces of the teeth, place the bristles on top of the teeth, press down firmly, and vibrate the brush back and forth with short strokes.

The inside, or lingual (tongue-side) surfaces, are brushed in a similar manner to the outside surfaces, except that you may find it easier to hold the brush in a vertical, rather than a horizontal position, especially

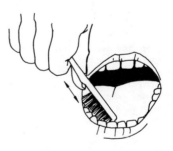

*It is often easier to hold the brush vertically to clean the inside teeth surfaces in the front of the mouth.*

in the front of the mouth, where the dental arch is curved. But the idea is still the same: push the tips of the bristles directly into the crevice where the teeth meet the gums, and then vigorously vibrate the brush so that plaque is cleaned out.

**Flossing Is Also Important** ● It is impossible to get the brush into the interproximal surfaces between the teeth, unless you have large spaces there. Normally the teeth are touching each other. You will therefore need dental floss to get these interproximal surfaces clean. But please be very careful. You should really get some professional help, if you haven't already, in learning how to floss without slashing your gums. You can use either waxed or unwaxed floss—the choice is up to you.

Take out a three-foot piece of floss and wrap it around the middle finger of each hand. Then, using the first finger and thumb as a guide, *gently* ease the floss through the contact area between each tooth and insert the floss as far down as it will go between the gum and tooth. Be careful not to snap the floss through the contact area between the teeth as this might injure the gum. Instead, gently tease it through, by sawing it in and out as you carry the floss down to the gum.

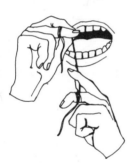

*Wrap the dental floss around the middle fingers, as shown here, and carefully guide it through the space between each tooth.*

Now hold the floss snugly around the tooth and bring it up and down several times. As the floss becomes ragged, wind it around one finger and off the other. This method removes plaque from between the teeth. This is an important area to keep clean every day, because most cavities and gum problems start in this area. Many people think that the purpose of using floss is to remove just the food that gets stuck between the teeth. These food particles may cause bad breath, but they do not cause cavities or gum disease. Plaque does. Even if you don't eat for a day, plaque will still accumulate in your mouth. Therefore, you should floss every day, whether or not you get food stuck between your teeth.

It's a good idea to use a methodical approach when brushing and flossing so that no surfaces of any teeth are missed. I suggest starting both brushing *and* flossing behind the last upper tooth in the back of the mouth, on the right side. Most people neglect cleaning the area behind the last tooth in the mouth and, as a result, often have deepened gum crevices in this area which require gum surgery to reduce the crevice depth and allow for proper cleaning. Move along the back of your teeth until you reach the left side of your mouth, and repeat the procedure on your bottom teeth. Then go back to the same upper right tooth and scrub the biting surface. When you have cleaned all the biting surfaces, you are ready to brush the gum crevices over the front of your teeth.

It's best, as I said, to do this very methodically, because each tooth has five surfaces that must be cleaned: front, back, top or biting surface, and two sides. If you are lucky enough to have all your adult teeth, you have 32 of them in your mouth, and 32 times 5 equals 160 surfaces! You can't reach all of them if you are going to be casual about it.

After you are done brushing, you can floss your teeth. Or, if you wish, you may floss them first. The important thing is to remove all your plaque by brushing and flossing properly at least once a day. Brushing after every meal is not necessary, but may be helpful for some people.

**Fine Tuning Your Plaque Control** • Some plaque may remain on your teeth even after diligently applying all of the rules for effective brushing. Therefore, after you wiggle the bristles of your toothbrush into the gum crevice, you may find it helpful to roll the brush towards the biting surfaces of the teeth in order to get them completely clean. In other words, you wiggle and then you roll. This might sound like a new dance craze, but it's actually a variation on Bass's brushing technique called the "Modified-Bass."

I strongly urge you to get some professional assistance in learning how to set up your own program of plaque control. The scientific evidence linking plaque to dental disease became available only recently. It will take time for this information to reach the entire dental profession. Many dentists already have excellent plaque-control programs in force, but they are in the minority. If your dentist does not have such a program, ask him if he knows of another dentist who does. Your local dental society may be of help. Every area has one—get the number from your dentist or look it up in the phone book. Or you can write directly to the American Society for Preventive Dentistry at 435 N. Michigan Avenue, Chicago, Illinois 60611.

**Diet Is Also Important** ● Diet, of course, plays a vital role in maintaining the health of the oral tissues. While it is essential for everyone to get all he needs of vitamins and minerals, so far as your dental health is concerned, what you *don't* eat is just as important as what you do eat. Avoid all refined sugar to the greatest possible extent. Table sugar is especially damaging when eaten in sticky snack foods between meals. The bacteria in plaque use the sugar to produce an acid which causes tooth decay and can rot your teeth right out of your mouth. People who eat few sugar-containing foods tend to get fewer cavities. The opposite is true for sugar lovers.

Another good reason for avoiding refined sugar is that an excess of sugar actually causes *more* plaque to form on your teeth. The more plaque you have, the more gum damage you may get.

## You Can Do What No Dentist Can

Now, let's briefly summarize the outstanding points of this approach to preventing tooth loss with oral hygiene. First, get yourself a toothbrush with soft nylon bristles, rounded and polished, with a small head which can easily fit in the corners of your mouth. Place the bristles directly into the gum crevice, at a 45-degree angle to the teeth, and press firmly while wiggling the top of the brush back and forth. Then roll the brush down along the tooth surface to complete the job.

Brush methodically, making sure to get the back of the teeth and the biting surfaces, as well as the front. Complete the job with gentle flossing, being careful not to lacerate your gums. Finally, rinse your mouth out thoroughly with water.

Remember, it's never too late to help yourself to better health. I have seen cases where a patient's gums have been bleeding for 30 years or more, with gradual loss of the gum tissue and subsequent loss of teeth, where the degeneration was halted within a week's time by the careful application of the techniques described here.

Remember, too, neither a dentist nor a periodontist can stop or prevent periodontal disease and bone loss from ruining your mouth. But *you* can prevent this disease, and probably keep your teeth for the rest of your life, by plaque control, proper diet, and professional help when needed.——*S.M.F.*

# Nutritional Cement for Loose Teeth

The right kind of oral hygiene is important in keeping the gums firm and strong enough to maintain their grasp on the teeth. But recent work in the laboratory and clinic shows there may be a deeper reason for tooth loss—as deep as the jawbone, to be exact.

While it's true that the teeth are supported by the gums, their roots are actually anchored in bony sockets on the crests of the jawbone. In advanced periodontal disease, these sockets shrink away from the teeth, and that is the main reason why 20 million Americans haven't got a single natural tooth left in their mouth.

The most widely held view today is that the direct cause of the bone recession is inflammation produced by bacteria which gained entrance through diseased gums. But there is another theory which says that the bone loss comes *first*. And that the cause of the bone loss is poor nutrition, not poor oral hygiene.

When Lennart Krook, D.V.M., Ph.D., and Leo Lutwak, M.D., Ph.D., and other researchers at Cornell University examined the jaws and several other bones from recently deceased patients who had periodontal disease, they found evidence of osteolysis, a deep-seated bone resorption (*Cornell Veterinarian,* July 1972). Here is where calcium plays a crucial role. Normally 99 percent of the calcium in the human body is found in the skeleton, while the remaining one percent circulates in the blood and other extracellular fluids. If the level in the blood should dip (as a result of the dietary calcium deficiency, for example) the blood must "borrow" some of this mineral from the bones.

In the cases that Cornell researchers examined, this "borrowing" had been going on for so long that the jawbones had lost considerable mass, and actually shrank. Other bones besides the jawbone were affected. "Bone loss caused by enhanced osteolysis was present in all bones from all subjects," the researchers reported. But "the bone loss was most severe in the jawbones, then in ribs and vertebrae, and least in long bones (such as arms and legs)."

The doctors theorize that as the jawbone recedes, movement of the loosened teeth injures adjacent gum tissue, causing inflammation and bleeding.

"It thus appears," they conclude, "that periodontal disease in man is probably a manifestation of generalized osteoporosis." Osteoporosis is the malady that makes bones porous, brittle, and fracture-prone with advancing age, particularly in women. Too low an intake of calcium is a major contributing cause.

## Teeth Gain Firmer Hold With Extra Calcium

What effect would extra calcium have on patients with periodontal disease? To find out, Drs. Krook, Lutwak and others selected ten patients—five men and five women—with ages ranging from 29 to 45 (*Cornell Veterinarian,* January 1972).

Taking a nutritional background survey, the researchers discovered that nine of the ten patients had daily calcium intakes of only 400 mg. or less. The Recommended Dietary Allowance for calcium for adult men and women is set at 800 mg. But the average intake of all ten patients was just 325 mg.—"a rather severe calcium deficiency," according to Dr. Krook and his colleagues.

For the next 180 days, the patients received 1,000 mg. of calcium a day in the form of calcium gluconolactate and calcium carbonate supplements. "All patients had gingivitis (gum inflammation) and bleeding at the start," the researchers noted. But after just six months of treatment, inflammation was improved in all cases and gone in three. Pockets along the roots of the teeth were recorded in eight patients before the study. In every case, pocket depth was reduced at the end of the treatment. Eight patients initially reported loose teeth. By the end of the study, tooth mobility was reduced in all but one. In one case, the teeth were now found to be completely firm in their foundations.

Even more impressive was what the investigators discovered when they examined X-rays of the patients' jaws. In seven of the ten cases, alveolar bone increased in amount and bony pockets along the roots of the teeth were partially filled in. *Healthy new bone had actually been deposited while the subjects were receiving additional calcium.*

Summing up their findings, the researchers concluded that "The clinical response to calcium therapy in periodontal disease was excellent. The radiologic examination showed that the osseous [bony] lesions are reversible. The improvement in amount of alveolar bone was remarkable, considering the relatively short period of treatment."

In addition to the effect on alveolar bone, the investigators reported that calcium supplementation caused two other "noteworthy changes": Blood pressure tended to decrease in the patients, and their serum cholesterol levels also dropped. Quite a bonus from a therapy aimed exclusively at achieving a healthy mouth!

In still another study reported in the *Israel Journal of Medical Sciences* (7: 504-505, 1971), Drs. Lutwak, Krook and others found that calcium supplementation does more than reverse the effects of bone resorption by depositing new tissue on bone surfaces. It can even make the *interior* of existing bone denser and stronger. Ninety patients with mild periodontal disease were selected, and their jawbone density measured by a special technical process called photon densitometry. Then one group received a gram of calcium every day for 12 months, while another group received a placebo. At the end of this period, the placebo group showed no change in bone density. But those who took calcium supplements regularly showed a significant increase in bone density of approximately 12.5 percent.

## Rx: 1,100 Mg. of Calcium, Plus Magnesium and Zinc

As a result of these and other experiments, Drs. Krook and Lutwak now believe that most adults need at least 1,100 mg. of calcium a day to protect against periodontal disease and osteoporosis.

And if you're going to increase your calcium intake, you might want to consider magnesium and zinc supplements as well. "Because it is known that the requirement of magnesium and zinc increases with increased dietary calcium," the pair note, "we propose that treatment of periodontal disease should include, in addition to increased calcium intake, increases in magnesium and zinc."

Recently a registered nurse from St. Louis wrote and told us that "Fifteen years ago, I received the diagnosis of osteoporosis of the anterior region of the lower jaw. . . . Though I improved my dietary calcium intake substantially over the years, X-rays continued to show little change in my bone condition. However, for about the past three years I have been taking bone meal and dolomite tablets, as well as A and D perles, twice daily. I was pleasantly surprised to learn that a recent dental film revealed almost complete recalcification of the area!"

## Good Oral Hygiene and Calcium and Other Minerals

If you use the Bass technique, which Dr. Feldman described earlier, you are doing the best you can to protect your teeth from an external point of view. It's something like applying fresh coats of paint to a house to prevent the underlying structures from being attacked by the elements.

But when you add calcium and other minerals to your diet, you're protecting your teeth from the inside as well. We should add that vitamin C is also of special importance in gum health, and that a number of people have told us that their gums stopped bleeding after they increased their intake of this vitamin. The combination of good oral hygiene and good nutrition—including the avoidance of sugary snacks—is an unbeatable one for total oral health.

# Toothache

Temporary relief from the pain of a common toothache may be achieved by removing—if you can—food debris from the cavity and applying oil of clove. The *Merck Manual* notes that "The clove oil may be mixed with zinc oxide powder to form a thick paste; this will afford longer relief and prevent the accumulation of food debris in the cavity."

If you don't have any clove oil—which you might be able to buy from an old-fashioned pharmacy—try using whole cloves. Steep them for a while in some hot water or honey to get the essential oil mobilized, and keep the clove in your mouth next to the aching tooth, rolling it around so that the oil contacts the tooth.

Other herbal oils said to be good for curing toothache are those obtained from sassafras and cayenne (red hot peppers). Apply with a swab.

Particularly useful for pain following an extraction is a wash of hot water and Epsom salts.

Recurrent toothaches, or an abscess under the tooth, are good indications for some definitive dental care. A woman recently asked me if I knew of any alternative to root canal therapy and I had to answer that the only alternative I knew from personal experience was agony.

# Ulcers

Stomach or gastric ulcers could profitably be studied as a case history in medical blundering. For years, a bland diet was prescribed for ulcers and, although some doctors still prescribe such a diet, there is no good evidence at all that bland foods are better for ulcers than any other kind of foods.

Antacids have also been used, but even their value has now been shown to be largely imaginary. Melvin L. Butler, LTC, M.D., and Harvey Gersh, CPT, M.D., in a study published in the *American Journal of Digestive Diseases* (September 1975) describe a controlled therapeutic study in which patients hospitalized with gastric ulcers were given either antacids or a placebo (dummy) liquid. The two doctors, both associated with the Gastroenterology Service at the Tripler Army Medical Center in Honolulu, found that there was no difference at all between the two groups in their rate of healing. They further suggest that the mere act of being hospitalized seems to create the kind of psychosomatic "atmosphere" which is necessary for most ulcers to heal, regardless of what kind of medication is or isn't used.

As for restrictive diets, they say that "The role of diet in the treatment of ulcer disease in general is probably of little importance. Except for evidence of stimulation of acid secretion by nicotine and alcohol, there is no scientific basis for a rigid dietary regimen in ulcer disease. 'Spicy' foods have not been shown to affect the gastric mucosa in any major way, and people who eat highly seasoned foods do not suffer an increase in gastric ulcer. We feel it is sufficient to advise patients with gastric ulcers to avoid only those foods that tend to give them 'heartburn' or pain."

It turned out in their study that even the suspicion that nicotine causes damage may not be true, because "the continuance of smoking did not appear to influence the rate of healing of gastric ulcers."

What all this means is that rather than go through life taking antacids (which can seriously upset the body's metabolic balance), people with ulcers should regard them as possibly symptomatic of stress. That doesn't mean that long psychotherapy is necessarily indicated, but it does point to the fact that chronic tension may well be involved in the cause of many ulcers. Relaxation, using a technique such as meditation or biofeedback, may help a lot. A few visits to a psychotherapist would also seem to be a logical step for a serious ulcer that may lead to surgery.

## Zinc Reported Helpful

One very encouraging finding about the healing of ulcers appeared in the *Medical Journal of Australia* on November 22, 1975, written by Dr. Donald J. Frommer, of the Department of Gastroenterology at the Prince of Wales Hospital in Sydney.

Ten ulcer patients were given 90 mg. of zinc (as zinc sulfate) three times a day, while eight other patients took a placebo. The patients in both groups were comparable in all respects, including the initial size of the ulcer. Neither patients nor doctors knew who was receiving the zinc and who was receiving the placebo until all the results were in. And those results showed that "Patients taking zinc sulfate had an ulcer healing rate three times that of patients treated with placebo. . . . Complete healing of ulcers occurred more frequently in the patients taking zinc sulfate than in patients treated with placebo. The placebo group contained more patients whose ulcers did not heal at all, than the group taking zinc sulfate. No side effects from zinc sulfate were noted."

Significantly, Dr. Frommer adds that "There was no evidence of zinc deficiency in any of the patients." That is an important observation because most of the studies which have been done with skin ulcers suggest that speedier healing is observed only in those patients who are actually low or deficient in zinc.

Dr. Frommer points out that zinc can accelerate the healing of gastric ulcers to a degree similar to that seen with a drug known as carbenoxolone. Zinc, however, has at least two advantages: "lower toxicity and cheapness." The drug, he says, has "a much higher frequency of serious side effects," and is about 10 times more expensive than zinc. Zinc sulfate, he notes, can sometimes cause mild gastric upset. But this can be avoided if the supplements are taken with food.

## Stress Ulcers and Vitamin A

There is a particularly severe form of ulcer known as a stress ulcer, which typically occurs in patients who have experienced severe injuries, such as large burns. In such cases, it's been shown that vitamin A offers very important protection. However, the vitamin A must be administered directly into the bloodstream in a water-soluble form, because in these states of stress, the body is apparently unable to mobilize vitamin A stores from the liver. It must also be given in very large amounts—several hundred thousand units. In such cases, a relative of the injured person should immediately talk with attending physicians, because stress ulcers can be very damaging and cause the loss of a great amount of blood.

# Ultrasound Therapy For Stiff Joints

A Pennsylvania businessman recently suffered a knee injury in an automobile accident. At the age of 50, he was still very athletic. But in the accident, the knee capsule had been lacerated.

"An injury of that type often means a permanently stiff knee, limping, and seriously restricted physical activity," says Richard N. Steigerwalt, chief physical therapist at the Allentown-Sacred Heart Hospital Center. "Frankly, we didn't expect him to achieve even 90 degrees of knee flexion." A normal individual has flexion of 135 degrees.

For more than two months, the executive underwent three-times-weekly treatments with ultrasound, a therapy commonly employed in physical therapy departments across the country, yet little known by the general public. Sometimes it does nothing. Sometimes it works virtual miracles. Usually, it helps.

Combined with strengthening and stretch exercises, the ultrasound therapy not only produced the 90-degree flexion the therapists hadn't anticipated, but more. By the time the executive discontinued treatment, satisfied with the results, he had achieved a flexion of 115 degrees. Today, he is back playing tennis several times a week—and a good game at that!

The device that helped him is not much bigger than the prover-bial bread box. On its face are a few simple dials and gauges. Attached to a cord running into the unit is a transducer similar in appearance to a small bathtub shower spray extension. At the "spray nozzle" end is a solid chrome plate about the size of a silver dollar. Instead of spraying water, the transducer sprays out a steady stream of sound waves, at a frequency so high that they are inaudible to the human ear.

In actual use, a gel is first applied to the surface of the body which is to be treated. When the transducer is placed against the injured part, the gel keeps the sound waves from being lost in air, which will not transmit them. The gel carries the waves directly to the skin.

## Sounds That Can Destroy or Massage

What happens when the current of an ultrasonic machine is turned on depends on the frequency of the sound waves being produced and the power or intensity of those waves. For therapeutic use, the frequency is usually set at about 800,000 to one million cycles per second, some 40 times higher than the 20,000 cycles per second which are the normal limits of our hearing. Increasing the *intensity* of the sound waves is like turning up the volume on a radio. If we could hear ultrasound, the increasingly intense or powerful waves would sound louder, just like music on the radio with the volume control turned way up.

In medical use, the relative intensity of the ultrasound waves is of critical importance.

At one end of the scale, surgeons are now using special devices with intensities on the order of 1,000 watts per square centimeter (WSC) to perform very difficult and detailed surgery in parts of the body inaccessible through traditional surgical approaches.

For nonsurgical uses, far lower intensities are used. Instead of destruction, what takes place is more like a gentle massage. The device used to treat the Allentown executive with the damaged knee was designed specifically for physical therapy, and could not have produced more than three WSC—a small fraction of the intensity used in surgery. That particular patient received two WSC for eight minutes, three times a week.

## Arthritis, Tendinitis, and Bursitis

And at proper intensities and frequencies, ultrasound may be the most effective therapy now available for people suffering from arthritis, tendinitis, bursitis, and related ailments. Evidence to that effect was presented as far back as September, 1965, when John L. Echternach, M.S., described his research with 73 patients in the *Journal of the American Physical Therapy Association.*

Typical was one 58-year-old man who came to Echternach complaining of shoulder pain. Movement of the shoulder was so limited because of the pain's severity that he was unable to work. A month later, he was free of pain, back at work, and had achieved an almost normal range of motion.

Another man, this one 47 years old, suffered from calcific tendinitis, a condition in which calcium forms along a tendon, irritating it and limiting its ability to stretch.

For a week, the man was treated with hot packs and exercise. When that failed, ultrasound was used. Twelve treatments later he had only minimal pain, regained normal flexion, and said he felt greatly improved. An X-ray examination showed that the calcification had disappeared.

All in all, Echternach said that 87 percent of his patients showed favorable results through ultrasound therapy. Of those suffering bursitis, 64 percent achieved good results. Echternach's definition of good is quite conservative: "Patients were considered to demonstrate good results if they exhibited normal range of motion (equal to the uninvolved shoulder), had minimal or no pain, and were able to return to full duties at work." Others might term that *excellent* results.

Fair results were experienced by 24 percent of the bursitis cases. Only 12 percent had poor results.

Of the patients suffering tendinitis, almost half (48 percent) showed good improvement on the ultrasound therapy.

All of which means that "a trial of ultrasound therapy would be indicated in both acute and chronic phases of shoulder disability," even though chances of success are higher if the ailment is treated as soon as it develops, rather than a long while later.

## Chronic Arthritic Pain Can Also Be Helped

A more detailed study of patients with *chronic* arthritis was reported in the April 1970 issue of *Physical Therapy* by James E. Griffin, Ph.D., and his colleagues. They studied 120 patients, ranging in age from 28 to 73. Most were over 50. All were suffering from chronic osteoarthritis or similar joint disease involving the shoulder, spine, hip, thoracic or lumbar vertebrae, or knee.

Dr. Griffin's study is important not only because it shows the potential effectiveness of ultrasound in treating ailments that are otherwise often untreatable, but also because it shows the necessity for precisely right frequency levels.

Dr. Griffin divided his patients into two groups. Each received three treatments a week for three weeks, at essentially the same intensity—1.5 to 2.0 WSC. The only difference was that one group received the ultrasound treatment at 89,000 waves per second, while the other received one million waves per second.

A surprisingly high degree of success among those receiving lower frequency treatments was reported: 63.5 percent showed significant improvement, 28.8 percent reported partial improvement, and only 7.7 percent remained unimproved.

Among those who underwent the higher frequency treatment, only 30.3 percent were improved, 41 percent partially improved, and 28.7 percent unimproved.

This finding that lower frequencies are more effective confirms similar conclusions in studies with animals. It also offers an explanation for the fact that some researchers have not experienced any particular success using ultrasonic therapy on patients.

Why success at the lower frequencies? Says Dr. Griffin: "The superior pain-relieving effects of low-frequency ultrasound in shoulder, vertebral, hip, and knee lesions are assumed to be the result of the greater depth of penetration of this frequency."

## Three Ways in Which Ultrasound Helps

The ability of ultrasound to penetrate deep into body tissue, reaching the desired target, is one of three important characteristics which make it so useful in physical therapy.

Besides relieving pain and stiffness, the penetrating waves may offer added benefits to those suffering acute arthritic pains and forced to resort to the potentially dangerous corticosteroids. A study by Dr. Griffin, Echternach, and two of their colleagues published in the July 1967 issue of *Physical Therapy,* shows that corticosteroid ointment driven through the tissue to the site of injury by an ultrasonic device was tremendously more effective than corticosteroids given by hypodermic. Hopefully, ultrasound will significantly reduce the amount of corticosteroids given orally—reducing potential adverse effects.

Ultrasound's second characteristic is that it produces heat as the sound waves rub against cell molecules and cause them to vibrate. "Heat has often been the basis of treatment for arthritic ailments," says Steigerwalt. "Traditionally we've used heat packs, infrared, similar approaches. But their effectiveness was significantly limited because such modalities rarely penetrate to any degree beneath the skin. Ultrasound can penetrate into the joint, and in acute cases, that's what's needed."

Heat, it seems, increases metabolism. And that may bring about any number of desirable effects. It could increase production of natural lubricants in the joint, reduce swelling, break down undesired and painful calcium formations, and increase blood supply.

Ultrasound's third characteristic is that it massages the painful tissue. This may relax muscles that are in spasm, causing agonizing pain to tendons and ligaments. If it relaxes the muscles constricting blood vessels, blood flow will increase and this will have a positive effect.

Probably through its capacity to massage, ultrasound also depolymerizes—loosens the glue in long-chained protein molecules so these tissues become more flexible. Thus, tendons and muscles that are under spasm and acutely painful, making motion impossible, can become flexible once more.

## The Gray Lining on a Silver Cloud

But the silver cloud of ultrasound therapy has a gray lining. For all its medical value, research into ultrasonic therapy (as well as diagnosis and surgery) is not nearly adequate. And standards are practically nonexistent.

We do not know, for example, precisely the most desirable levels of intensity and frequency for treating an ailment of the shoulder as compared to the hip or the back—nor how many minutes the treatment should ideally last. We *do* know that excessive exposure, even to the relatively low frequency physical therapy device, can produce a very painful burning sensation to bone surfaces, which absorb the heat of the ultrasonic waves far more readily than do the soft tissues.

We do *not* know what permanent damage can be caused, and at what levels—although with the physical therapy machines, long experience has suggested no danger.

The degree of inefficiency in some ultrasonic machines is nothing short of appalling. Writing in the July 1974 issue of *Physical Therapy,* Harold F. Stewart, Ph.D., and his colleagues describe a survey conducted by the Bureau of Radiological Health of the Food and Drug Administration in the St. Petersburg, Florida, area. Investigators reviewed information on ultrasonic therapy units found in hospitals, clinics, medical centers, nursing homes, private offices, and health spas. In the words of Dr. Stewart and his associates, "Eighty-five percent of the units surveyed had indicated output levels that differed from the actual measured output values by more than 20 percent for at least one power setting." Of these, about 25 percent radiated more ultrasound than indicated and 60 percent produced less ultrasound than indicated.

Dr. Stewart says, "The most striking result of the survey was that the ultrasonic therapy units were, in general, out of calibration; some had outputs much higher than indicated, and others produced less ultrasound than indicated."

## What's Needed in the Future

Ultrasound is no toy. It is an immensely valuable and potentially destructive therapeutic tool. And those who use it in the St. Petersburg area told the investigators through answers to a questionnaire where ultrasound ought to be going.

—An interlocked timer should be included in all ultrasonic therapy equipment so that the machine will shut off after the desired treatment is complete.

—Some degree of knowledge regarding ultrasound, its frequencies, intensities, effects on tissue, etc., are essential to those who use it. Labeling, providing this information, should be required for each device.

—Information should be available indicating what size area of the body is being treated by the ultrasonic transducer at any given time. Thus, the therapist will have a better chance to avoid both excessive treatment by accidentally overlapping, and insufficient treatment by missing areas he had assumed were being exposed to ultrasound.

—Probably most important, standards must be set for both the timing devices used on ultrasound equipment and the accuracy of frequency and intensity calibrations.

Standards such as these, along with a great deal of concrete research into precisely how and why and under what circumstances ultrasound does what it does—those are the factors on which ultrasound's future depends. Today, it usually helps. Tomorrow, given greater precision and knowledge, it could be a major factor in reducing the need for drugs.

# Urinary Incontinence

Frequent, excessive, or uncontrollable urination is only symptomatic and thorough medical evaluation is always needed to try to find the cause, which may be anything from diabetes to nervousness. Once there has been medical treatment and the problem persists, we can only refer to the world of folk remedies. Unfortunately, folk remedies are abundant for obstructed urination but skimpy when it comes to urinary incontinence. Dr. George Zofchak, an herbalist, told us that St.-John's-wort is a specific for this problem.

One anecdote is possibly worth passing along. A reader who suffered from bladder incontinence for five years, and urinated every hour or two during the day and had to get up as often as five times a night, told us that she stumbled across the solution to her problem in the form of cherry juice.

Previously, she had tried various home remedies and had been to a doctor who prescribed hormones which did not help. For no particular reason, she drank a bottle of cherry juice during the course of one week and was surprised to realize that her bladder trouble was much improved. After that, she took it regularly and the problem all but disappeared. She said that she buys cherry juice concentrate from a health food store and uses one tablespoon in a glass of water each morning.

# Urinary Problems

Clearing up urinary problems requires not only excellent medical attention, but frequently persistence and some imagination, because medicine is sometimes not enough. Metabolic or environmental conditions often play an unsuspected role in urinary problems, as demonstrated by the facts that inflammation may be present without unusual amounts of bacteria, or a lot of bacteria may be found in the urine but no infection or even inflammation.

A good example of some of the "surprises" that are constantly showing up in urological research is the finding that milk—perfectly pure milk—can cause urinary infections in girls and probably women as well. That particular story is unfolded in the pages of the August 1973 issue of *Pediatrics* by P. Z. Neumann, M.D., and colleagues, of Canada. Dr. Neumann provided additional information at a meeting of urological specialists held in Toronto that same year.

To begin with, you have to appreciate the fact that recurring urinary tract infections are as frustrating to doctors as they are painful and debilitating to the victims. In a small number of cases, the problem is caused by a physical obstruction in the tract, which can be remedied by surgery. In most cases, there is no obstruction, and although the infection can be temporarily beaten down with antibiotics, it proves to be persistent in some 50 to 60 percent of all cases. And the repeated use of antibiotics, particularly in young children, is something that all conscientious doctors try to avoid —if possible.

The Canadian doctors, who see thousands of children in their practices, noticed that an extraordinarily high number who had urinary tract infections also had chronic constipation. While constipation is seen in a general population of pediatric patients at the rate of about 15 percent, the Canadians noticed that in those who had urinary infections, 34 percent of one group and 42 percent of another group were either constipated or had otherwise abnormal bowel habits.

The doctors selected 45 children who had a history of urinary tract infection and abnormal bowel habits as well. One of the first things they discovered was that in no case did the parents volunteer the information to doctors that their children were constipated; this fact had to be solicited by the doctors. That helps explain why the relationship between the two conditions had not previously been recognized.

Careful examination of the children showed that none of them had physical obstructions of the urinary tract. However, many of them had a dilated colon typical of the damage wrought by chronic constipation.

All 45 children were put on a four-pronged regimen. Antibiotics were given for six weeks to wipe out the infecting organisms. Parents were then instructed in proper bowel training techniques, consisting essentially of sitting the child on the toilet with feet on the floor for proper leverage for 30 minutes after each meal. A successful bowel movement at one sitting would eliminate the next two. To start the program off, a bowel stimulant and lubricant were also given to the children during the first six weeks.

It turned out, though, that the most important part of the regimen was the dietary advice. And this, the doctors say, consisted of "essentially the exclusion of milk and milk products." The reason we say it was apparently the most important factor is that in the nine cases where the regimen failed to prevent a recurrence of urinary tract infection, the most common finding was that bowel habits had not been normalized, "usually resulting from persistence of large milk intake," the doctors declared.

## Milk Elimination Very Effective

In the other 36 children where the recommended dietary regimen was followed, *there was not a single recurrence of infection.* The overall success rate was therefore 80 percent. But in those cases where bowel function was normalized, primarily by means of diet modification, the success rate was 100 percent.

Although these results were very gratifying, the researchers decided to make certain that the success of their treatment was in fact produced by the elimination of constipation. After a year had gone by, they told the parents of 18 of the 45 children to forget about the diet and bowel habits they had previously followed. The result, after another year, was that the 18 children had a total of 16 urinary tract infections, or a recurrence rate of 88 percent.

Eventually, all the children were put back on the regimen, and the incidence of reinfection dropped to nearly zero, with the exceptions always associated with the return of constipation.

That was quite a triumph, because as the doctors point out, the only other way to achieve this kind of success is to administer antibiotics "constantly."

At this point, we have to answer two questions. First, why

should constipation cause urinary infection? And why would reducing or eliminating dairy products end constipation?

The first question is answered by the doctors themselves, who explain that when the rectum is full, particularly in the small pelvic space of a child, there can be great pressure on the neck of the bladder. This in turn causes a back up or retention of urine, which creates the right conditions for the multiplication of bacteria. Because of the presence of the ovaries, the pelvic region of a girl is even more crowded, and this may be one reason why these infections are more common in girls than boys (and women than men).

As for how these infections get started, one medical text states that the large bowel is considered to be the major source of bacteria, although it has not yet been established precisely how the germs get from the large bowel into the bladder.

The answer to why milk can cause constipation seems to be that when children fill up on milk, they do not get enough of the bulk they need to establish good bowel function. Neither milk nor cheese nor ice cream contains even a trace of fiber.

Do these findings have relevance for adults? When Dr. Neumann reported on his work at a meeting of urologists, one of the doctors present said that there was, indeed, an association between constipation and urinary tract infections in adults.

Of course, it's possible for an adult to be constipated even if he or she does not drink a great deal of milk. The best way to solve the problem is to avoid laxatives completely and simply make sure you get an adequate amount of fiber and fluids in your daily diet. Many people find the most convenient way to do this is to take several tablespoons of bran each day, mixed with cereal or yogurt.

## Full Bladder Bad

Bad bladder habits as well as bowel habits can also lead to recurring urinary infections, according to Dr. Jack Lapides. At the meeting of the Utah State Medical Association in Salt Lake City in 1972, Dr. Lapides, head of the Urology Section at the University of Michigan, made one of the more interesting statements I have read about health. "If Women's Lib is seeking a cause," Dr. Lapides said, "I can think of none more worthy or important than encouraging females to urinate more frequently" (*Family Practice News,* December 15, 1972).

The urologist said that holding urine in too long distends the bladder and sets up the right conditions for infection. Sometimes the problem is created by what is called "an infantile bladder," in which pressure is built up very quickly.

At least two other habits may be involved in causing or preventing the clearing up of urinary infections in women. One is the habit of using toilet paper in such a way that the tissue is drawn up in the direction of the vagina. The bacteria found in fecal matter are also frequently found in urinary infections, and wiping in this manner is decidedly unwise.

### Sexual Habits Important

Sexual habits may also play an important role in chronic urinary infections. Dr. Saul Kent, writing in *Geriatrics* (July 1975), points out that "infection may occur during various kinds of sexual activity. The infective organisms may be introduced into the urethra by manual or oral stimulation of the vagina or clitoris during foreplay, or the vulva, urethra, or bladder may be irritated during intercourse."

He adds that "The anterior 'high-riding' position of the male partner during intercourse may heighten clitoral stimulation but can also cause excessive irritation to the adjoining urethra. . . . Post-menopausal women tend to have weakened urethral and vaginal walls because of estrogen deprivation, which may predispose them to trauma during intercourse and to lower urinary tract infection. They also have diminished vaginal lubrication and a more constricted, shorter vaginal barrel and thus are more susceptible than younger women to mechanical irritation."

In addition to drug therapy, Dr. Kent recommends that "it may be helpful for the patient to flush out the lower urinary tract by urinating as soon as possible after intercourse. Intake of extra fluids may be helpful in this regard. A shower before and after intercourse may decrease the number of organisms in the periurethral area. The male-superior position for intercourse is probably not advisable when recurrent infection is a problem, because this position exerts extra stress on the urethra."

Fletcher C. Derrick, Jr., M.D., of the Medical University of South Carolina at Charleston, wrote in *Postgraduate Medicine* in March 1975, that "I instruct women with recurrent infection following intercourse to place a pillow under their hips during intercourse.

This prevents the thrusting and massaging action of the penis against the urethra. A rear approach instead of the male-on-top position eliminates massage of the urethra and may prevent recurrent infection. Also, sufficient foreplay is important to allow the lubricating juices of the vagina to flow."

Dr. Derrick also points out that "A few women who take oral contraceptives experience increased susceptibility to urinary tract infection and have recurring infections or vaginitis. Discontinuance of the Pill very often stops further recurrence. Tampons and douches occasionally appear to contribute to recurrent infection, and the patients should be advised to stop their use."

The urologist adds that a woman may cause a man problems, instead of vice versa, by passing along bacteria from her vagina into his urethra. "Temporary use of condoms may result in a cure."

## Vitamin C Can Help

Another approach to controlling urinary infections is to increase the acidity of urine. At the Veterans Administration Hospital in St. Louis, a group of five doctors who work with spinal cord injury patients said in a letter to the *Journal of the American Medical Association* (April 21, 1975) that as a routine procedure, all these patients "received doses of ascorbic acid [vitamin C] of or more than 4 gm./day [4,000 mg. daily] to enhance urinary acidity." (Actually, the reason they wrote that letter was not to make a case for vitamin C, but to refute the suggestion that taking large amounts of vitamin C causes a deficiency of vitamin $B_{12}$. Their letter went on to state that although ten patients had been taking high doses of ascorbic acid for more than 11 months, all had perfectly normal $B_{12}$ levels and three were actually above the "high normal" level.)

Vitamin C can also help when inflammation but not infection is present. That is the case in urethritis—irritation of the male urethra —caused by phosphatic crystals. Dr. Stephen N. Rous, Chief of Service in the Department of Urology at the New York Medical College—Metropolitan Hospital Center, said in an article in the *New York State Journal of Medicine* (December 15, 1971) that 12 men suffering from this painful disorder were checked and found to be free of any infection or damage that might be causing their misery during and after each urination. Each man was then given three grams (3,000 mg.) of vitamin C for four days. Result? "Complete relief of symptoms," Dr. Rous said.

The urologist explained that the irritating phosphatic crystals had apparently formed in the urine because of insufficient acidity. The large dose of vitamin C proved to be a safe way of introducing enough acidity to force the crystals back into solution.

It is interesting to note at this point that what cured Dr. Rous's patients and protected the patients at the St. Louis Hospital was the "wasted" vitamin C, the part that could not be used by the body and spilled into the urine. But far from being wasted, as some "authorities" insist it is, the excess vitamin C in their urine was exactly what these men needed to protect or restore their health.

A number of PREVENTION readers have told us various ways in which they seem to have overcome recurrent urinary problems. One woman who read about acidifying the urine with vitamin C said that her husband had been taking ampicillin for months due to a chronic bladder infection, but when he began taking vitamin C together with the medicine four times a day, the infection swiftly cleared up.

## Folk Remedies

Folk medicine has it that vinegar will acidify the urine, but the information I've seen about the manner in which vinegar is metabolized by the body indicates that this effect is at best unlikely and perhaps impossible. Cranberries are believed by at least some doctors to be able to acidify the urine. A woman told us that she had been suffering with chronic bladder infections for more than 40 years and nothing helped for very long. She even tried canned cranberry juice, but it did nothing. What did help her, she said, was grinding up *fresh* cranberries in the food chopper. She mixed some of the cranberries with yogurt and added a little honey and began eating some every day. This regimen, she told us, has kept her free from infections for a full year. (Just as we were going to press, medical tests confirmed that both cranberry juice *and* vitamin C are effective in acidifying the urine, and therefore helpful in preventing recurrences of urinary infection. When cranberry juice and vitamin C are taken together, the acidifying effect is even greater than when taken individually.)

Still another reader, a registered nurse, told us that she discovered she was able to abolish her cystitis, or bladder infection, by taking six tablets of dolomite with plenty of water several times a day. This worked, she said, after her doctor's prescription, a sulfonamide drug, failed to do the trick. Since then, she said, she had two more recurrences and each time took dolomite and water. "Both times it completely cleared within a day. My sister had the same results when she recently got cystitis."

The pods of kidney beans are apparently also very helpful in relieving some cases of urinary retention and irritation. However, only the fresh pods seem to work, and the tea made from them must be rapidly used. So the only way to get the benefit from this folk remedy is to plant kidney beans. In any event, a surprisingly large number of readers with urinary problems told us that they tried taking kidney bean pods and found that it worked amazingly well. One gave these instructions for making tea:

> Pick the beans from your garden, remove the pods, and put about two ounces of pods in four quarts of water and boil slowly for four hours. Strain carefully, let cool, strain again if necessary, and drink one glass every few hours. When the brew is more than 24 hours old, it may lose all its potency.

Judging from the letters we received, there is something in kidney bean pods which stimulates copious urination and often relieves pain.

There are a surprisingly large number of traditional herbal remedies for urinary retention, gravel, and other urinary problems. Apparently, most of these herbs work by stimulating urination, although some may have other properties as well. Generally, teas are made from these herbs in the usual manner, and two or three herbs are usually combined in the tea. In the approximate order of their traditional popularity, these herbs include bearberry (uva-ursi), corn silk (pulled from sweet corn), couchgrass, broom, buchu, cubeb berries, cleavers (goosegrass), dandelion root, parsley, and horseradish. Strawberries, asparagus, fresh watermelon, cherries, and a tea made by simmering watermelon seeds in water for half an hour are also valued for their diuretic effect.

See also KIDNEY STONES and URINARY INCONTINENCE.

# Varicose Veins

Varicose veins are a lot easier to prevent than they are to cure, but it's likely that many of the preventive steps will also help improve, or at the very least halt the progress of already existing varicosities.

One generally unappreciated finding about varicose veins is that they may be very closely linked with constipation. A recent analysis by British physicians established a solid statistical link between the two conditions, and on theoretical grounds, it is not difficult to understand why this is so.

Very simply, veins in the lower legs develop varicosities as a response to a backup of blood. Normally, most of the blood returning to the torso from the legs passes through deep veins, but when the blood backs up to the extent that they can't return it, it tries an end-run through superficial veins, and the result is those streaks of blue.

Constipation enters the picture because it necessitates straining at stool, and the straining blocks off veins used for the return of blood from the legs. Measurements taken with sophisticated instruments indicate that the resulting pressure can increase more than you might think.

So, number one, don't be constipated and don't strain. (See CONSTIPATION.)

Another cause of the sluggish return of blood from the legs is simply lack of exercise. People were made to walk, and the act of walking turns the calf muscles into what has been called a "second heart," with the contractions of this powerful muscle pushing blood upwards. When you don't walk, you aren't getting the benefit of this pumping action. When you sit in a chair for hours at a time, the situation is worse, because the pressure of the chair against the back of your legs may further reduce circulation. Finally, many people who do walk don't get the full benefit of this exercise because they wear high-heeled shoes that interfere with the full and natural contraction of leg muscles.

At every opportunity, go barefoot or wear flat shoes or negative-heel shoes, and give your legs a workout. It's also a good idea to periodically elevate your legs, as many doctors will recommend, but compared to active exercise that gets your feet, ankles, and calf muscles working, this is merely a stopgap measure.

Drs. Evan and Wilfrid Shute have reported many cases of varicose veins improving with vitamin E supplementation, usually in amounts ranging between 400 and 800 I.U. daily. It's their theory that vitamin E helps open collateral circulation in the legs which takes some of the pressure off the varicosities. In France, some doctors have reported gratifying results with bioflavonoid supplements.

When varicose ulcers develop, vitamin E can be applied directly as well as taken orally. A warm (not hot) poultice made from the mashed roots of the comfrey plant are also said to be helpful by some who have used them. If you wish, you can make an ointment which includes vitamin E and some strong brew made from the comfrey root. Oral supplements of zinc, 30 to 50 mg. a day, may also speed the healing of varicose or any other kind of ulcer. The healing of leg ulcers in people who are on cortisone therapy can be greatly helped by direct application of vitamin A in ointment form, as well as oral vitamin A.

# Vision Problems

There are relatively few natural therapies for visual problems that have been developed to the point where I would consider them "practical" enough to describe in detail here. One exception, of course, is that vitamin A is the specific and essential therapy for night blindness, or greatly diminished ability to see in dim light. If this condition is allowed to progress, the result can be permanent blindness. In some parts of the world, vitamin A deficiency is, in fact, the leading cause of blindness, particularly among children. These children need protein as well as vitamin A, because the vitamin A can't be used without sufficient protein.

Another example of a very specific natural therapy for a visual problem is elimination from the diet of all foods containing a sugar known as galactose. Some children are born with an enzyme deficiency and develop cataracts because their bodies cannot properly metabolize this sugar. Such cases need strict medical attention and a highly restricted diet which eliminates, among other things, milk and other unfermented dairy products; processed foods which may contain milk or milk sugars; legumes such as soybeans, peas, and lima beans; beets; liver; brains and sweetbreads.

For cross-eyed children, doctors may prescribe "orthoptic" exercises. Directions and guidance are needed from a doctor or visual therapist, and I will not describe these exercises here.

Although there are reports in the medical literature describing other natural therapies for more common visual disorders, these results seem not to have been duplicated by other investigators and in some cases involve procedures that are potentially dangerous. However, I feel I should mention one relatively well-known "therapy" for myopia, which is the system of exercises and "sunning" developed and popularized by William Horatio Bates, M.D., during the 1920s. His ideas were taken up by others and several books have lauded his techniques. Whether or not there is really anything to the Bates method, I cannot say, except that after studying the literature, pro and con, I doubt it. If you want more information on the Bates technique, you might want to read *Do You Really Need Eyeglasses?* (Hart, New York, 1974) by New York psychotherapist Marilyn B. Rosanes-Berrett, Ph.D.

Meanwhile, optical engineering has been producing a variety of new devices, including electronic night vision scopes which amplify available light even in near-total darkness. Ophthalmologists are doing some very interesting things with soft contact lenses, sometimes placing special medications under the lenses. Another promising lens is one which prevents ultraviolet radiation from the sun from reaching the eye and is said to halt the progression of myopia in children, sometimes even bringing about an improvement.

A small number of optometrists have been also using new approaches, including different kinds of spectacle and contact lenses to retrain or even reshape eye structures. Although good results are claimed, these treatments are still experimental and may be relatively expensive.

One of the major challenges in the vision field is diabetic retinopathy, which afflicts many thousands and is essentially atherosclerosis of the blood vessels in the eye's retina. Although it might be expected that a lifestyle and diet designed to improve microcirculation might help this condition, not much has been accomplished except for a few unduplicated studies. On the other hand, an optimal diet is advisable in any case, since eye problems are only part of the challenges facing the diabetic, and a good diet will help protect his health in general. Such a diet includes polyunsaturated oils such as safflower or wheat germ oil, calcium, plentiful amounts of lecithin derived from soybeans, and the full range of other nutrients.

# Visualization Therapy

**by Grace Halsell**

Visualization is in many ways similar to hypnosis except that the patient is conscious. By itself, visualization is not considered to be a definitive therapy for any medical disorder, but it is being increasingly used in conjunction with other therapies.

O. Carl Simonton, M.D., a specialist in oncology, the science of tumors, says results can sometimes be "truly amazing" when a cancer patient allows his mind to participate in his treatment.

Dr. Simonton, formerly chief of radiation therapy, David Grant USAF Medical Center, Travis Air Force Base near San Francisco, and now in private practice in Forth Worth, Texas, recalls that his first patient might have been considered by some as a "hopeless" case.

"He was a 61-year-old man with very extensive throat cancer. He had lost a great deal of weight (down to 98 pounds) and could barely swallow his own saliva and could eat no food."

Dr. Simonton, at that time serving his residency at the University of Oregon Medical School, recalls: "I told him how, through mental imagery, we were going to attempt to affect his disease. I had him relax three times a day, mentally picture his disease, his treatment, and the way his body was interacting with the treatment and the disease, so that he could better understand his disease and cooperate with what was going on. The results were truly amazing.

"He was an ideal patient because he was completely willing to cooperate. I taught him to relax and mentally picture his disease," Dr. Simonton relates. "Then I had him visualize an army of white blood cells coming, attacking, and overcoming the cancer cells. The results of treatment were both thrilling and frightening. Within two weeks his cancer had noticeably diminished and he was rapidly gaining weight. I say it was 'frightening' because I had never seen such a turnaround; I wasn't sure what was going on and I didn't know what I would do if things went sour. But they didn't go sour. The man had a complete remission.

"Like most cancer patients that I have treated, Bill had suffered an emotional stress not very long before the cancer became apparent —in his case, it was a serious loss on the stock market.

"Generally, a patient with an advanced cancer is depressed, even morbid. But from the start, Bill began to 'visualize' himself as being well; his picture of the future was positive, bright." He was able to take further radiation treatments, and, "even during the therapy his mental attitude was so strong that it enabled him to have the strength to go fishing every day.

"His attitude—and his recovery—was beyond anything I had

ever seen," Dr. Simonton says. "The surprising thing was not that he got over his malignancy so much as that he did so without any side effects from the treatment. He very much enjoyed life while he was being treated. He then used the same procedure to get over arthritis that had bothered him for many years, and then he got over his sexual impotence. He had been sexually impotent for 20 years, since his retirement. I've seen him recently, and he's still very sexually active."

Dr. Simonton believes that "You are more in charge of your life—and even the development and progress of a disease, such as cancer—than you may realize. You may actually, through a power within you, be able to decide whether you will live or die, and if you choose to live, you can be instrumental in choosing the *quality* of life that you want."

In addition to the 61-year-old man, Dr. Simonton's other dramatic successes have included:

—A 55-year-old woman with advanced anal cancer, completely well in six weeks. Today, three years later, X-rays show only a slight loss of pigment in the area.

—A 12-year-old boy with a large scrotal cancer, that dramatically shrank in two weeks.

Dr. Simonton, whose wife, Stephanie, works as a cotherapist with him, said his training as an M.D. had taught him "statistics and facts" about cancer—that, for instance, it can happen to any one of us, at any age—but that developing cancer himself, when he was 17, first prompted him to look within himself for possible causes.

He later learned that investigators in the last 20 years have identified certain characteristics that may make one prone to malignancy.

## The Personality of the Cancer Patient

"Some personality characteristics of the cancer patient that other scientists have identified as significantly different than noncancer patients are: (1) a tendency to harbor resentment and an impairment in his ability to express hostility, (2) a tendency towards self-pity, (3) difficulty in developing and maintaining meaningful, long-term relationships, and (4) a poor self-image." In addition, a sense of basic rejection, either by one or both of his parents, consequently develops the life history pattern seen so commonly in the cancer patient.

But, the doctor quickly adds, "We are not like ships without rudders to be blown about. We can change our course, largely determine the quality of our lives. Just as Drs. Meyer Friedman and Ray H. Rosenman in *Type A Behavior and Your Heart* (Fawcett World Library, New York, 1975) point out that the problems of personality in heart disease are changeable, so I strongly feel that the cancer personality is changeable.

"One very large factor contributing to heart disease is the person's response to stress. The same is true with cancer patients. It is not stress, as such, but how you deal with it."

Dr. Simonton teaches his patients first of all that cancer is *not* synonymous with death. Rather, that all normal people generate cancer cells and that the immunization process in the body ordinarily attacks these cells and destroys them to maintain health. Failure of the immunization process can lead to tumorous growth; restoration can lead to recovery.

A cautious medical man who shies from words such as "cure" and "healing," Dr. Simonton acknowledges that if a person will cooperate, his or her chances of recovery are improved. Not only is the "belief system" of the patient important, but the "belief system" of his family and the "belief system" of his physician also play a critical role in the patient's response.

"Most physicians are not aware that their own thoughts about the treatment and the patient's own ability influence the outcome, but they most definitely do," Dr. Simonton said. "Expectancy of teachers influences children, and on down the line.

"Real problems come when the physician's 'belief system' parallels that of the initial 'belief system' of the patient: that the disease comes from without; that it's synonymous with death; that the treatment is bad; and that the patient has little or nothing that he can do to fight the disease."

The cancer specialist says, "I think of myself as a coach, making the patient aware of what he is doing, so he can begin to change, in a way that is more productive. Sometimes you sit on the sidelines and think: if one would just dribble the ball this way, and shoot it that way he would make the basket, but he doesn't—he does it a different way, and he trips and falls.

"It would be impossible for me to know a patient only from

what the patient tells me. I can only know him by the way he lives his life.

"For instance, a patient with lung cancer *says:* 'Cure me of this malignancy.' But he continues to smoke. I want to say: 'That's foolish. Why are you smoking?' because I told myself: if I were this man, I would stop smoking. I would do those things I understood to do, in order to get well.

"I had so many lung cancer patients who refused to stop smoking that this was what got me involved in this whole area of the role of the mind in cancer therapy."

The Simontons say that helping the patient to restore himself to a healthy life is a "subtle area." Stephanie Simonton remarks:

"If you want to understand—and it took me awhile to grasp it—how difficult psychotherapy is when you're ill, try an experiment. The next time you have the flu or a cold, ask yourself that very difficult question, 'Why did I need this? What purpose does it fill?'

"If we are going to believe that we have the power in our own bodies to overcome cancer, then we have to admit that we also have the power to bring on the disease in the first place. With those patients who are willing to stay with us and persist, we invariably find that the cancer has filled some emotional need.

"We try to stress that there is a difference between being responsible for your cancer and being an object of blame. We all from time to time create a sickness to solve an emotional conflict. The cancer victim is no more to blame for participating in the development of his cancer than is the person who comes down with a cold to avoid a stressful situation at the office. We all have emotional needs that are very real and very concrete and if these are denied, life loses its meaning. Our body can even begin to seek the end of our life. We stress not that our patients should feel guilty, but that they have emotional needs that are not being met."

## A New Self Image

Both Dr. Simonton and his wife attempt to offer patients new emotional responses and new self-images.

"Over and over again, we have seen that the cancer patient has certain recurrent character traits. One of them is a low self-image. There is also a great tendency to hold resentment and a marked inability to forgive. There is also a tendency to self-pity and a poor ability to develop and maintain meaningful, long-term relationships. And, many times, the cancer is triggered by the loss of a serious love object."

Mrs. Simonton stresses the necessity of a reason for living. "We had two patients at the same time. One man quit work, just 'gave up' on living. The second was a 59-year-old man whose lung cancer had spread into the brain. Early in his treatment this man came to realize the problems that had caused life to lose meaning. He started to spend more time with his family, and, I remember his saying one day, 'You know, I had forgotten to look at the trees. Now I'm looking at trees and flowers again.'

"The first man went downhill very fast—and died. The second man has shown improvement, is getting stronger, healthier."

Dr. Simonton thinks that we often underestimate the wisdom of our bodies. He begins to encourage patients to have positive images by showing them a series of slides that illustrate "some of the best results I've seen, with some of the least side effects to the treatment. This is so the patient might see the potential of his or her body, both in getting rid of the disease and in the minimal reaction to his or her treatment."

The Simontons' patient-training program of relaxation, meditation, and visualization helps the patient "to understand where he is in life, and allows him the freedom to change his course, however he or she chooses to do so. If a person wants to die, far be it from me to stand in his way. What I would choose to do is to allow the person to see that he has a choice in whether he lives or dies, and the *quality* of life that he has. That he, in truth, has much more to do with that than anyone else. My purpose is not so much to change a person's beliefs but to give him an awareness of the beliefs that he currently possesses, and allow him the freedom to change them if he so chooses."

## Visualizing Success

Those who wish to change their beliefs and improve their self-image are given a cassette tape to play three times a day. The recorded voice of Dr. Simonton speaks reassuringly. "Take a deep breath, and blow it out, and as you blow it out, mentally say 'relax'. And now if you have cancer, I want you to mentally picture your disease, the way it seems to you. . . . It may look like a cauliflower;

it may look like a piece of hamburger with strands going out into other areas; it may seem like a water-filled balloon full of liquid. However it seems to you is perfectly fine but force yourself to create this mental picture.

"Now, if you're receiving radiation therapy, I want you to mentally picture your treatment. Picture the treatment as a beam of millions of tiny bullets of energy coming down, hitting all the cells in the area. The normal cells have a great ability to repair the minimal amount of damage done. The cancer cells are much less able to repair this damage, so they die. This is the whole purpose of the treatment. Mentally see this happening. . . . Picture the cancer shrinking. . . ."

The taped voice continues: "If you're receiving pills by mouth, see yourself taking those pills and them dissolving in the stomach and then going into the bloodstream. See them flowing around to where the cancer is. . . . They are poison to the cancer cells and—they die. . . . See the cancer shrinking as the white blood cells are indeed coming in and picking up the dead and dying cancer cells. . . ."

Dr. Simonton urges that "if you're having pain in an area, mentally project yourself into that area that is causing the pain. Cause your mind to flow to that area in a more or less inquisitive nature, wondering what's causing that and participate in the process —allowing yourself to become more in touch with your body in those things that are going on within yourself. . . . Feel happy for the realization of your ability to participate in your own illness and in your own health."

## Not a 'New' Discovery

Dr. Simonton says he has no "new" discoveries, that he is following in the footsteps—and convictions—of others. He quotes these sources, among many others, who have encouraged and inspired him:

—Eugene P. Pendergrass, M.D., former president of the American Cancer Society, who, in 1959 told the Society, "There is solid evidence that the course of the disease in general is affected by emotional distress. . . . It is my sincere hope that we can widen the quest to include the distinct possibility that within one's mind is a power capable of exerting forces that can either enhance or inhibit the progress of this disease."

—Psychotherapist Lawrence LeShan, who identified a life history pattern associated with patients who develop cancer.

—Dr. Bruno Klopfer of the University of California in Los Angeles, who was able to predict tumor growth on the basis of psychological data only.

—Over 200 articles in medical literature, Dr. Simonton adds, "conclude that there is a relationship between malignancy and emotions and stress."

Dr. Simonton says that early in his career, "I went on a very unusual search—a search to find out how to teach attitude, or the will to live. Some of the experts teaching attitude, I soon found out, are in the sales field. Here you can tell the attitude of the salesman by his results in income. The methods centered largely around positive thinking and imagery.

"During the time of exploring these areas, I came upon the terms 'autogenic' and 'biofeedback'. The principles of biofeedback were just coming into their own. I found two allies; one was a pediatrician, and the other a neurologist. . . . As we started to apply the biofeedback principles to ourselves, amazing things started to happen. In attempting to obtain the desired EEG [brainwave] or EMG [muscle tension] results, we found that relaxation was not as easy as we had supposed, but we did eventually gain some control over our blood pressure, temperature, and other physiological processes of the body. As we talked to other investigators who were working in these areas, it seemed that it would be equally as easy (or difficult) to gain control over the immune mechanisms, which is an exceedingly big factor in cancer.

"People say I have had phenomenal success. That's true and it's not true. It's true when patients completely cooperate with the program. It's not true when you consider the number of patients I treat who will not cooperate."

Far from being dogmatic about his approach, Dr. Simonton says, "We use words such as 'spontaneous remission'. But none of us fully understands what happens if there is a cure.

"I am attempting to put the person back in charge of his own direction. Our whole society is geared toward someone else assuming responsibility, which I think is a very unhealthy state. I want the patient who comes to me to realize that he shares responsibility for his own situation and for his own course. We then can work together toward achieving a healthier life for him."

# Vitiligo

Vitiligo is characterized by patches on the skin where pigmentation is absent. Way back in January of 1945, a study appeared in the *Virginia Medical Monthly* suggesting that the B vitamin PABA can help. A group of 48 people ranging in age from 10 to 70 years were given 100 mg. of PABA three or four times daily, in addition to a tablet containing all the other B vitamins. The rate of improvement was slow, so injections of the vitamin were begun, along with two daily oral tablets. Within two months, the white areas had turned pinkish, and after six months, all 48 people were reportedly free of the colorless patches.

Some 30 years after that study was published, we received a letter from a woman in California who had an extremely severe case of vitiligo. It began quite suddenly as light patches on the inside of her wrists and as the years passed, took over larger areas of her body "until I was completely devoid of all pigmentation of the skin." She consulted a great number of dermatologists and other specialists who sent her to medical laboratories for innumerable tests. The results indicated there was nothing that could be done for her.

Her condition was greatly worsened by excruciating burning sensations which occurred during menopause and may have also been associated with her vitiligo.

Finally, after reading about an English doctor who was successfully treating vitiligo with the B complex, she began to take this supplement, as well as an array of other vitamins and a generally well-balanced high-protein diet.

In a month's time, the burning sensations that had virtually crippled her had been greatly relieved, and as more time passed, she noticed that the natural pigmentation was beginning to return to her arms. On one arm, there were islands of new pigmentation scattered from her upper arm to the wrist, while on the other arm, normal and healthy pigmentation stretched from wrist to elbow.

Another woman took a different approach, after deciding that vitiligo was in some way related to the destruction of the natural acid mantle which the skin should have. She said that she would crush five 100 mg. PABA tablets, dissolve them in one-quarter cup of hot (not boiling) water, and mix them with one cup of pure mayonnaise. She would then anoint the affected areas after every washing of the hands or body. The purpose of the PABA, she said, was to screen out harmful sun rays, rather than to supply the vitamin to the body. At any rate, it worked for her, curing the condition in several months, after many doctors told her there was no cure for vitiligo.

# Warts

The simplest and probably most effective natural way to get rid of warts that I know of is to apply vitamin E directly to the darn thing and keep applying it once or twice a day until it falls off or disappears. Many people have found it most convenient to saturate the gauze portion of an adhesive bandage, apply it over the wart and change daily. It may take anywhere from one week to several months to achieve results.

Curiously, I have never come across a single word in the medical literature about applying vitamin E to warts. But many readers have sent in letters to PREVENTION describing what often seems to be astonishing success, and when others try it, they too write in about "amazing" results. So the therapy is kept alive; a true folk remedy.

Typical of many letters we have received is one from a woman in Bowie, Maryland, who described at length an experience with a dozen plantar warts her 10-year-old son had on the ball of his foot. Three times a day over a period of two months, the woman faithfully broke a 100 I.U. vitamin E capsule and rubbed the contents on her son's foot. That seemed to stop the warts from spreading but it did not make them go away.

On the advice of her father, a retired osteopathic physician, the woman began giving her son a daily dosage of 800 units of vitamin E as well as the topical applications. After just two days, "a definite change was taking place in the many warts on his foot. They seemed to be separating. After five days they all turned black under the skin, but they were still there. After one week I could feel that the hard mass or lumps under the skin had disappeared and it was not at all painful to press on the warts; however, they appeared to look the same except for being black.

"After 10 days all the smaller warts were peeling off or coming out of the skin and after 12 days the larger warts came out leaving several holes in his foot where they had been. At the end of two weeks time and 800 I.U. vitamin E per day, the warts were completely gone and his foot was completely healed with the skin as smooth as though there had never been any warts at all."

Now, it is true—and I am the first to admit it—that most warts which are less than a year old will go away by themselves. And although a virus seems to be involved with the appearance of warts, there is unquestionably a psychological factor at work in many cases. For this reason, I would suggest that warts which prove resistant to other modalities may respond dramatically to the ministrations of a hypnotist. But sometimes you needn't be exactly hypnotized in order to get results.

Robert Rodale, editor and publisher of PREVENTION, told me that as a young boy he developed some ugly-looking warts on his arm, and his father, J. I. Rodale, took him to a doctor. The doctor, apparently a wise old bird, looked at the warts and told young Robert that if they did not go away within two weeks, he was going to have to burn them off. To the child's mind, the idea of having his skin burned was a horrifying prospect.

Two weeks later, all the warts had vanished.

I should add, though, that the action of vitamin E on warts seems to be rather more than a placebo effect, as a number of readers report that warts on their pet dogs went away after application of the vitamin.

Vitamin E is not the only natural cure for warts. An old Indian method, which a woman from Ontario, Canada, told us "really works," is to "go out and pick a dandelion two or three times a day and put the milk from the cut end on the wart." The woman said that she got rid of her warts "in no time after they grew back again after having them burned off."

This anecdote brings up an important point. Many people probably imagine that having warts burned off or surgically removed by a doctor is the swiftest and most reliable method to rid yourself of warts.

Not true. The fact is, as any honest dermatologist will tell you, that warts which are "destroyed" have an amazing propensity to return over and over again, no matter how many times they are treated, often spreading or growing in the process. This does not seem to happen with vitamin E or other natural methods.

Another reader took the advice of the mystic, Edgar Cayce, who suggested putting warm castor oil on gauze and applying three times a day for half an hour. The reader reported that Cayce's method got rid of 14 warts on both hands in two months.

Daniel Hyman, M.D., of Suffern, New York, told *Modern Medicine* in 1975 that the appearance of warts on the body most frequently signals a shortage of antibodies that can reject the invading virus. Working on the theory that sulfur-containing amino acids "are essential for development of the antibodies toward the polyoma virus group," Dr. Hyman said that he gave a large number of patients desiccated liver tablets, because of their high content of these particular amino acids in the most efficacious form. He found that "excellent response was obtained in treating warts in institutionalized individuals given three desiccated liver tablets TID [three times a day]." He adds that these particular individuals "were so retarded that they did not know they had warts or that they were being treated for warts. Therefore, all psychological factors were removed from this trial. . . ."

It seems, then, that a good antiwart regimen would include nine tablets of desiccated liver a day, a goodly amount of vitamin E orally, and the same vitamin applied regularly to the wart.

## Aloe Plant May Help, Too

If this doesn't work, you may be interested in knowing about a combination herbal-abrasive technique described to us by Dr. Karl-Heinz A. Rosler, of the University of Maryland School of Pharmacy. Dr. Rosler, who holds a Ph.D. in pharmacognosy, and is therefore highly knowledgeable about herbs, said that as a youth, he suffered acute embarrassment from warts on his hands. He tried an emery nail file and worked on the warts until they almost bled but had to stop because they became so inflamed.

The warts stayed with him for many years. Then, he was told by a neighbor that the juice of the aloe plant, famed as an anti-inflammatory agent, could be useful in getting rid of warts. What the neighbor had done was to deliberately burn his wart with a match and then apply juice from the aloe leaf, so the inflammation would disappear along with the wart.

Dr. Rosler said that by coincidence, at about this time, a Ph.D. wrote a paper saying there is nothing beneficial in the aloe plant. Nevertheless, Dr. Rosler told us, "I decided to try a little folk medicine on myself. I again filed the warts back and applied the juice from a fresh aloe plant, and this did keep down the inflammation, to such an extent that the next day I was able to continue filing—and I filed the warts flat, applying the aloe juice each day. I soon had all of the warts filed down to nothing, and they never reappeared."

# Yeast Infections

Yeast infections, as they are commonly known, are not truly caused by yeasts. Perhaps the most common cause is an organism known as *Candida albicans,* which is a yeastlike fungus. An infection caused by this organism is properly known as candidiasis.

Like a number of other organisms which can become troublesome—or even highly dangerous—*Candida albicans* is frequently found on the skin or mucous membranes of perfectly healthy people. It rarely becomes an infectious agent until some predisposing factor is present. But then, even when the fungus is eradicated by medication, it often returns unless that underlying environmental or metabolic factor is normalized.

Diabetes is one such predisposing factor, but far more frequently, candidiasis erupts in the wake of antibiotic therapy. Excessive sweating or moisture may also invite infection, and the wearing of pantyhose is believed to create highly favorable conditions for a vaginal infection. (Undyed cotton underwear is recommended.)

Small cracks or other injuries of the skin also invite trouble. Vitamin deficiencies, notably of the B complex, may also be responsible for infections which are difficult to eradicate.

Because there is always some danger—slight, but real—that these infections can worsen and even become systemic, they should be treated by a doctor. However, many women find that the prescribed medications either do not work or that the infection returns as soon as the medication is stopped. Fortunately, a great many women have found purely natural therapies which succeed in stopping the recurrence of these infections.

The most effective therapy seems to be a concentrated form of *Lactobacillus acidophilus* culture. Jonathan V. Wright, M.D., of Kent, Washington, wrote in PREVENTION (January 1976), that "Women at our offices with a diagnosed yeast infection are given 'antiyeast' medicine and asked to follow this with applications for several nights of *Lactobacillus* mixed with yogurt. Once this is done, and the *Lactobacilli* are established, the yeast almost never returns (until the next antibiotics!). The yogurt-*Lactobacillus* mixture should be introduced in exactly the same way as the 'antiyeast' medication. If the medication applicator is unsuitable, then a plastic syringe with the end cut off, obtainable at most pharmacies, will do very well."

Dr. Wright added: "As an aside—with *very early* vaginal infections, frequent applications of yogurt and *Lactobacillus acidophilus* will solve the problem with no medication needed."

The acidophilus culture can also help when eaten. One woman told us in a letter that she suffered from *Monilia* (*Candida*) for over seven years, and visited five gynecologists, none of whom were able to cure it. A sixth doctor finally did manage to subdue it, but a month later, when the woman had to take an antibiotic, the vaginal infection came back. At that point she began taking frequent doses of acidophilus culture in pill form, plus plain yogurt, and that cured the infection.

The B-complex vitamins also seem to be helpful, even in cases where it's doubtful that an absolute deficiency of these vitamins exists. In one case, a woman told us in a letter that she had suffered with a yeast infection for four years and had spent considerable money on doctors, but to no avail. "I even went in the hospital for a D and C which was costly. Also, I had a bladder infection which the doctor said stemmed from this vaginal fungus. But none of the medication they gave me got rid of the itch and inflammation." After all that, the woman read a letter from another reader who had beaten a similar problem with B vitamins, and she began taking two B-complex tablets each day, one with breakfast and one with dinner. All her symptoms vanished within a few days.

# Yoga Therapy

**by Theodosia Gardner** *

Yoga is one of the oldest (5,000 years) yet newest forms of healing therapy. No longer regarded as the theatrics of Indian fakirs sitting on spikes, the amazing results of yoga are now being studied scientifically.

All over the world, teams of doctors are researching the results of yoga. At the I.C. Yogic Health Centers in Bombay and Lonavla, India, detailed records are kept of patients treated for diabetes, respiratory ailments, digestive complaints, and obesity. In Krakow, Poland, Dr. Julian Aleksandrowicy, Director of the Third Clinic of Medicine, has examined the effects of yoga postures on the composition and quality of the blood. (With 10 percent less oxygen inhaled in the headstand pose, there was found to be 33 percent more oxygen utilized in the blood.) At the Veterans Administration Hospital in Sepulveda, California, Dr. Barbara Brown, researching brain waves of yogis, said, "Eventually, most diseases may be treated by establishing healthful brain wave patterns, either by self-training or by mechanical means."

Mind over matter? Such research led Dr. Elmer Green of the famed Menninger Clinic to India for investigation of yogic mind control. And Dr. Eugene P. Pendergrass, past president of the American Cancer Society, in his presidential address said, "There is solid evidence that the course of the disease [cancer] in general is affected by emotional distress. . . . Within one's mind is a power capable of exerting forces which can either enhance or inhibit the progress of this disease."

In a study of 152 cancer patients over an 18-month period at Travis Air Force Base, California, Dr. Carl Simonton, M.D., reports, "Those patients with a positive attitude had good responses and those with negative attitudes had poor responses. Only two did not fall into the predicted categories." His techniques combine traditional cancer therapy with relaxation (see *Complete Breath, Corpse Pose*)

---

* Theodosia Gardner is a longtime student and former teacher of yoga. Based in Ormond Beach, Florida, most of her time is currently taken up with writing, illustrating, painting, and metal sculpture.

and visualization ("seeing yourself get well"). For a more complete discussion of visualization, see VISUALIZATION THERAPY.

People in every walk of life whose lives are under constant strain and who must maintain a high level of mental and physical fitness have discovered the value of yoga's effectiveness. In New York, an investment broker relates how yoga had restored his health after the collapse of his career. A harpist with the San Francisco Symphony speaks of his increased stamina and creative energies. A Florida dentist who feared he'd die at 52 from accumulated tensions has gained a new lease on life. And in Los Angeles, former Mayor Sam Yorty attributed his dynamic energy to daily yoga exercises.

Teachers of handicapped children now use breathing techniques (*Complete Breath, Corpse Pose, Mountain, Sun Salutation* poses) to increase oxygen consumption, improving attention span, memory, and learning capacity in retarded brains. A nurse in an intensive care unit of a big hospital in Oakland, California, declares, "We treat overdose suicide attempts with yoga respiration to prevent pneumonia from setting in."

Basically, yoga teaches that a healthy person is a harmoniously integrated unit of body, mind, and spirit. Therefore, good health requires a simple, natural diet, exercise in fresh air, a serene and untroubled mind, and a spirit full of awareness that man's deepest and highest self can be recognized as identical with the spirit of God. The law of yoga is the law of life.

## The Primacy of Relaxation

Yoga therapy begins with relaxation. Living in an age of anxiety, we are often unconscious of our tensions. With normal bodies, why are we depressed, tired, prey to disease? Because tension is invisibly draining away our health energies!

Ruth Rogers, M.D., of Daytona Beach, Florida, who has made a 10-year study of yoga therapy, says, "In understanding the healing process, relaxation is of supreme importance. You feel pain, and you don't want to move, so you tighten up. You're tense. Your muscles contract, constricting the blood flow. Swelling begins. More circulation is cut off, creating a vicious cycle. There's more pain, more tightening, more stiffness, more swelling. . . . This is also what happens in many back problems." She adds: "But if you can relax, fresh blood can circulate nourishment to the afflicted tissues and relieve pain-loaded nerve endings. Healing can begin."

Dr. Rogers reports, "A woman came to me suffering from headache, blurred vision, and nausea. All due to extreme tension. We treated her by rubbing the occipital bones at the base of the skull, by yoga eye exercises, the *Shoulder Stand,* the *Corpse Pose,* and the *Complete Breath.* Her symptoms all disappeared."

A nurse in a pediatric hospital reports, "We teach our asthmatic children the *Complete Breath.* We put a little plastic duck on their abdomens and tell them to watch the duck float up and down on the tummy waves. It not only quiets their fears but gives them more air and strengthens their lungs."

A 65-year-old patient of Dr. Rogers was nervous and unable to sleep. She complained that her mind raced all night. After practicing the *Complete Breath* several times a day, meditating on peacefulness and calm, she was able to sleep until morning. For additional relaxation, she practiced the *Knee to Chest,* the *Sun Salutation,* the *Shoulder Stand,* and the *Corpse Pose.*

If you practice yoga postures, you are strengthening the body. If you control your breathing, you are creating a chemical and emotional balance. If you concentrate your mind in affirmations, you are practicing the power of prayer. But if you synthesize all three, you are entering the most powerful mystery of healing: the basic harmony of life.

"The benefits of the postures are greater," says Dr. Rogers, "if the patient concentrates on the healing action where it is happening. In other words, you should mentally see the affected area as receiving fresh blood circulation, oxygen, and physical massage. A diabetic should visualize the healing energies to the pancreas, near the stomach. A rheumatic can concentrate on the release of synovial fluid. Synovial fluid is a lubricant and also disperses waste matter which can cause stiffness at joints."

## A Guide From India

Most of the following common disorders, scientifically treated at the Yoga Research Laboratory at Lonavla, India, have also been treated successfully by Dr. Rogers. Each posture should be preceded by relaxation and deep breathing. Directions for each posture are given later.

Asthma: *Corpse Pose, Mountain, Shoulder Stand, Fish, Complete Breath.*
  Visualization: Lung expansion, renewed strength.

Backache: *Corpse Pose, Locust, Plow, Knee to Chest.*
  Visualization: Fresh circulation to nourish back muscles.

Bronchitis: *Mountain, Shoulder Stand* (drains out secretions), *Fish, Locust.*

Cold: *Lion, Shoulder Stand.*

Constipation: *Corpse Pose, Fish, Twist* (loosens spine), *Plow, Knee to Chest* (reinvigorates liver, spleen, intestines), *Posterior Stretch, Uddiyana, Yoga Mudra.*
  Visualization: Increased circulation to tone intestines.

Depression: *Yoga Mudra, Shoulder Stand, Plow, Corpse Pose.*
  Visualization: New energy from increased oxygen, pending new joyous activity.

Diabetes (not a cure!): *Corpse Pose, Shoulder Stand, Plow, Twist* (flexing the spine stimulates nerve impulses to pancreas, massages the pancreas), *Kneeling Pose.*
  Visualization: Activation of thyroid gland (*Shoulder Stand, Plow*) which affects the whole metabolism. See healing energies of fresh circulation to pancreas.

Emphysema: *Complete Breath, Locust, Grip, Shoulder Stand.*
  Visualization: Healing circulation to lungs.

Eyestrain: *Neck and Eye Exercises.*
  Visualization: Absorb invisible energy from the air ("prana") into the eyes.

Flatulence: *Knee to Chest.*

Headache: *Corpse Pose, Neck and Eye Exercises, Shoulder Roll.*
  Visualization: A summer blue sky. No thoughts.

Indigestion: *Corpse Pose, Mountain, Locust, Shoulder Stand, Plow, Twist, Posterior Stretch, Cobra, Uddiyana.*

Insomnia: *Corpse Pose, Mountain, Locust, Shoulder Stand, Posterior Stretch, Cobra.*
  Visualization: Blue sky. *Enjoy* the yoga. No thoughts.

Menstrual Disorders: *Shoulder Stand, Plow, Fish, Uddiyana, Cobra, Posterior Stretch.*

Neurasthenia: *Corpse Pose, Mountain, Shoulder Stand, Posterior Stretch.*

Visualization: Energy-giving fresh circulation.

Obesity: *Locust, Shoulder Stand, Plow, Posterior Stretch, Cobra, Yoga Mudra, Bow, Sun Salutation.*

Piles: *Fish, Shoulder Stand, Plow.*

Prostate: *Kneeling Pose.*

Rheumatism: *Mountain, Shoulder Stand, Twist, Knee to Chest, Posterior Stretch.*

Visualization: The dispersal of waste matter causing stiffness at the joints.

Sciatica: *Shoulder Stand, Knee to Chest, Grip, Kneeling Pose, Twist.*

Sexual Debility: *Shoulder Stand, Plow, Uddiyana, Kneeling Pose, Twist, Complete Breath.*

Visualization: Youthful vigor from fresh blood circulation.

Sinus: *Neck and Eye Exercises, Corpse Pose, Shoulder Stand.*

Skin Diseases: *Sun Salutation.*

Visualization: A general physical tone-up, regulating and balancing any irregularity.

Sore Throat: *Lion.*

Visualization: Constriction of blood vessels in the throat; the relaxation brings fresh circulation to sore area.

Varicose Veins: *Shoulder Stand.*

Wrinkles: *Shoulder Stand, Yoga Mudra.*

Dr. Rogers states, "All people, young and old, can benefit from yoga. I have a six-month-old baby who comes to my classes with her parents. And the elderly can avoid that hunching effect that often accompanies old age. They can do the *Mountain,* the *Corpse Pose,* the *Knee to Chest,* and the *Complete Breath.*"

Of a serious emphysema patient, Dr. Rogers said, "Yoga therapy most definitely prolonged her life. . . . She is alive to this day! The lung fluids were drained by what we call a *Reverse Posture.* She lay on the bed, carefully sliding off until her head was resting on the floor, her hips and legs remaining on the bed. She relaxed her arms and shoulders. Coughing occasionally while breathing slowly cleared her lungs of draining fluids. We found that she had no colds, was stronger, and had better breathing. She also practiced the *Twist,* the *Shoulder Stand,* and the *Grip* to expand and strengthen the lungs."

## Posture Instructions

Before eating, either morning or late afternoon, spread a blanket on the floor in a well-ventilated room. Wear loose clothing. As a general rule, the backward-bending postures should be balanced by forward-bending poses.

Never force or strain in yoga. These postures should be performed slowly, meditatively. Yoga postures are meant to be held in dynamic tension, not to be confused with vigorous calisthenics which deplete energy, accumulate body toxins, and forcefully constrict blood flow.

**Bow** ● Lie flat on your stomach, grasping the ankles. Inhale. Lifting legs, head, and chest, arch the back into a bow. Retain breath, then exhale and lie flat. Repeat three or four times.

More advanced: While in the *Bow* position, rock back and forth, then from side to side. Slowly release and exhale.

*Reported benefits:* Massages abdominal muscles and organs. Good for gastrointestinal disorders, constipation, upset stomach, sluggish liver. Reduces abdominal fat, aids in rectifying hunchback.

(Not for persons suffering from peptic ulcer, hernia, or cases of thyroid or endocrine gland disorders.)

**Cobra** ● Lie on the stomach, toes extended. Place the hands, palms down, under the shoulders on the floor. Inhaling, without lifting the navel from the floor, raise the chest and head, arching the back. Retain the breath, then exhale while slowly lowering to the floor. Repeat one to six times.

*Reported benefits:* Tones ovaries, uterus, and liver. Aids in relief and elimination of menstrual irregularities. Relieves constipation. Limbers spine. Excellent for slipped disks.

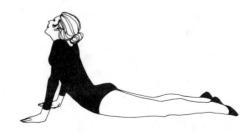

(Not recommended for sufferers from peptic ulcer, hernia, or hyperthyroid.)

**Complete Breath** • Crowded city living, air pollution, and sedentary jobs are helping to increase respiratory ailments. Tight clothes encourage shallow breathing and cramp the lungs. The purpose of the *Complete Breath* is to fully expand the air sacs of the lungs, thereby exposing the capillaries to the maximum exchange of carbon dioxide and oxygen.

1. Lie down, loosening clothing. Place hands on the abdomen, resting fingertips lightly on the navel. Breathing through the nose, inhale and expand *only* the abdomen. (Watch the fingertips part.) Exhale and contract the abdomen. (The fingertips will meet.) Practice this *Abdominal Breath* slowly, without strain, 10 times.

2. Place the hands on the rib cage and inhale, expanding *only* the diaphragm and the rib cage. (Watch the fingertips part.) Contract and slowly exhale. Practice this *Diaphragm Breath* 10 times.

3. Placing the fingertips on the collarbones, inhale *only* in the upper chest. The fingers will rise, indicating a shallow breath. This is how we usually breathe. Notice the insufficiency. Now, raise the shoulders for more air. Exhale and practice the *Upper Breath* 10 times.

4. Finally, placing the hands, palms up, beside the body, put these three breaths together. Inhale, expanding the abdomen, the diaphragm, and the chest, in a slow, wavelike movement. Hold. Exhale in the same order, contracting the abdomen, the diaphragm, and the chest. Repeat these instructions to yourself as you adjust the *Complete Breath* to your own rhythm. Concentrate on what is happening: you are increasing the expansion of the terminal air sacs in the lungs. Notice how slow, deep breathing makes you calm, yet fills you with energy! Very logically, yoga links a long life with proper breathing.

*Reported benefits:* Increases vitality, soothes nerves, strengthens flabby intestinal and abdominal muscles.

**Corpse Pose** • Lie down on your back, in a quiet place. Place the arms beside the body, palms upturned. Heels slightly apart. *Breathe* *slowly and deeply, feeling a sense of calm relaxation come over your whole body. Concentrate on loosening all tensions.*

The following variation will increase your ability to relax:

1. Slowly inhale through the nostrils (always breathe through the nostrils since the tiny hairs strain out impurities), and tense the ankles, feet and toes. Hold the breath while you tighten the muscles. Exhale and relax.

2. Slowly inhale and contract the kneecaps, calves, ankles, feet and toes. Hold and tighten. Exhale and relax.

3. Slowly inhale, contracting all the muscles, tissues, and organs of the abdomen, pelvic area, hips, thighs, kneecaps, calves, ankles, feet and toes. Hold the breath and tighten the muscles. Exhale and relax.

4. Inhale. Tense the neck, shoulders, arms and elbows, wrists, hands and fingers, chest muscles, lungs, etc. down to the toes. Hold and tense. Exhale and relax.

5. Inhale and contract the hairs on the head, the scalp, the tiny muscles of the face, brain, eyes, ears, forehead, and squint the eyes, wrinkle the nose and mouth, tighten the tongue, constrict the throat, and tighten the whole body. Hold and feel the terrible tension. Exhale and relax. Now, let the strain melt into the floor. Feel heavy. Enjoy the support of the floor. Sense the tingling of fresh circulation, the new muscle tone, and emotional calm.

*Reported benefits:* Stimulates blood circulation and exercises inner organs. Alleviates fatigue, nervousness, neurasthenia (a general worn-out feeling), asthma, constipation, diabetes, indigestion, insomnia, lumbago. Teaches mental concentration.

**Fish** ● Lie down on your back. Prop up your body on your arms and elbows. Let your head slowly fall backwards. Raise your chest, arch your back, and as you slide your elbows back down, rest the top of your skull on the floor. Rest the weight on the head and buttocks.

Relax, palms up, arms beside the body, releasing all facial, neck, and shoulder tensions. Using *Abdominal Breath* (see *Complete Breath*) breathe slowly and deeply. Hold the pose 30 seconds or longer. Replacing the elbows beside the body to catch the weight, lift your head slowly, then slide down gently into a prone position. Relax.

More advanced: Sit cross-legged. Bend backwards, using support of elbows until crown of head touches floor. Hold onto big toes with fingers. Keep back well arched. Practice *Abdominal Breath.*

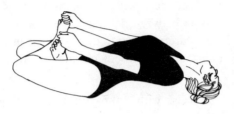

*Reported benefits:* Relieves constipation, bronchitis, asthma; corrects posture defects; alleviates stiffness in spine; stimulates thyroid and parathyroid glands. Also relaxes the neck and beautifies the neckline. (Since the *Fish* relieves chest congestion, it should always follow the *Shoulder Stand,* which constricts the chest.)

**Grip** • Sitting on the heels, raise the right hand. Bring it slowly behind the shoulder, touching the spine at the shoulder blades. Slowly bend the left arm behind the back from the bottom, and join the hands. Hold, then repeat with the other side.

*Reported benefits:* Proper execution develops the capacity of the thoracic cage, helps prevent bursitis and the formation of calcium deposits at the shoulder joints. Benefits emphysema and asthma.

**Knee to Chest** • Lying on the back, bring the knees to the chest. Grasping the folded knees, rock gently back and forth. (This relaxes and massages the spine.) Lower legs. Inhale and bend the right knee to the chest, pulling it into the chest with interlocked fingers. Retain the breath and raise the head, touching the knee with the nose. Hold for a count of 10. Exhale and lower the head almost to the floor. Repeat five times, then change legs. Exhale as the head is lowered to the floor. Straighten right leg, lower slowly to the floor. Repeat with left leg. Now, draw up both legs, touch nose to knees. Hold with breath. Exhale and relax.

*Reported benefits:* Relieves stiffness and soreness of back and extremities, constipation, diabetes, flatulence.

A 28-year-old student hurt his back while laboring as a construction worker. While waiting for his surgical operation, he practiced the *Knee to Chest* pose, particularly the rocking movement. Also practicing the *Abdominal Breath* (see *Complete Breath*), he gradually was able to do the *Sun Salutation* pose. His back improved to the point where he finally canceled the operation.

**Kneeling Pose** • Sit on heels, with a straight back. Relax. Separate feet and slowly sink in between, letting the buttocks touch the floor, doing this slowly and carefully, not to damage knee ligaments.

*Reported benefits:* Increased circulation to prostate gland or uterus.

**Lion** • Sitting on heels, with palms on knees, stiffly fan out the fingers. Lean slightly forward over the hands. Protrude the tongue as far as possible, contract the throat muscles, and roll the eyeballs upward. Completely exhale, saying "Ahhhhhhh." Repeat four to six times.

*Reported benefits:* Helps to relieve sore throat. Stimulates circulation to throat and tongue.

**Locust** • Lie face down, chin on floor. Clench fists, press arms and knuckles down under the groin. Inhale. Using the lower back muscles, raise one leg towards the ceiling. Hold. Exhale and relax. Repeat with other leg. Repeat two or three times, according to capacity.

More advanced: While in pose, raise *both* legs. A strenuous pose.

*Reported benefits:* Relieves problems of abdomen and lower back.

(Not for those with hernia or back problem in acute stage.)

**Mountain** • Sitting cross-legged, stretch both arms up towards the ceiling in a prayerlike pose, fingertips together. Stretch up and breathe deeply and slowly five to ten times. Exhale and lower arms.

*Reported benefits:* Strengthens lungs, trunk, and abdominal muscles. Purifies bloodstream, improves digestive system, tones nervous system. Prevents the stooped look of the aged.

**Neck and Eye Exercises** • Sitting upright, nod head forward slowly, three times. Nod to the left shoulder three times. Nod to the back three times, letting the mouth fall open. Nod to the right shoulder three times. Slowly roll the head clockwise three times, then reverse.

Inhale. Shut eyes tightly. Hold position with breath. Exhale, open eyes wide and blink rapidly 10 times.

Opening eyes wide, look in a slow circle. Repeat in opposite direction. Now, look diagonally. Next, look up and down 10 times.

Rub palms together vigorously. Close eyes and cover with palms. Take five very slow deep breaths, visualizing new energy and brightness into the eyes.

*Reported benefits:* Relieves headache and eyestrain; improves eyesight. Relaxes neck and shoulder tensions.

**Plow** ● Lie on the floor on your back. Slide arms under buttocks for support. Raise the legs, slowly swinging the feet over behind the head until the toes touch the floor. Rest the arms beside the body with palms down. Concentrate on relaxing the shoulders, arms, and hands. The legs should be straight. Slow the breathing. Rounding the back is very good for tight back muscles.

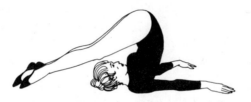

Don't worry if you can't touch behind the head. You can let the knees rest on the forehead. As you relax and practice the *Abdominal Breath* (see *Complete Breath*), you will be massaging the abdominal organs. Meantime, your back muscles will slowly become limber. Inhale and round the back. Roll out slowly. Exhale and lie prone. Relax.

If there is discomfort in the back, rock in the *Knee to Chest* pose. *Never force any yoga movement or hold it if it hurts.*

*Reported benefits:* Relieves headache, hangover, sinus and nasal congestion. Benefits diabetics. Slimming.

Dr. Rogers states, "Rolling out of this one slowly, rounding the back, is very good for displaced vertebrae."

**Posterior Stretch** ● Sit on floor, with the left leg outstretched, the right heel tucked into the crotch. Inhale and reach arms overhead.

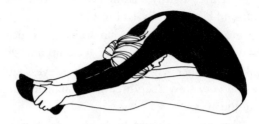

Hold the breath, drop forward, reaching the arms toward the left ankle, the head to the knee. (If you can only grasp the calf, do that, and relax, breathing slowly.) Concentrate on the muscles as they slowly lengthen, and inch down lower. Close your eyes. Release any discomfort in a sensation of relaxation. Hold one minute. Inhale, raise up, arms overhead, and exhale as you lower the arms to the side. Repeat with opposite leg. Repeat with both legs outstretched.

*Reported benefits:* A powerful massage to the abdominal organs. Improves digestion and elimination through the forward-bending movement; relaxes tensions in the back. Brings fresh circulation to face, firming tissue and improving color.

(Not for slipped disks.)

**Shoulder Roll** ● Sitting or standing, roll shoulders loosely forward in a circular movement, five times. Reverse.

For a bigger stretch, roll one shoulder at a time.

*Reported benefits:* Relieves headache, fatigue, tension, neckache.

A dentist reported, "After bending over patients all day, I found that the shoulder exercises cure my neck and back strain. I can practice these in between patients."

**Shoulder Stand** ● Lie on back, on floor. Slide arms under buttocks. Inhale and slowly raise the legs. Lift the trunk, hips, and legs to a vertical position. Resting the elbows on the floor, support the back with the hands. The chin is pressing into the chest, the legs vertical, like a candle. Hold this pose for as long as comfortable, no longer than 15 minutes. Breathing slowly and evenly will help to steady the legs. Concentrate on the thyroid gland in the neck which yoga experts say is stimulated.

*Reported benefits:* Reduces excess fat; stretches the spine and muscles of the legs, back, abdomen, and neck. Tones up the nervous system; improves circulation.

(Not for people with high blood pressure, enlarged liver or spleen.)

**Twist** • Sit on floor with legs outstretched. Bend the left leg under 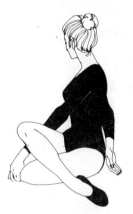 the right thigh. Bring the right foot across the left leg, placing the foot on the outside of the left knee. The left hand grasps the toes of the right foot from outside the right knee. Inhale and swing the free right arm to bend across the lower back, lower palm turned outward, the trunk and head twisted right around. Hold the pose for as long as is comfortable, increasing to two minutes. Repeat to other side. Work into the *Twist* easily and gradually.

*Reported benefits:* Massages stomach, kidneys, liver, pancreas. Said to help emphysema patients.

(Not for those with back operations.)

**Uddiyana** • Stand with feet apart, knees slightly bent. Lean forward, arching the back, hands on thighs. Exhale all air. Suck abdomen back against the spine. Hold for several seconds. Relax and repeat, all within one exhalation. Work up to 20 repetitions with one exhalation.

*Reported benefits:* Alleviates constipation, indigestion and stomach problems. Good for obesity, diabetes, hepatitis.

**Yoga Mudra** • Sitting cross-legged, exhale and lean forward to touch the floor with the forehead. Place arms behind the back, one hand grasping the opposite wrist. Hold the pose. Inhale and slowly return to sitting position. Practice up to 15 minutes.

*Reported benefits:* Gives energy, massages colon and intestines, relieves constipation. Good for complexion.

**Sun Salutation** • Finally, for people with limited time, the *Sun Salutation* exercises every muscle, joint, and all major organs. The name itself means to give prostrations to the internal sun as well as to the external sun, the creative life-force of the universe, which the yogis believe to radiate *inside* as well as outside the body.

1. Stand erect, feet together, palms prayerlike in front of the chest. Feel awareness of the whole body.

2. Inhale deeply, raise arms overhead, hands apart, leaning back.

3. Exhale, bending forward, legs straight.  Touch the ground or try to, but *don't strain*.

4. Not moving hands nor the left foot, bring the right leg back as far as possible, bending the left leg.  Support weight on both

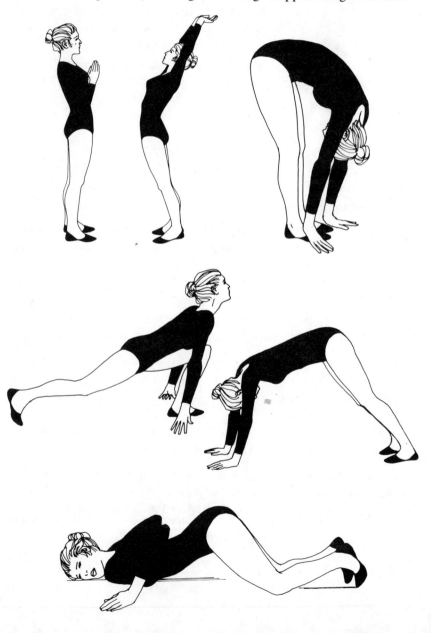

hands, left foot, right knee, and toes of the right foot. Tilt the head back, look up. Inhale and retain breath.

5. Place the left foot next to the right, raise the abdomen, making the body a triangular arch. Place the head between the arms. Try to keep the feet flat. Exhale.

6. Hold breath. Lower body to floor, keeping abdomen and hips off the ground.

7. Inhale and raise body in *Cobra* position, looking up.

8. Exhale, resume position 5.

9. Inhale, bring left foot forward, and lower right knee as in position 4.

10. Exhale, resuming position 3.

11. Return to position 2, raise the hands while inhaling.

12. Exhale and return to position 1.

*Reported benefits:* Positions 1. and 12. Establish state of concentration and calm. Positions 2. and 11. Stretch abdominal and intestinal muscles, exercise arms and spinal cord. Positions 3. and 10. Aid in prevention, relief of stomach ailments. Reduce abdominal fat. Improve digestion and circulation. Limber spine. Positions 3. and 9. Tone abdomen, muscles of thighs and legs. Positions 5. and 8. Strengthen nerves and muscles of arms and legs. Exercise spine. Positions 6. and 7. Strengthen nerves and muscles of shoulders, arms, and chest.

## A Basic Daily Program

Daily yoga practice is a good investment in health. Twelve minutes a day will purchase a toning of the muscles, improve the digestive, circulatory, and respiratory systems, as well as increase energy-giving oxygen consumption to the nerves and brain. The following exercises will provide a well-balanced program, supplemented, of course, by any other postures particularly good for your needs.

First Day: *Complete Breath, Knee to Chest, Cobra, Sun Salutation, Corpse Pose.*

Second Day: *Complete Breath, Shoulder Stand, Plow, Sun Salutation, Corpse Pose.*

Third Day:  *Complete Breath, Bow, Cobra, Posterior Stretch, Corpse Pose.*

Fourth Day and On:  Repeat sequence.

Good health is not just a blessing, but an inner virtue, which has its source in the courage of the soul. Therefore, take a big breath, pick up thy bed of nails, and walk into a fresh life of health and self-mastery!

# Index